Pelvic Pouch Procedures

Pelvic Pouch Procedures

Phillip E. Thomas MB, ChB, FRCS
Research Fellow and Tutor in Surgical Gastroenterology, University Department of Surgery, Manchester Royal Infirmary, UK

T. Vincent Taylor MD, ChM, FRCS
Consultant Surgeon and Reader in Surgery, University Department of Surgery, Manchester Royal Infirmary, UK

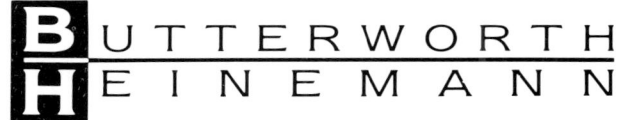

Butterworth-Heinemann Ltd
Halley Court, Jordan Hill, Oxford, OX2 8EJ

 PART OF REED INTERNATIONAL P.L.C.

OXFORD LONDON GUILDFORD BOSTON
MUNICH NEW DELHI SINGAPORE SYDNEY
TOKYO TORONTO WELLINGTON

First published 1991

British Library Cataloguing in Publication Data

Thomas, P.E.
  Pelvic pouch procedures.
  1. Man. Pelvic region. Surgery
  I. Title   II. Taylor, T. V. (Thomas Vincent)
617.55.59

  ISBN 0 7506 1250 9

Library of Congress Cataloging in Publication Data

Thomas, P. E.
  Pelvic pouch procedures/P.E. Thomas, T.V. Taylor.
    p.   cm.
  Includes bibliographical references and index.
  ISBN 0-7506-1250-9 : $47.59
    1. Colectomy. 2. Ileostomy. 3. Rectum--Surgery.
  I. Taylor, T. Vincent.   II. Title.
    [DNLM: 1. Anastomosis, Surgical--methods.
  2. Colectomy. 3. Ileostomy. 4. Rectum--surgery.
  WI 520 T461p]
  RD549.T53   1991
  617.5'54--dc20
  DNLM/DLC   90-15151

Phototypeset by Scribe Design, Gillingham, Kent
Printed and bound by Hartnolls Ltd, Bodmin, Cornwall

Foreword

Excising a diseased large intestine and yet maintaining transanal faecal continence has long been a goal of gastrointestinal surgeons. Only in recent years, however, has the goal been realized. The pelvic pouch procedures have now allowed proctocolectomy with preservation of transanal defecation and reasonable faecal continence, at least for patients with ulcerative colitis and familial adenomatous polyposis.

The authors of this superb book trace the background and need for the continence-preserving procedures, the early surgical attempts at achieving continence, and the emergence and later refinements of the pelvic pouch operations. They review the history and physiology of continence, the alterations produced by disease and operation, and the ability of the pelvic pouch procedure to maintain the anatomy and physiology. The pelvic pouch provides a satisfactory 'neorectum', and the preserved anal sphincters maintain a living barrier to faecal loss. The complications of the operations and the physiologic and metabolic consequences of the procedures are described well enough to provide the reader with abundant ammunition to combat them effectively. The last chapter appropriately projects the reader into the future.

This book is a timely, up-to-date, cutting-edge publication that brings together a vast amount of material in a well-organized, lucid way. It documents a quantum leap in gastrointestinal surgery that emphasizes not only the abolition of disease, but the restoration of health and a reasonable quality of life. Continued growth and further applications of the pelvic pouch procedures will undoubtedly occur.

Surgeons, gastroenterologists, other medical personnel, students, and above all, patients owe much to the authors who have provided this milestone. We are now better equipped to continue the way.

Keith A. Kelly, MD
Professor and Chairman,
Department of Surgery,
Mayo Clinic and Mayo Medical School,
Rochester, Minnesota, USA

Preface

The last decade has witnessed a revolution in the surgical treatment of several diseases of the colon and rectum. Initially, much effort and enthusiasm was expended on finding alternatives to the permanent ileostomy, be it conventional or continent. At the forefront of such effort has been the quest for a satisfactory neorectum. Supported by important new developments in our understanding of the mechanisms of anorectal continence, surgical ingenuity over the last 40 years or so has culminated in the use of reservoirs constructed from the terminal ileum, and anastomosed to the anal sphincter mechanism. Admirable persistence by a few, often in the face of severe learning curves, ultimately brought many reports of successful results with such procedures. Encouraged by this success, attempts are now being made to widen the indications for such sphincter preservation. Such intestinal pouches, constructed from the colon itself, have now been utilized after rectal excision for malignant disease.

Whilst this is now an accepted alternative to permanent ileostomy, many surgeons have been reluctant to recommend this form of treatment to their patients. Early reports of the pelvic pouch procedure documented difficult surgical techniques and often serious complications. There can be little doubt that such complications are becoming not only less frequent, but also more successfully managed when they do occur. This has allowed many more patients to retain their pouches, when excision may have once been the only surgical option. Subsequently, restorative proctocolectomy has become the treatment of choice for many patients requiring proctocolectomy.

The early chapters of this book document the history of the surgery of ulcerative colitis and adenomatous polyposis. Subsequent chapters detail the technical, clinical and pathophysiological details of ileal pouch–anal anastomosis. Each section details a very specific area, commencing with relevant physiology, and moving on to discuss changes after pouch construction.

The book is copiously referenced, with references from as recently as July 1990. Hence it is hoped that it will provide an up to date source of reference for surgeons already performing this procedure. However, it is also hoped that it will prove to be particularly useful to surgeons aiming to commence this work. It will also be valuable to surgeons undertaking the new Intercollegiate examinations in General Surgery of the British Royal Colleges, and for the American Boards in Coloproctology.

Special thanks are due to Sandra A. Roe, University of Manchester, for preparing the artwork.

P.E.T.
T.V.T.

Contents

1

Surgery for ulcerative colitis – historical perspective

Surgery for inflammatory bowel disease has been practised for almost a century. During this time the surgery of ulcerative colitis has passed through a series of interesting innovations. Indeed, the last decade has witnessed something of a revolution in the surgical management of 'benign' disease of the colorectal mucosa, principally ulcerative colitis.

Despite there being varying interpretations of indications for surgery, some 15–50% of patients with colitis will ultimately require it at some time (Cattel, 1948; Waugh, Harp and Spencer, 1964). The likelihood of the necessity for surgery in any one patient is particularly related to the severity and distribution of their disease. The aetiology of relapse in ulcerative colitis remains debatable (Riley *et al.*, 1990). It has been found that, of patients suffering with distal proctitis alone, 2% would come to surgery. Corresponding values for other subgroups were: 5% for those with left-sided disease, and 30% for those with an extensive colitis (Ritchie, Powell-Tuck and Lennard-Jones, 1978). Similar figures have been reported by others (Leijonmarck, Persson and Hellers, 1990). It has been suggested that distal colitis may represent a different or modified disease process to that involved in the more extensive variant of the disease (Jenkins, Goodall and Scott, 1990).

Colonic irrigation and the conventional ileostomy

Initial experience with the creation of intestinal stomas was obtained in the management of large bowel obstruction, and as such has been used for some two hundred years. However, towards the end of the last century Mayo Robson employed colonic irrigation through a left iliac sigmoid colostomy in a case of severe ulcerative colitis (Figure 1.1). The stoma was apparently closed upon remission of the inflammation (Mayo Robson, 1893). Shortly thereafter, both Keetle and Weir irrigated the colon via a catheter inserted through an appendicostomy (Figure 1.2). This form of stoma avoided intestinal leakage. In addition,

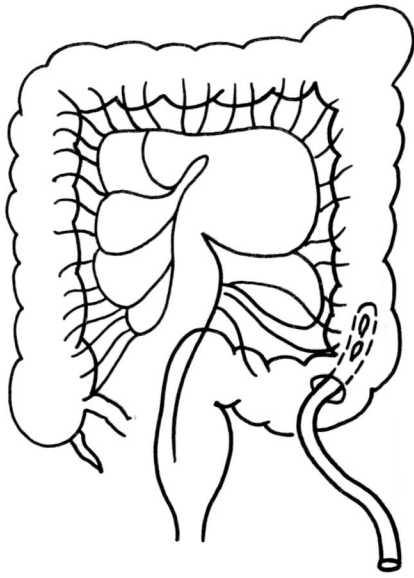

Figure 1.1 Irrigating sigmoid colostomy

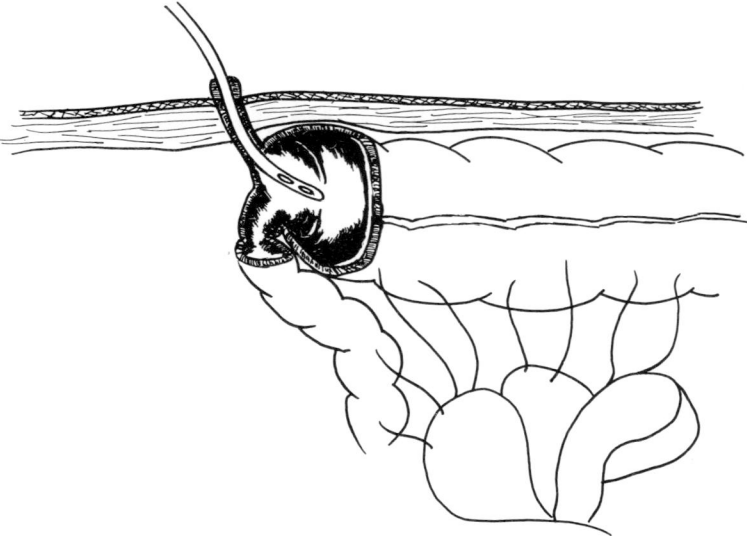

Figure 1.2 Appendicostomy

closure was facilitated by simple appendicec-tomy. As a result, and because of its simplicity, appendicostomy remained the surgical treat-ment of choice in ulcerative colitis until the 1940s (Corbett, 1945), but it did not adequate-ly defunction the colon.

Over the following years it was reasoned that not only was colonic irrigation important, but in addition the inflamed large bowel should be completely rested. Consequently, Brown cre-ated a flush ileostomy for diversion, and added a tube caecostomy for irrigation (Figure 1.3).

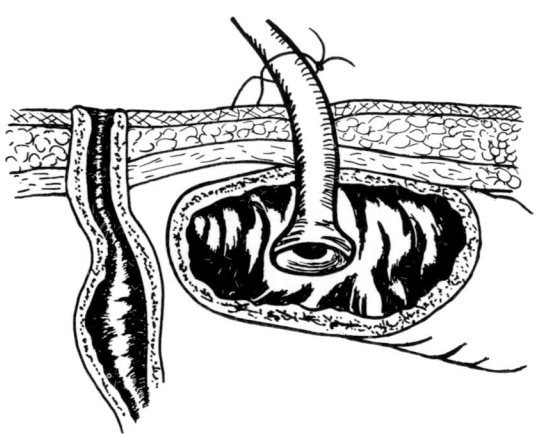

Figure 1.3 Tube caecostomy (after Brown, 1913)

In this first description of the use of faecal diversion in inflammatory bowel disease the attractiveness of the odourless ileal effluent was stressed, but it was also falsely asserted that ileal contents did not induce skin irritation (Brown, 1913). Conversely, some workers accepted the role of faecal diversion, but remained unconvinced as to the efficacy of colonic irrigation in these disorders (Hurst, 1935). No doubt the relatively unscientific nature of the differing irrigating fluids fuelled this scepticism. Irrigations varying from saline to boracic acid had been employed by various surgeons with varying results. For workers antagonistic to colonic irrigation, ileostomy remained their only surgical option. Further, once created, such stomas were rarely closed, irrespective of whether colectomy had been performed or not.

Ileostomy remained however very much a salvage procedure performed in almost mori-bund patients. Indeed, its use was considered by many to constitute a disaster, chiefly due to the many aesthetic and social adaptations required from its recipients. Complications continued to be common and problematical, often made worse because of the lack of satisfactory stoma appliances. In these early years, patients had to suffer the indignities of wearing abdominal corsets, into which cups were incorporated to collect the ileostomy

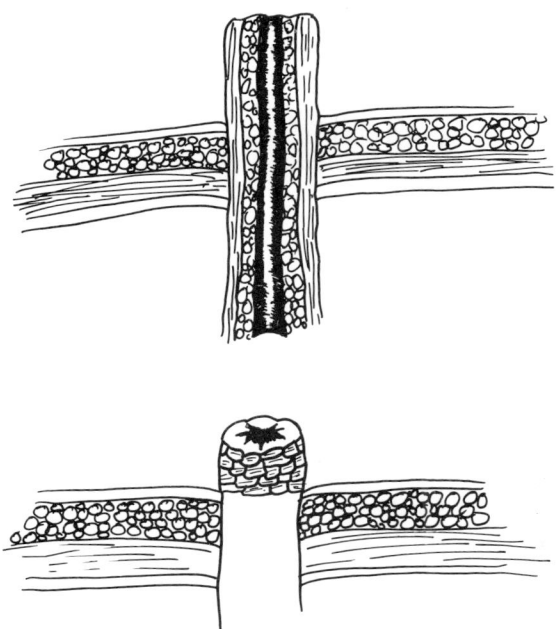

Figure 1.4 Skin-grafted ileostomy (after Dragstedt, Dack and Kirsner, 1941)

effluent. Skin excoriation was inevitable and frequently severe.

In an attempt to produce a more satisfactory stoma, Dragstedt described the use of a skin-grafted ileostomy. The distal ileum was protruded, and covered with a split-thickness skin graft, depicted diagrammatically in Figure 1.4 (Dragstedt, Dack and Kirsner, 1941). This resulted in a mature ileostomy from the outset (see below), and hence reduced considerably the dehydration and other electrolyte disturbances associated with ileostomy dysfunction. Understandably, graft failure was common, and even when the graft did survive, it tended to wear out within the first 5 years of its construction. The technique however did result in functional improvement, and gained some popularity in the USA.

A major advance in stoma care came in 1944, when the Koenig-Runtzen bag was described (Strauss and Strauss, 1944). It consisted of a slender rubber bag, with a circular facepiece. The latter was reinforced with a rubber-covered metal disk incorporating an opening to accommodate the intestinal stoma. An adhesive sealed the facepiece to the peristomal abdominal skin. Leakage was considerably improved, and the appliance remained in place during emptying.

Such new improved appliances were not, however, a panacea for patients requiring an end-ileostomy. Repeatedly, the postoperative period was complicated by severe abdominal pain and excessive ileostomy output; the latter commonly posed serious electrolyte problems in patients already suffering hypoalbuminaemia. This high output state occurred in up to 60% of patients, in whom there was a mortality of 5% (Warren and McKittrick, 1951). Crile and Turnbull (1954) subsequently showed that the aetiology of these phenomena was infection of the exposed serosa of the ileal spout, resulting in contraction and retraction; a process termed 'maturation'. However, the process did not stop when mucosa to skin healing had taken place, and stricture formation was all too common.

In time, Dragstedt's skin-grafted ileostomy fell into disrepute due to poor graft survival, resulting in high rates of stoma revision. Another solution to exposure of the ileal serosa to effluent was described in 1949, when Brooke used the method of partial intussusception of the ileal spout upon itself to provide serosal cover (Figure 1.5). Brooke's eversion technique has become standard surgical practice ever since (Brooke, 1952). This major breakthrough successfully prevented both stomal stenosis and the excessive output states, so commonly a previous cause of morbidity.

A small number of workers, most notably those from the Cleveland Clinic, still accept that there is a role for a diverting loop ileostomy combined with 'simple', so-called 'blow-hole' colostomies to facilitate bowel

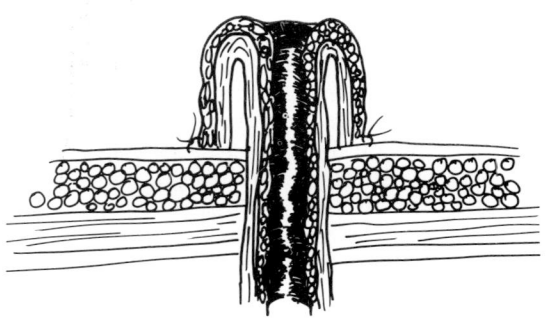

Figure 1.5 Brooke everted ileostomy

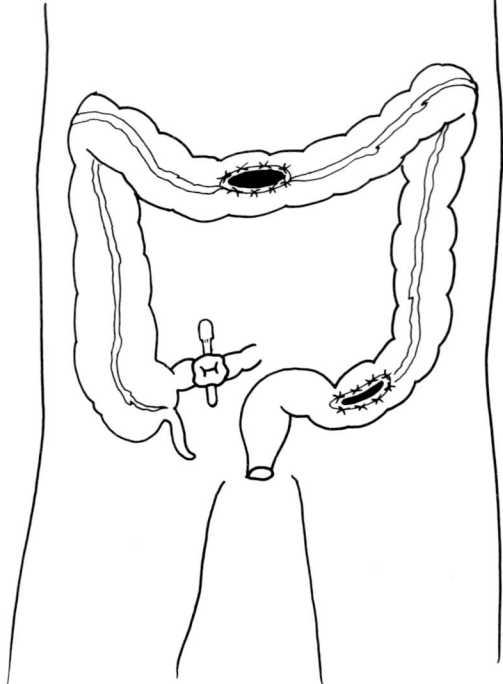

Figure 1.6 'Blow-hole' colostomies

decompression without resection in extremely severe cases of toxic dilatation (Figure 1.6). This has been found to be particularly useful if toxic dilatation is complicated by a sealed colonic perforation (Turnbull *et al.*, 1970; Fazio, 1980). There is excellent evidence that there is probably no role for segmental colonic excisions in ulcerative colitis. Patients thus treated by rectal or rectosigmoid excisions, with the formation of sigmoid or transverse colostomies, have almost inevitably required further colonic resections sooner rather than later. In almost all cases, recurrent colitis is the indication for such resections (Stahlgren and Ferguson, 1959; Varma *et al.*, 1987).

The major technical problems with conventional end-ileostomy had therefore been solved by the simple but ingenious Brooke ileostomy. Results of surgery improved, and whilst complications are still not rare, their incidence and severity have diminished. Like most surgical complications these can be divided into those occurring in the early postoperative period, and those appearing at a later date. Early complications are predominantly related

to difficulties with fluid balance and excoriation of the skin. Later complications are far more numerous, and tend to be of a mechanical nature, such as ileostomy retraction, stenosis, prolapse or parastomal herniation. It soon became obvious that, for several reasons, ileostomy formation without colectomy was inadequate for many patients. Most notably failure to thrive, a persistent anal discharge, failure of systemic non-gastrointestinal manifestations to subside, and, latterly, the realization of the potential for colonic malignancy have prompted surgeons to undertake synchronous colonic excision in addition to stoma formation.

Over the past approximately 40 years, most patients requiring surgery for ulcerative colitis have therefore been treated by proctocolectomy and formation of a permanent Brooke everted end-ileostomy. This is often quoted as being the 'gold standard' against which all other operations for colitis must be compared. The procedure is simple and has a low mortality, however, in addition to the complications occurring after formation of a Brooke ileostomy, several other specific features of total proctocolectomy must be discussed.

A persistent perineal sinus may occur in between 25% and 35% of cases (Watts, de Dombal and Goligher, 1966; Pemberton *et al.*, 1987). Goligher has identified that females, and patients taking a prolonged preoperative course of steroids, were at greater risk of this complication. Whether perineal drainage, increased anal skin excision or the severity of colitis also predispose to sinus formation is less obvious. Pemberton and colleagues found that the incidence of perineal sinus formation was only 20% after colectomy for polyposis. Interestingly, they also found that it occurred with equal frequency in patients with either ulcerative colitis, Crohn's disease or cancer.

Intestinal obstruction is also relatively common after colectomy, with incidences of between 5% and 15% in major series (Hughes, 1965; Watts, de Dombal and Goligher, 1966; Daly and Brooke, 1967; Ritchie, 1971). The aetiology is frequently a twisting or kinking of the bowel, an adhesive obstruction, small intestinal volvulus, or incarceration in the parastomal gutter. It has been suggested that retention of the diseased rectum predisposes to ileal kinking, and hence that this complication is more frequent after ileorectal anastomosis or subtotal colectomy with ileostomy (Hughes, 1965).

As already stated, immediate maturation of the ileal stoma using Brooke's technique of eversion was a most significant advance in this field. However, in spite of the dramatic reduction in the necessity for stomal revision, peristomal skin irritation continues to be a significant problem. Indeed, up to 60% of patients may report skin irritation, if only intermittently. This represents a challenge to those charged with the supervision of these patients, and is a problem which can be refractory.

Disturbances in male sexual function after rectal excision are not infrequent, particularly after proctectomy for malignant disease. In this group of patients such dysfunction may occur in as many as half to two-thirds of patients. Avoidance of wide dissection of the mesorectum, as is necessary during cancer operations, has facilitated an improvement in these results. Stahlgren and Ferguson (1959) recorded that three-quarters of their patients had 'normal' sexual function, whilst 20% had some degree of impotence and/or ejaculatory difficulties. Importantly, age was found to be particularly significant, with older patients accounting for almost all of these complications. However, as will be described in Chapter 5, the technique of close perirectal dissection is now almost universally utilized in proctectomy for benign disease, hence avoiding damage to the pelvic autonomic nerves. This results in a further significant reduction in the incidence of neurogenic complications such as impotence and/or retrograde ejaculation. Corman has recently stated that none of 76 male patients has experienced sexual difficulties after rectal excision (Corman, Veidenheimer and Coller, 1978). Whilst neuropathic disturbances should be avoidable, the effect of the stoma itself on the sexual activities of the patient are less easily obviated. Social and psychological problems are not infrequent. Embarrassment secondary to the physical characteristics of the stoma and its effluent are understandable, particularly if they have an excessively negative effect on the patient's partner. Interestingly however, conversion of a conventional ileostomy to a continent stoma often has little effect on this problem. This may suggest that, rather than the effluent being the source of embarrassment, the stoma itself is the culprit.

Sexual dysfunction in female patients has been less well described. There is anecdotal evidence that fertility may be slightly reduced after proctocolectomy. However, statistics are hard to find, and even harder to interpret. Certainly, there are many women who have successfully conceived, and undergone a normal vaginal delivery after this procedure.

Therefore, proctocolectomy and permanent ileostomy formation has become a well-established procedure in patients requiring colectomy for ulcerative colitis. However, the attendant problems associated with the perineal wound prompted the development of techniques which obviated the necessity for such an extensive perineal dissection.

Other methods of rectal excision

Conservative proctocolectomy

Throughout the development of proctocolectomy, the perineal dissection was often found to be associated with episodes of hypotension. Consequently, methods have been devised which allow for excision of the diseased rectum whilst retaining some or all of the anus and its sphincters. Initial attempts at such surgery were aimed at retention of both the internal and external sphincters along with the mucosa of the lower anal canal (Figure 1.7). Fallis and

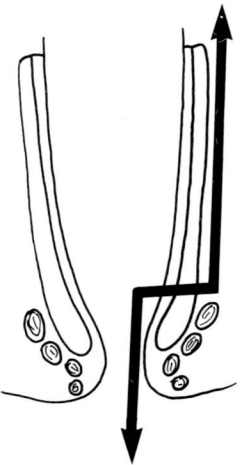

Figure 1.7 Conservative proctocolectomy

Barron described their initial experience with this technique in 1953. Their favourable experience prompted others to recommend this procedure, termed 'conservative procto-colectomy', for patients requiring rectal exci-sion for inflammatory bowel disease (Deane and Celestin, 1983). In these younger patients, this had the advantage of not only avoiding the perineal wound, but also preserving the perineum with its supportive capacity. This is of particular importance in the female, where loss of pelvic support for the vagina can occur.

Doubt has recently been cast upon the efficacy of conservative proctocolectomy (Tal-bot, Ritchie and Northover, 1989). Assessing 23 patients retrospectively, uncomplicated healing occurred in only 13%. In spite of pelvic drainage, almost half developed some degree of anal discharge, whilst 40% had an infected pelvic haematoma. Of 14 patients who de-veloped pelvic sepsis, only one healed spon-taneously. In the other 13 patients, treatments such as curettage, anal sphincterotomy, and anal canal excison were attempted. Whilst anal excision was successful, sphincterotomy proved to be disappointing, and precluded subsequent reconstruction. Only two patients with persistent sepsis proceeded ultimately to ileal pouch–anal anastomosis.

The technique of conservative proctocolec-tomy has also been modified by retaining a long denuded rectal cuff, as utilized by some surgeons during restorative proctocolectomy (see Chapter 5). Whilst encouraging results have been reported with this technique, it has failed to gain widespread acceptance (Fonkals-rud and Ament, 1978; Hulten, 1983).

Intersphincteric proctectomy

In 1977, Lytle and Parks described their technique of 'intersphincteric proctectomy', depicted diagrammatically in Figure 1.8. This dissection, performed from below, results in the preservation of an intact external sphincter and levator ani. In the majority of patients, the perineal wound is closed primarily.

After this form of surgery, more than 50% of perineal wounds will heal primarily. Of the rest, some 60% will heal within the first postoperative year. Should pelvic sepsis de-velop, perineal drainage through the external sphincter is usually adequate. This re-emphasizes the advantage of intersphincteric

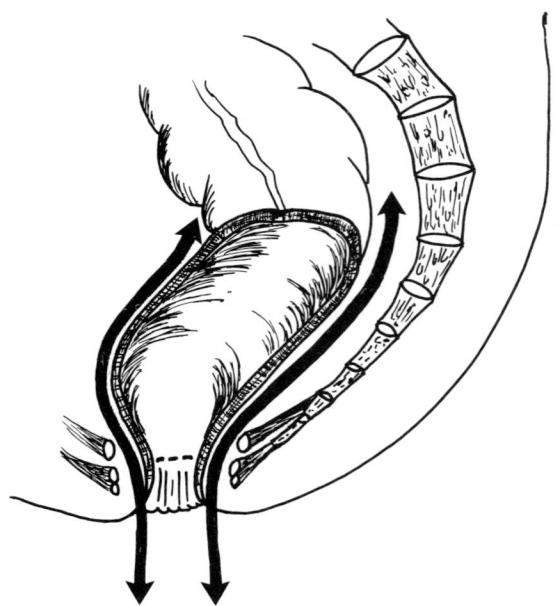

Figure 1.8 Intersphincteric proctectomy

proctectomy over conservative proctectomy, in which such drainage is rarely adequate (Leices-ter, Ritchie, Wadsworth *et al.*, 1984).

So what roles, if any, do these modifications to standard proctocolectomy have? They have traditionally been advocated in the manage-ment of patients in whom a precise diagnosis of ulcerative colitis cannot be made, and in whom Crohn's disease cannot be excluded. In addi-tion, those patients found to have a rectal carcinoma have been considered for such conservative procedures. However, as will be discussed in Chapter 5, most patients with indeterminate colitis can undergo primary restorative proctocolectomy with ileal pouch construction. Even the presence of a carcino-ma in the mid to high rectum need not preclude such a policy. In those patients who are unsure as to the desirability of pouch construction, such operations offer them the opportunity of subsequent pouch–anal anastomosis. In parti-cular, if there is a particularly severe proctitis, with or without carcinoma, these procedures are to be preferred if the patient declines restorative proctocolectomy, but wishes to retain this option. Clearly, any form of subtotal colectomy with rectal preservation would be contraindicated in this situation. In addition, in those patients who decline pouch–anal anastomosis and are prepared to accept permanent ileostomy from the outset, we would favour a more conservative procedure. In such circumstances, we would advocate the use of intersphincteric proctectomy. It holds the advantages of more predictable perineal healing, more easily treated sepsis should this occur, and easier pouch–anal anastomosis should this be desired.

However, in spite of the developments in both rectal excision and conventional ileostomy just described, several surgeons were turning their attention to preserving intestinal continuity. Numerous options were available, but it was ileorectal anastomosis following colectomy which was initially favoured.

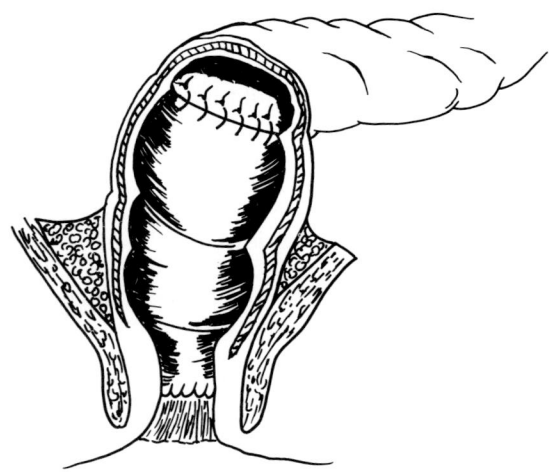

Figure 1.9 Ileorectal anastomosis

Ileorectal anastomosis

In 1903, Lilienthal was the first to perform ileosigmoid anastomosis for ulcerative colitis. Over the next 25 years or so reports of similar procedures were to be found in the literature, if somewhat sparsely (Reinhoff, 1925; Arn, 1931). This new technique was considered to be a significant innovation from the aforementioned procedures of appendicostomy, caecostomy or loop ileostomy, which tended to be performed only in last minute dire circumstances. However, further advances, and general acceptance of the above, were slow in coming. In 1943 Devine described his extraperitoneal ileosigmoid anastomosis. This he created in stages, the patient's condition improving after the initial ileosigmoidostomy. Subsequently, the diseased colon was removed. The experiences of others with this technique, or modifications thereof, were varied; many patients requiring conversion to permanent ileostomy (Corbett, 1952; Gabriel, 1952). It was later suggested that retention of the sigmoid colon might have an adverse effect on the final functional result (Mayo and Broders, 1957; Goligher, 1961). Consequently, true ileorectal anastomosis was adopted (Figure 1.9).

Goligher's report highlights differences between the results obtained with ileorectal anastomosis in patients with 'diffuse' colitis as compared to those with 'segmental' colitis. It is likely that many of the latter were in fact cases of Crohn's colitis. Of the 22 patients discussed,

excellent results were seen in cases of 'segmental colitis', but poor results were recorded in those with 'diffuse colitis'. This was early confirmation that ileorectal anastomosis was not equally efficacious in all cases of inflammatory bowel disease.

In the UK, the main protagonist of ileorectal anastomosis has been Aylett (Aylett, 1960). His operative mortality was 5.4%, and only four patients required conversion to a permanent ileostomy because of incontinence or rectal fistula formation. More than 90% of patients were restored to health, and the number of bowel movements per day was six or less in 80% of the series. This is an important observation, in that after a successful ileorectal anastomosis, bowel function is usually as good, and often better, than after other more modern procedures used in ulcerative colitis. In addition, this procedure has the other advantage of avoiding a rectal dissection; with its attendant risk of reducing sexual function.

Not all have held Aylett's enthusiasm for the procedure. As stated by Goligher, their main objection was that as the rectum was always involved in ulcerative colitis, leaving this disease in place was bad in principle, and that the long-term risk of cancer developing in the rectal stump was a serious problem (Goligher, 1971). In fact, it had even been suggested that the risk was the same as if the colon had not been removed. At this stage it is worth considering this cancer risk in some detail.

Malignant degeneration within an inflamed rectum was first described by Crohn and Rosenberg in 1925. However, it was Bargen who, in 1928, documented his experience with 17 cases of colitis-associated carcinoma, and proposed that the two conditions were related. Since then, the increased risk of carcinomatous change in ulcerative colitis has been extensively investigated and reviewed (Counsell and Dukes, 1952; Slaney and Brooke, 1959; Edwards and Truelove, 1963; Nefzger and Acheson, 1963; MacDougall, 1964; Lennard-Jones *et al.*, 1977, 1990). These surveys have led to the universal acceptance of a predisposition to cancer, but its magnitude has been a matter of some controversy. In particular, it is likely that the risk was overestimated initially.

Whilst differing forms of study, particularly those involving retrospective surveys of hospital records, have made accurate cross-interpretation of such data extremely difficult, most workers accept that the annual risk of malignancy is approximately 20-fold in patients who have a 20-year history of colitis, compared to those whose history is less than 5 years (Edwards and Truelove, 1963). These workers also found an incidence of 7.2% in patients with a pancolitis compared to only 1.3% in those patients whose disease was predominantly distal. Similar results have been reported by MacDougall (1964). Lennard-Jones, however, described a far less gloomy picture, with only two cancers being confirmed after 838 patient-years of exposure to colitis in 169 patients (Lennard-Jones *et al.*, 1977).

In their series, Edwards and Truelove calculated a three-fold increased risk of malignancy if colitis commenced in the first decade of life, as compared to its commencement in the second two decades. No cancers were detected in patients developing colitis after the age of 60 years. Similar figures have been described by others (Edling and Eklof, 1961). This latter report documented that this phenomenon is not related to increased 'exposure' to colitis; they noted that the duration of 'precarcinoma colitis' was similar in those patients developing colitis both before and after the age of 15 years.

It is often reported that colitis-associated carcinomas behave aggressively. It is likely, at least in part, that this arises from a delay in diagnosis due to the concomitant disease, and not an accelerated aggression in these tumours,

per se. The symptoms of ulcerative colitis and colon cancer may be indistinguishable. This may result in a higher initial staging. Slaney and Brooke (1959) calculated a 5-year survival of 18.6% in 358 cases of colitis-associated carcinoma, which naturally raised the question of prophylactic surgery; its necessity, its extent and its timing. Slaney and Brooke (1959) also showed that simple defunctioning of the large bowel provided inadequate protection against the risk of cancer. In addition, 11 of their 304 cases had occurred in patients who had undergone subtotal colectomy and ileostomy formation, the carcinoma developing in the retained rectal stump. This 'stump' carcinoma had also been found in three patients after colectomy and ileorectal anastomosis. Clearly retention of any diseased bowel held a risk of the subsequent development of cancer.

Part of the answer again came from St Mark's Hospital (Lennard-Jones *et al.*, 1977). Experience in the follow-up of patients with extensive colitis using regular rectal and colonic biopsies taken at endoscopy, showed that if good collaboration could be obtained between clinician and pathologist, then the search for epithelial dysplasia could be very helpful in monitoring malignant potential. In particular, even in patients in whom their colitis had not warranted early surgery, 2-yearly colonoscopy and biopsy performed after a 10-year history of the disease revealed a cumulative incidence of carcinoma of 3% at 15 years. Corresponding values at 20 and 25 years were 5% and 9% respectively (Lennard-Jones *et al.*, 1990).

In the 31-year period between 1953 and 1984, 125 patients had undergone subtotal colectomy and ileorectal anastomosis at St Mark's Hospital (Hawley, 1985). This followed the introduction in the 1970s of an active policy to undertake this operation in suitable cases. There were 11 deaths, only four of which could be ascribed to the operation or recurrent disease; importantly there was one death due to carcinoma of the colon, and one due to carcinoma of the rectum. Twenty-eight per cent of patients have subsequently undergone rectal excision, and one patient has a permanent ileostomy with the rectum left *in situ*. The reasons for rectal excision invite further scrutiny.

In 18 of the 33 excisions, unsatisfactory functional results in terms of frequency and continence were the reasons for conversion to ileostomy. Early postoperative technical failures were quoted in five patients, whilst bleeding was the reason in one patient. Significantly, six patients required proctectomy for severe dysplasia, and in two of these small areas of invasive carcinoma were found. Carcinoma has been diagnosed in a further three patients at follow-up. Only one of these patients has died of carcinoma. Functional results were satisfactory, with bowel frequencies of six or less in a 24-hour period in more than 80% of patients. This is in line with previously quoted results (Newton and Baker, 1975). Only 4% had a regular nocturnal bowel action. Urgency and soiling were not a significant complaint, although almost 20% had had at least one episode of faecal soiling in the last 12 months. Fifty per cent had to take regular medication to decrease the frequency of bowel action, and almost 10% took occasional medication to control rectal inflammation.

Further support for the long-term safety of ileorectal anastomosis has recently been provided by Leijonmarck and colleagues. Of 486 patients who underwent colectomy for ulcerative colitis between 1955 and 1984, 12% underwent ileorectal anastomosis. Of these, 86% were elective procedures. Overall, 94% of these ileorectal anastomoses were performed as one-stage operations. Mean follow-up was 13 years. Importantly, whilst more than half of the patients required subsequent rectal excision, 75% of such excisions were for recurrent inflammation. The remaining excisions were equally divided between other miscellaneous complications and dysplasia. There were no carcinomas in this series (Leijonmarck *et al.*, 1990). In addition, functional results were better than those reported after ileal pouch–anal anastomosis.

Whilst debate continues as to the advisability of ileorectal anastomosis in ulcerative colitis, it became obvious that there are certain physiological consequences to this procedure. Most of these result from the retention of the diseased rectum. The inflamed rectal mucosa may demonstrate altered absorptive characteristics. Whether this is clinically significant is questionable.

Using the techniques described in Chapter 8 for assessing pelvic pouch compliance, rectal reservoir capacity and compliance have been assessed after ileorectal anastomosis (Mignon and Bonfils, 1985). A series of 29 patients were compared with normal controls and patients with colitis up to 5 years after ileorectal anastomosis. Measuring the maximal tolerated volume, this was found to be closely correlated with both rectal compliance and bowel frequency. Importantly, for equivalent degrees of inflammation, rectal compliance was improved in the postoperative group compared to the colitics who had not undergone colectomy. Indeed, in the former group, it had improved to a level similar to that recorded in the normal controls.

Unfortunately, there is little information regarding the function of the anal sphincters in ulcerative colitis. Studies have been performed after colectomy for either colitis or Crohn's disease, especially during a period of defunctioning of the rectum by subtotal colectomy with sigmoid mucous fistula formation (Henriksen and Anthonisen, 1972). Anal sphincter function was found to decrease with increasing post-defunctioning periods. Encouragingly, this function tended to improve with time after sigmoid colectomy and restorative ileorectal anastomosis. However, poorly functioning anal sphincters were associated with a less satisfactory result after this procedure. In addition, the formation of a stiff, non-compliant, contracted 'microrectum' is encouraged by prolonged periods of defunctioning. Consequently, if colectomy with mucous fistula formation is performed, early ileorectal anastomosis is to be recommended. It is likely that such restoration of intestinal continuity should be performed within 6 months of the initial colectomy. However, the development of microrectum occasionally may be witnessed within 3 months of colectomy. It has also been suggested that a demonstrably reduced anal sphincter strength need not be a contraindication to ileorectal anastomosis. However, many surgeons would not recommend any form of sphincter-saving surgery under such circumstances.

Several surgeons, most notably Aylett and French surgeons, have felt able to advocate ileorectal anastomosis in the over 90% of colitics requiring colectomy (Aylett, 1953; Mignon, Bonnefond and Vilotte, 1974; Ribet, Wurtz and Paris, 1981). The majority of these workers consider significant disease of the anal sphincters to be a contraindication to ileorectal anastomosis. In addition, malignant disease of the rectum, rectal stenosis or the small non-compliant microrectum would also preclude this procedure. In the rare group of patients who have severe rectal bleeding, this form of restorative surgery is best avoided. However, most exponents of this procedure do not consider severe rectal inflammation to be of significant prognostic importance. Indeed, rectal inflammation frequently subsides after ileorectal anastomosis (Aylett, 1953). Overall, approximately 10% of patients therefore would be deemed unsuitable for ileorectal anastomosis based upon these criteria. Alternatively, even amongst surgeons who feel that there is a role for this procedure in ulcerative colitis, only 10% of patients have been deemed suitable for ileorectal anastomosis (Farnell, van Heerden and Beart, 1980).

There can be little doubt that some surgeons have reported extremely acceptable results with ileorectal anastomosis in ulcerative colitis. However, it must be appreciated that this has not been the experience of all. Such discrepancies may, at least in part, be explained by the greater experience of these surgeons with this technique, and by the numerous technical features which some have incorporated into the operation. Many surgeons perform a one-stage colectomy with ileorectal anastomosis. Those surgeons with most experience with this technique tend to advocate two-, or even three-stage procedures. Whatever the logistics, the restorative anastomosis is almost always covered by a temporary loop ileostomy. To extend this argument, whilst these surgeons do not consider severe rectal inflammation to preclude ultimate ileorectal anastomosis, they tend not to perform a primary anastomosis in these circumstances. Most would undertake colectomy with sigmoid mucous fistula formation. Thereafter, irrigation of the sigmoid colon and rectum is instigated, and ileorectal anastomosis performed secondarily. Finally, many advocate the use of anastomosis at the level of the sacral promontory; therefore performing what is virtually an ileosigmoid anastomosis. Anastomoses performed lower, such as below the peritoneal reflection, may be associated with less satisfactory functional outcomes.

A final important consideration regarding ileorectal anastomosis relates to the patient with what can be termed 'indeterminate colitis', in whom a precise pathological diagnosis excluding Crohn's disease cannot be made. In this group the results of ileorectal anastomosis have been generally thought to be superior to any form of reservoir construction. However, doubt has recently been cast upon this by the Mayo clinic group who, with their large experience of this problem, are now prepared to offer such patients the option of ileal pouch–anal anastomosis (Pezim et al., 1989). The authors' own limited experience with indeterminate colitis treated by J-pouch–anal anastomosis has not been so encouraging, with two pouches subsequently requiring excision because of poor continence. Others have found perineal complications to be more common in this group of patients (Koltun et al., 1990).

In that small subgroup of ulcerative colitics in whom there is relative rectal sparing, there may be a role for ileorectal anastomosis. That recurrent proctitis may subsequently necessitate either the potentially more complicated pouch–anal anastomosis, or formation of an ileostomy (be it incontinent or otherwise), need not be deemed to constitute a failure of ileorectal anastomosis. So long as the patient accepts that regular endoscopic follow-up is required, and that should either symptoms or dysplasia demand subsequent rectal excision, then the initial performance of ileorectal anastomosis might be justified. The benefits are that the procedure is easily performed; in many surgeons' hands does not require a temporary ileostomy (Hawley, 1985); and is further associated with few complications, a reduced hospital stay, and a shorter period of convalescence. In addition, on the whole nothing irrevocable has been done with regard to the subsequent performance of sphincter-saving procedures. Hence, the patient might benefit for several years from a simple procedure, whilst still keeping all his or her options open.

Ileorectal anastomosis can be considered to be a safe conservative operation in selected patients with ulcerative colitis, and it has certain advantages over some of the alternative sphincter-saving procedures. By careful cancer monitoring a cancer mortality of less than 1% should be readily attainable. Indeed, with improved techniques and experience of such surveillance, it may be that even earlier stages of 'pre-cancer' dysplasia may become recognizable. Should this be the case, there may ultimately be a resurgence of interest in ileorectal anastomosis. Therefore, this risk of cancer need not be considered a contraindication to the performance of ileorectal anastomosis after colonic excision for ulcerative colitis. Further, the use of ileorectal anastomosis is not contraindicated in the older age group, so long as adequate sphincter function can be demonstrated. To date, elderly patients have usually been deferred from ileal reservoir procedures, although this trend may be altering.

However, many surgeons, including ourselves, have not felt able to include ileorectal anastomosis in their repertoire for colitics requiring surgery, preferring complete excison of the diseased colorectal mucosa. Whilst the majority have continued to perform proctocolectomy with ileostomy formation, a few have attempted to improve the lot of their patients by constructing continent ileostomies. Certainly, in spite of skilful construction of conventional stomas, and the use of satisfactory stoma appliances, the patient may still face many problems. Even if the patient makes an acceptable physical and emotional adaptation to his new circumstances, both personal and/or ethnic reasons may make those around him unable to do so.

The continent ileostomy

It is well recognized that mechanical stimulation of the small intestine results in increased motor activity. This results in an elevation in intraluminal pressure, and bowel contents are propulsed distally. It is important therefore that any vessel required to act as a storage organ fulfills at least two fundamental criteria. First, the outlet of the ileostomy has to be continent but allow periodic evacuation of the effluent. Secondly, to avoid this valvular element leading to obstructive symptoms and ultimately to paralytic ileus, a capacitance vessel or reservoir has to be constructed.

During the 1960s, Professor Nils Kock had been accumulating considerable experience in the use of isolated intestinal segments to provide for bladder replacement after cystectomy. Various designs and modifications had been tried, utilizing both small and large intestine. Unfortunately, most early designs failed to remain continent, particularly at

night. However, through the physiological assessment of these intestinal 'bladders', Kock was able to describe the basic characteristics of such isolated intestinal segments (Eckmann *et al.*, 1964).

Several types of intestinal segments had been employed as bladder substitutes. Kock infused each configuration of reservoir with saline, and recorded the pressure profile of each type during filling. Such important initial basic work provided a fundamental scientific background for what might now be called 'pouchology'. In the V-type ileal bladder

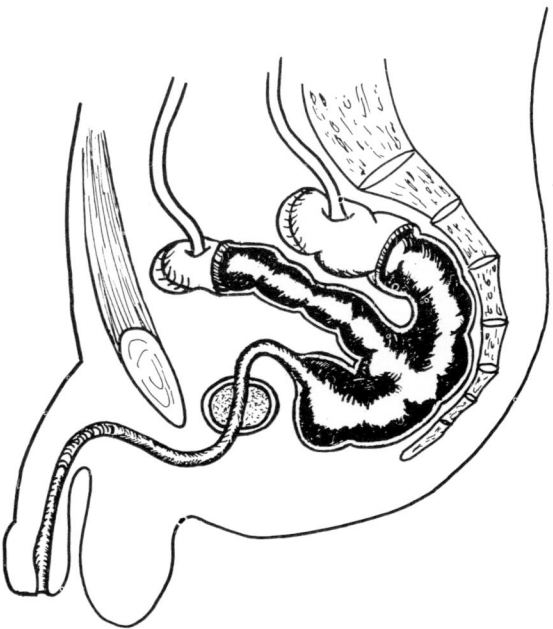

Figure 1.10 V-ileal bladder substitution

substitute (Figure 1.10), filling induced pressure waves with amplitudes greater than $100\,\text{cmH}_2\text{O}$. This resulted in leakage as the resistance of the urethral sphincter was overcome. Subsequently, an isoperistaltic segment of sigmoid colon was employed by anastomosing it to the urethra (Figure 1.11). The filling-pressure profile of this type of conduit revealed that leakage occurred at a filling volume of 150 ml, this being again associated with the generation of a high pressure. To be

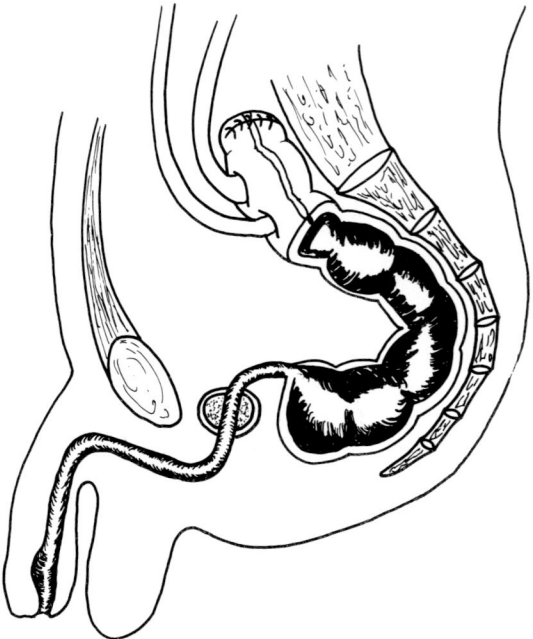

Figure 1.11 Sigmoid colon bladder substitution

suitable for utilization as a continent ileostomy, such a reservoir would have to have a capacity of approximately 500 ml in order to keep the number of evacuations to about three per day. In addition, the pressure generated at this volume must not be great.

The Tasker pouch (Figure 1.12) involved splitting an isolated ileal loop along its antimesenteric border, folding this into a U, and closing the U from side to side. Hence, this is analogous to the J-type reservoirs used for pelvic pouch construction. The filling-pressure profile of this vessel revealed high pressures only late in the record, at volumes greater than 200 ml. In patients with this type of reservoir used as a bladder substitute, leakage was only problematical at night.

In order to obviate even this late pressure rise, Kock designed his own doubly folded reservoir (Figure 1.13). He again utilized an ileal loop split along its antimesenteric border, which was similarly folded into a U. This time the U was folded along its transverse axis, with the ends of the U being anastomosed to the base of the U. The filling-pressure profile of

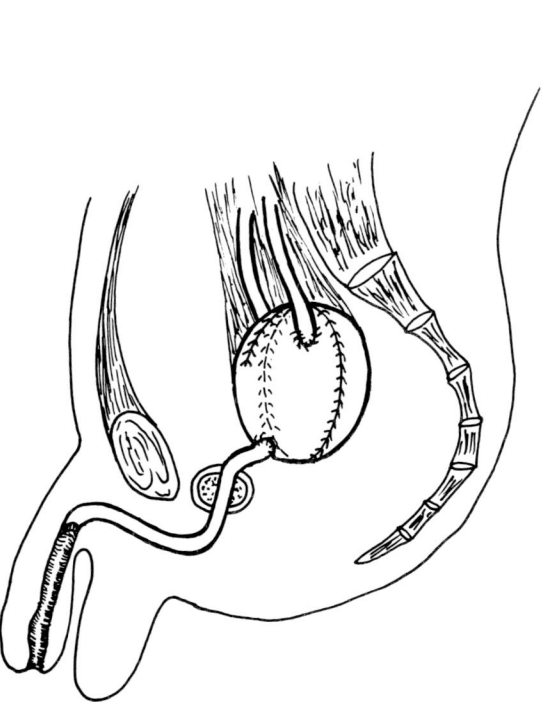

Figure 1.12 Tasker J-pouch bladder substitution

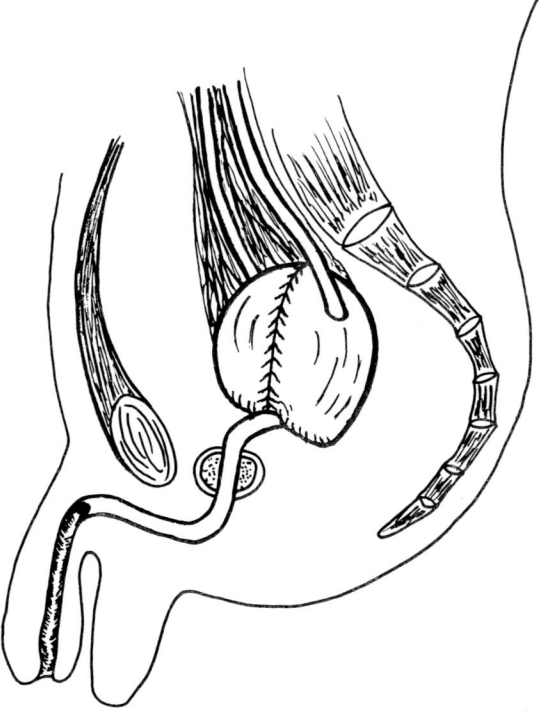

Figure 1.13 Kock pouch bladder substitution

this design showed a slow rise in basal pressure, but more importantly, very few pressure waves were seen. Clinical experience with this configuration used as a bladder substitute was very encouraging, with resulting capacities of between 300 and 600 ml (Faxen, Kock and Sundin, 1973). This reservoir therefore fulfilled the criteria for its utilization as a continent ileostomy. As with the ileal pelvic pouch, these pouches were emptied by a combination of a Valsalva manoeuvre and manual compression over the bladder substitute.

Kock's design of ileal reservoir was first employed as a continent ileostomy in 1967, utilizing the terminal ileum for its construction after proctocolectomy (Kock, 1969). Initially, one corner of the reservoir was taken out through the rectus muscle and sutured flush with the skin (Figure 1.14(a)). This method of providing continence was generally satisfactory. However, it was found that because

patients had no absolute control over faecal expulsion, many continued intermittently to use stoma appliances. However, long-term experience with this form of 'valve' has been shown subsequently to be generally satisfactory.

Kock subsequently turned to using varying lengths of either an anti- or isoperistaltic outlet segment to provide more certain and controllable continence (Figure 1.14(b),(c)). Results with this modification were extremely variable, usually in spite of an adequate reservoir capacity.

In 1972, a new valve was constructed, utilizing an intussusception of part of an isoperistaltic outlet segment (Figure 1.14(d)) (Steichen, 1977). This resulted in a leak-proof, one-way valve which allowed absolute control. Immediately postoperation, patients were completely continent. However a number of patients complained of leakage of gas and faeces through the stoma within a few months.

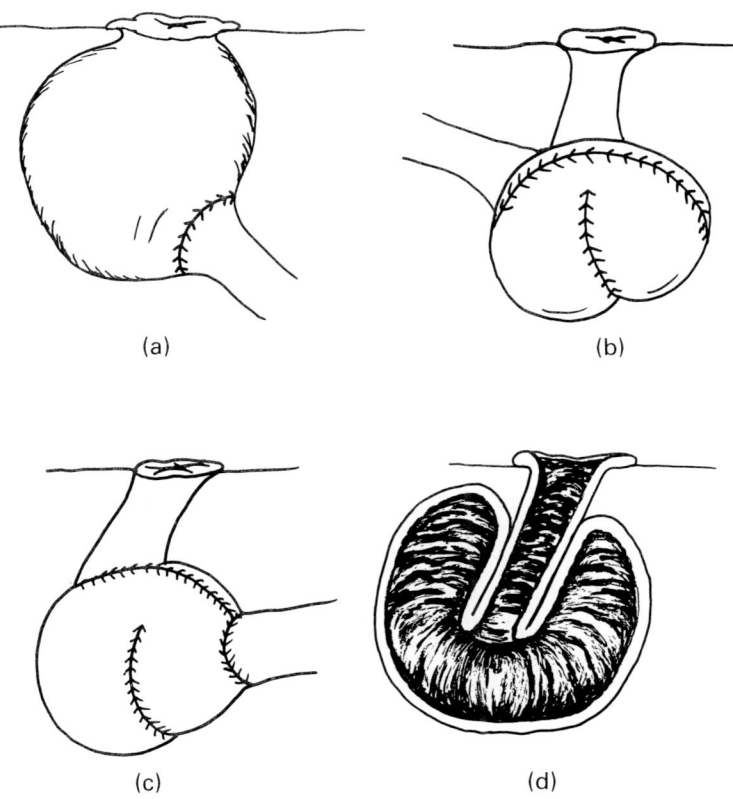

(a) (b)

(c) (d)

Figure 1.14 Valves used in the continent ileostomy

Associated with this was the complaint that catheter introduction through the valve also became more difficult. The reason for this was a partial or complete dessusception of the intussuscepted valve mechanism.

This dessusception usually occurred on the mesenteric side of the valve, where firm fixation of the intussusceptum was prevented by the bulk of the mesentery. Reservoir dilatation during the first 6 months after construction, results in an increase in the intramural tension at the site of suturing around the base of the nipple valve. This causes the two intestinal walls to tear apart, rendering the previously intussuscepted valve incompetent.

Numerous technical modifications were attempted, the evolution of which has been well described elsewhere (Kock, Darle and Hulton, 1977; Kock, Myrvold and Nilsson, 1980). Stable fixation of the intestinal walls could be achieved by longitudinal stapling of the valve (Steichen, 1977). Initially, staples were not applied directly to the mesentery for fear of jeopardizing the blood supply of the valve, but sliding on the mesenteric side still occurred. Fascial strips and other foreign materials were employed to prevent this slippage, but with little initial success. Four sets of staples were subsequently applied to the valve, including over the mesentery, after the latter had been stripped of peritoneum and fat (Madigan, 1976). Other techniques used to aid in valve fixation have included the subserosal injection of concentrated tetracycline solution, and extensive scarification of the serosa. Such techniques have helped to prevent sliding, and it was soon found that the longitudinal lines of staples became embedded in the muscular layer of the nipple, and were completely covered by regenerating mucosa (Kock, Myrvold and Nilsson, 1980). These modifications have reduced the rate of valve revision from approximately 50% to less than 10% (Dozois, Kelly and Beart, 1980; Gerber, Apt and Craig, 1983).

Whilst the technical modifications described have improved the results obtained with the Kock pouch utilized as a continent ileostomy, other techniques providing for a continent ileostomy have been described. Bokey has been predominant amongst workers attempting to obviate the need for such a complicated pouch construction. He has used a J-

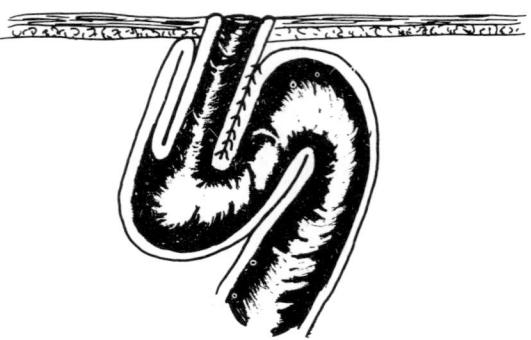

Figure 1.15 J-pouch continent ileostomy (after Bokey *et al.*, 1983)

configuration two-limb side-to-side reservoir for continent ileostomy formation (Figure 1.15) (Bokey *et al.*, 1983). In dogs, an 8-cm nipple valve was created within a 20-cm pouch. Ileostomy output decreased by 40% over the first three postoperative months. Compliance studies using saline infusion up to a volume of 600 ml failed to demonstrate the presence of large amplitude pressure waves. Importantly, the small intestine proximal to the pouch was not found to be dilated. Therefore, this easily constructed pouch showed all the performance characteristics of an acceptable capacitance vessel.

Bokey has also assessed the potential for providing a continent ileostomy without the construction of an intestinal pouch (Bokey, Hayward and Johnson, 1981; Bokey, 1984). In animal experiments a 10-cm segment of the terminal ileum was mobilized. The proximal 8 cm are retrogradely intussuscepted after threading a fascial strip through its mesentery. After intussusception, the fascia comes to lie around the base of the nipple valve, where it is stitched. The isoperistaltic last 2 cm of terminal ileum are brought to the skin surface as a flush ileostomy (Figure 1.16). A catheter facilitated postoperative decompression of the bowel lumen. Over the postoperative weeks, progressively longer periods were allowed between emptying of the terminal ileum. The postoperative course was usually uneventful, with decreasing ileostomy outputs. Contrast studies demonstrated that the terminal ileum had dilated, however the ileum proximal to this was of normal dimensions. Again, compliance

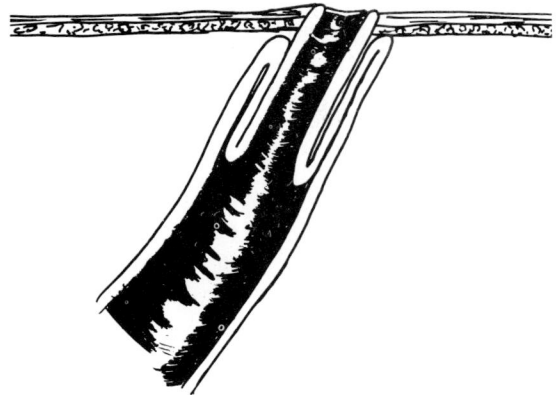

Figure 1.16 Continent ileostomy without pouch (after Bokey, Hayward and Johnson, 1981)

studies using saline infusion failed to induce high pressure waves. Histologically, there was evidence of muscular hypertrophy and mucosal inflammation within the dilated ileal segment. Initial clinical experience with this technique showed that valve desussception proved to be problematical, however the overall functional results appeared to be encouraging.

Whether the relative disadvantages of pouch construction warrant this new technique is debatable. Complications have, over recent years, become less common. However, there remain certain relatively specific complications of the continent ileostomy. Included amongst these are structural complications, such as stomal stenosis and mucous leakage. In addition, and importantly, there are several biological consequences of placing a closed capacitance vessel at the distal end of the small intestine. Significant amongst these is an increased effluent bacterial count, presumably secondary to stasis. Anaerobes, most particularly Bacteroides, are found in abundance, the effluent taking on a more 'stool-like' characteristic. Vitamin B_{12} may be malabsorbed from continent ileostomies, particularly in patients with evidence of bacterial overgrowth and/or excessive effluent output. A similar phenomenon is witnessed when bile salt absorption is assessed, and mucosal morphology is seen to alter within these intra-abdominal reservoirs, to a form that is recognizably more 'colonic'. All these biological changes are discussed in detail elsewhere in this book. Suffice to say, on the whole, changes witnessed after construction of a continent ileostomy are little different from those recorded after ileal pouch–anal anastomosis. In this sense, both are more representative of there being a closed, static loop at the end of the intestine.

There is little doubt that the continent ileostomy offers a better quality of life compared with the conventional ileostomy (Kock, Darle and Kewenter, 1974; King, 1975; Nilsson, Kock and Kylberg, 1981). Technical modifications have reduced the early and late complications to an acceptably low level. Kock's group have recently reported their long-term experience with the continent ileostomy in 36 patients, all of whom were followed up for at least 16 years. All were in excellent health. Gall stones had occurred in 22% of patients, however in only 8% had they appeared since construction of the continent stoma. Nephrolithiasis occurred in 17% of patients. There was no incidence of reservoir dysplasia in this group of patients, and few had any limitations on their social or work commitments. Interestingly, in spite of the fact that 11 of the 36 patients had Kock pouches constructed without the use of valves, 92% of patients were fully continent (Ojerskog *et al.*, 1990). Therefore, is there still a place for this procedure, and if so what role might it have in the management of patients requiring proctocolectomy?

Certainly, the operation does not eliminate the necessity for a stoma, though this is much less prominent and unsightly. According to Kock, his technique has many advantages over the ileoanal pouch procedure, including the lower frequency of evacuation and the absence of urgency. Many surgeons with an interest in this field have stated that ileal pouch–anal anastomosis has reduced the indications for procedures such as the continent ileostomy. The authors' consider that whilst the role for this procedure has undoubtedly diminished, in some respects its indications have become better defined. Certainly, there is now a 'snow-balling' tendency towards the maintenance of faecal continence. It is likely that in the near future, many more patients requiring colectomy for ulcerative colitis will be offered a pelvic pouch. For those patients for whom such a procedure is deemed inappropriate, there may be an obligation amongst surgeons to at least discuss the option of a continent ileostomy. It may be prudent initially to construct a conventional Brooke ileostomy, with a view to converting this to a continent stoma at a later date, should the patient so desire. Alternatively, many surgeons would be happy to construct such a stoma *per primum*.

In addition, with the rising popularity of pouch–anal anastomosis, it stands to reason that increasing numbers (but one would hope a decreasing proportion) of patients will require excision of their pouches. With the technical problems requiring further surgery on continent stomas now significantly reduced, the commitment that continence preservation justifies the performance of a pelvic pouch, surely also obliges surgeons to consider the continent ileostomy as an alternative to a more conventional incontinent stoma in this group of patients. Such conversion of a failed ileoanal pouch has been reported (Kusunoki *et al.*, 1990a) (see Chapter 6).

In the past, the continent ileostomy has obtained most of its protagonists from within the realms of colorectal specialists. Recent improvements with regard to valve construction, particularly with the use of linear stapling guns, has made this procedure much more accessible to other surgeons with less experience of the technique. It is interesting that exactly the same scenario has been witnessed with restorative proctocolectomy, with many surgeons now happy to take up this procedure, utilizing various stapling techniques.

The technical complexity of the continent ileostomy encouraged other workers to concentrate their efforts upon ways of allowing for periodic evacuation of a conventional stoma. Bokey's technique of creating an intussuscepted valve at the end of a conventional 'straight' ileostomy has been described above. In addition, the provision of an occluding continence valve has received attention, but has failed to gain widespread enthusiasm (Pemberton, Kelly and Phillips, 1985). Whilst initially devised for the malfunctioning continent ileostomy, its use has been extended to provide continence with the conventional ileostomy.

These technical modifications to the continent ileostomy have been a relatively recent event. The initial complexity of this procedure, coupled with the fact that patients still required an external stoma, encouraged surgeons to look for further alternatives. Based upon their contention that retention of the rectum, be it particularly diseased or otherwise, was undesirable, they felt unable to utilize ileorectal anastomosis. As a consequence of this, the search was on for a means of providing a satisfactory 'neorectum'.

2

Rectal replacement and the pelvic pouch procedure – historical perspective

As discussed in the previous chapter, some surgeons have considered that neither the creation of a permanent stoma, nor the retention of the potentially diseased rectum, represent ideal treatment options after colectomy for benign mucosal disease of the large bowel. For these workers, a means of providing a suitable 'neorectum' has had to be sought. This quest continues to the present day. However, enthusiasm was aimed initially at ileoanal anastomosis.

Ileoanal anastomosis

To date, ileoanal anastomosis has been practised for some 80 years. Initially performed to avoid permanent sigmoid colostomy after rectal excision for malignancy, most workers used an isolated segment of ileum interposed between the colon and the anal canal; the so-called 'ileocolorectoplasty' (Figure 2.1) (Vignolo, 1912; Stone, 1928; Quenu, 1933). Early results were marred by severe complications, such as pelvic abscess, anastomotic breakdown and sacroperineal fistula. In the preantibiotic period these were a source of numerous postoperative complications, including a significant mortality.

At the turn of the century, Hochenegg described distal mucosal proctectomy, combined with a coloanal pull-through anastomosis (Figure 2.2) (Hochenegg, 1900). He argued that rectal mucosal stripping would promote adhesions between the colonic serosa and the denuded rectal cuff. This modification significantly reduced postoperative morbidity and mortality, and was incorporated into the repertoire of many workers in this field (Vignolo, 1912). However, there were doubts as to the safety of the technique, particularly with regard to continence (Wangensteen, 1943; Goligher, 1951). It would be more than two decades before almost universal acceptance of its safety would be realized. To a great degree it was increasing knowledge of the mechanisms of anorectal continence which encouraged such acceptance (see Chapter 4).

The acceptance of mucosal proctectomy as a safe, powerful weapon in the armamentarium of the proctologist, allowed renewed vigour in the quest for sphincter preservation after radical surgery for mucosal disease of the large bowel. In 1933 Nissen had reported the case of a 10-year-old child with familial polyposis coli, in whom he performed the three-stage procedure of ileostomy, total colectomy and ileoanal anastomosis. An acceptable result was obtained, and this was the first occasion on which an ileoanal anastomosis had been performed for a benign disease. In spite of his encouraging results, few took up the mantle of ileoanal anastomosis. It was more than a decade before Ravitch and his team followed up this work with some of the most important contributions in this field (Ravitch and Sabiston, 1947; Ravitch, 1948).

Operating upon dogs, the terminal ileum was mobilized until it would reach the perineum. The intestine was replaced and the

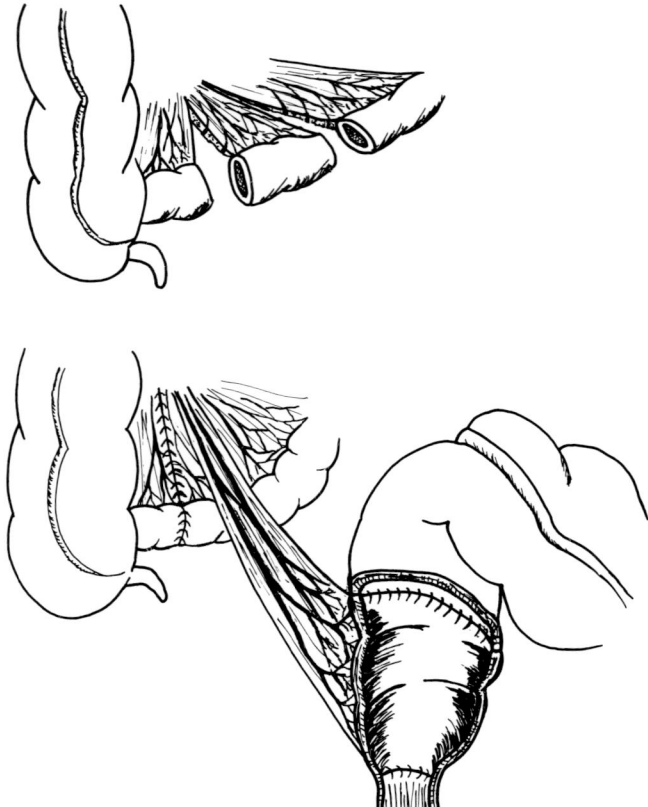

Figure 2.1 Ileocolorectoplasty

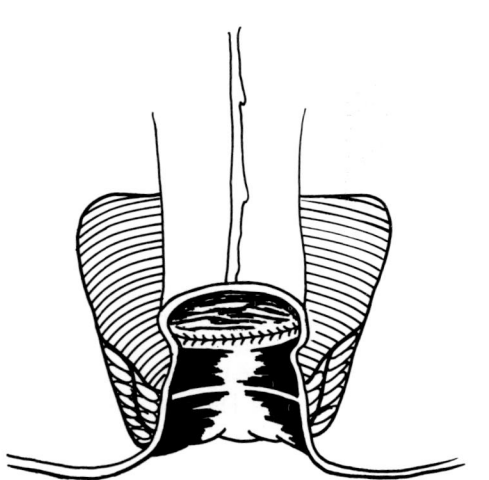

Figure 2.2 Coloanal sleeve anastomosis

abdomen closed. A circular incision was made in the mucocutaneous junction within the anal canal, and the dissection carried up submucosally. When a flap approximately 5 cm long had been developed the incision was continued through the outer rectal coats into the peritoneal cavity. This enabled the operator to deliver the then freed bowel through the intact sphincter. The outer coats of the rectum were then everted through the anus so that the rectal stump could be sutured to the ileum, serosa to serosa (Figure 2.3).

Using this technique, primary healing was satisfactory. Therefore, the procedure was offered to two patients (Ravitch, 1948). The first was a 28-year-old male, with a 12-year history of severe ulcerative colitis. Staged construction of an end-ileostomy, and later subtotal colectomy with mucous fistula, had resulted in little improvement. Consequently, the remaining colon and rectum were excised

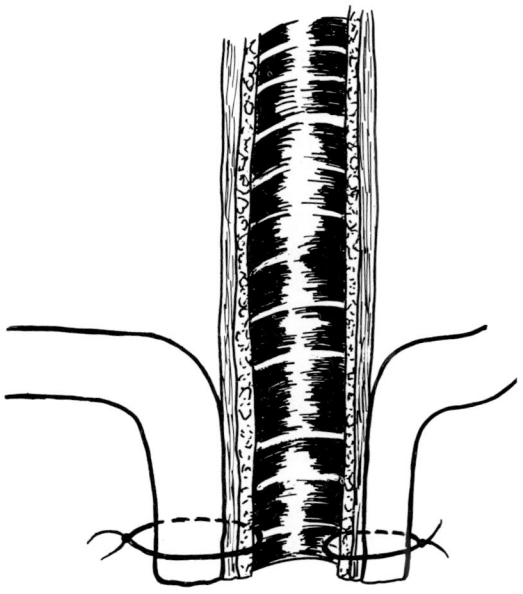

Figure 2.3 Everted ileoanal anastomosis

and the ileoanal anastomosis constructed as described. After a prolonged postoperative course, including relaparotomy for small bowel obstruction, he eventually made a remarkable recovery. By the fourth month satisfactory sphincter control had been gained, two formed stools were passed per day and the abdominal cramps had ceased. He put on 27 kg in weight.

The second case was a 36-year-old woman with an 8-year history of ulcerative colitis. Formation of a Dragstedt ileostomy lead to only slight improvement, so total colectomy and ileoanal anastomosis was performed. All wounds healed *per primam*, and her postoperative course was uneventful.

Five years prior to Ravitch's reports, Wangensteen had performed and documented this procedure in a schoolboy with ulcerative colitis. In this patient the 'temporary' ileostomy was closed after more than four and a half years with an acceptable degree of continence. However, daytime frequency and nocturnal diarrhoea necessitated early re-establishment of a permanent ileostomy (Wangensteen and Toon, 1948). It was Ravitch's success which renewed interest in the ileoanal anastomosis (Devine and Webb, 1951).

Unfortunately, postoperative complications associated with ileoanal anastomosis remained common. With a view to allowing the anastomosis to heal, and to decrease the incidence of postoperative sepsis, Goligher (1951) reported the use of the loop ileostomy (see Chapter 6). This form of protection became a standard incorporation with many (Schneider, 1955). Testimony to the importance of the staged procedure with a covering protective loop ileostomy is the fact that, for most surgeons, it has remained an integral part of ileoanal anastomosis.

Increasing clinical experience resulted in further refinements, some of which have passed subsequently into obsolescence. Some years earlier, it had been noted that the terminal ileal segment underwent dilatation (Best, 1952), no doubt due to partial obstruction of the small bowel by the tonically closed anal canal. In spite of this adaptation, excessive stool frequency and faecal incontinence were commonplace. Generally, this was considered to be due to the propulsive properties of the ileum eventually overcoming the anal sphincters. Therefore, techniques to solve this problem were devised, including division of the ileal circular muscle at several points on the circumference (Casanova-Diaz, 1954), or interposition of an antiperistaltic straight ileal segment above the anal sphincters (Bokey *et al.*, 1985).

General experience with ileoanal anastomosis demonstrated that less than one-third of the patients had what could be considered a satisfactory result in terms of continence, the ulcerative colitics seeming to fare worse than those patients with polyposis coli (Ravitch, 1956).

Further interest was prompted after Soave's report of his considerable success with mucosal proctectomy (Soave, 1964). His technique was adopted by many paediatric surgeons, but was not enthused upon by general surgeons of the day. The intricacy of this procedure, and the not insignificant complications discouraged many, and prevented widespread acceptance. However, interest was rekindled in the mid-1970s, after reports of improved results after ileoanal anastomosis. Safaie-Shirazi and Soper (1973) described their successful utilization of this procedure in four patients with familial polyposis. This was followed in 1977 by Martin's report of unprecedented success with the procedure in patients with ulcerative colitis and polyposis coli (Martin, Le Coultre and Schubert, 1977). In this series, 17 patients, 11–20 years of age, underwent colectomy and an abdominal rectal mucosal proctectomy, commencing at the peritoneal reflection. Endoanally, the rectal mucosa was divided 1 cm above the mucocutaneous junction and the ileoanal anastomosis completed. A covering loop ileostomy was constructed, and closed at 3–6 months following demonstration of complete healing of the anastomosis. There were no postoperative deaths, however these 17 patients had a total of 18 postoperative complications, including wound infection, pelvic infection, cuff abscesses, anastomotic strictures and bowel obstruction. Pelvic sepsis necessitated the construction of permanent ileostomies in two patients, neither of whom had been given temporary diverting ileostomies. The other patients with functioning ileoanal anastomoses had frequent watery stools for up to 1 year, after which all had complete control of between two and eight semiformed stools daily.

In spite of these complications, it must be stressed that these results were in marked contrast to those usually obtained with this procedure, the success of this group being due in no small degree to the meticulous and prolonged preparation of the rectal mucosa preoperatively. Their aim was a macroscopically disease free rectum at the time of operation. This was achieved by various degrees of intensive medical management, total parenteral nutrition or a preliminary ileostomy with subtotal colectomy. It was not uncommon for patients to undergo up to 2 months of total parenteral nutrition adequately to prepare the rectum.

Coran has similarly reported excellent results with straight ileoanal anastomosis. Whilst he originally advocated this procedure for young patients with pancolonic involvement with Hirschsprung's disease, it was later used with effect in ulcerative colitis and polyposis coli (Coran, Sarahan and Dent, 1983). Even during the early patients in this series, daytime continence was complete immediately after closure of the loop ileostomy. Admirably, even nocturnal soiling was unusual during this period, when bowel frequency varied between 2 and 20 motions per 24 hours. However, after 1 year this had reduced to a median of six motions per day. Nocturnal evacuation was infrequent. Perhaps surprisingly, one patient (2%) had significant perianal excoriation, which resolved after 1 year. Contrary to the experience of others, use of antidiarrhoeals and stool-bulking agents became less unnecessary 1 year after closure of the temporary ileostomy, such that few patients required their regular use. Only 12% of patients found the increased frequency associated with ileoanal anastomosis to be less preferable than their ileostomy (Coran, 1985).

Unfortunately, few other surgeons have been able to emulate Coran's remarkable results with the straight ileoanal anastomosis. In the majority of reported series, it soon became apparent that stool frequency remained problematical. It therefore became obvious that straight ileoanal pull-through anastomosis failed to satisfy one essential requirement for continence: the provision of an adequate reservoir. Subsequent efforts therefore began to be aimed at this next important factor.

Balloon dilatation

Telander from the Mayo clinic reported his favourable experience of using postoperative, but often preileostomy closure, balloon dilatation of a straight ileoanal anastomosis (Figure 2.4) (Telander and Perrault, 1981). Two weeks after endorectal pull-through, a balloon was used to perform gentle anal dilatations. These prevented the occurrence of stenoses at the ileoanal anastomoses. (In their subsequent pouch–anal anastomosis patients, they instructed the patients to perform gentle digital anal dilatations.) Over the 2–3 months of defunctioning, balloon dilatation of both the ileoanal anastomosis and the distal ileal 'neorectal' segment were performed. Both the volume and the duration of inflation of the balloon were increased daily. The former by 15 ml, the latter by 15 minutes. After 2 months, most patients were tolerating a balloon volume of some 100–150 ml over a period of 6 hours or so. Importantly, the procedure was stopped if either pain or anal bleeding ensued. Using this regimen, mean neorectal volume increased by 40% per month. The loop ileostomy was closed at about 3 months, after which the neorectal

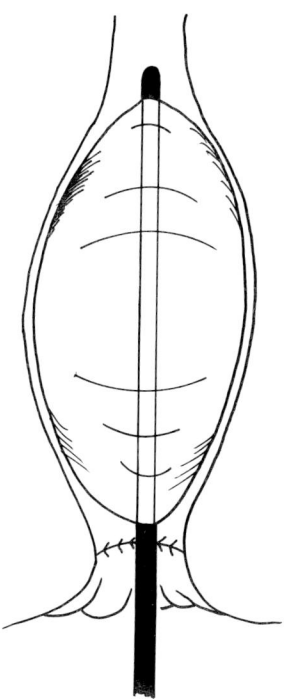

Figure 2.4 Balloon dilatation

first 3 months after ileostomy closure the former group had a bowel frequency of 10.5. The latter had a frequency of 6.4 per 24 hours. Comparable figures after 6 months were 8.7 and 5.8 respectively. Telander emphasizes that for the majority of patients, the cessation of their colitis and the maintenance of normal anal defaecation are more important than the precise values for defaecation frequency and minor problems with continence, such as soiling and nocturnal evacuation. This is an opinion with which we concur.

Whilst balloon dilatation may be inconvenient to perform at home, and for a minority of patients proves to be too difficult, no serious complications were attributable to it. Telander therefore concluded that this procedure could be recommended for young people requiring total colectomy. However, with the subsequently favourable experience with pouch–anal anastomosis reported from his colleagues at the Mayo clinic, Telander now utilizes this latter procedure in most of his patients. Hence, in spite of somewhat improved functional results, balloon dilatation of the straight ileoanal anastomosis has not proved popular with workers in this field.

volume increased by only 6.6% per month without balloon dilatation.

Results were satisfactory, there were no deaths, and apart from one case of vesicoenteric fistula in a patient subsequently shown to have Crohn's disease, pelvic infection was not a problem. In the 24 patients who had undergone closure of ileostomy, stool frequency decreased over a period of time, inversely proportional to the degree of dilatation of the neorectum. However, such frequency was rarely less than 5 per 24 hours, and more usually between 8 and 10 per day. Such dilatation could be promoted by deferring defaecation for as long as possible, and by taking regular exercise. Leakage was relatively common, and 25% of patients were classed as having only a fair or poor result. In spite of this, results were still an improvement on a straight anastomosis without dilatation. Importantly, comparing patients who underwent ileoanal anastomosis without balloon dilatation with those undergoing this procedure, in the

Ileal mucosal grafting

Although dilatation represented an advance, throughout the early years of experimentation with neorectal formation, workers were also assessing the feasibility of grafting ileal mucosa, as opposed to full thickness ileum, to the denuded rectum (Peck and Hallenbeck, 1964; Glotzer and Pihl, 1969; Peck, 1980).

Describing their technique used in five dogs, Glotzer and Pihl (1969) created a preliminary appendicostomy 2 weeks prior to definitive surgery. Subsequent preoperative preparation involved 3 days of colonic irrigation via this stoma. After infiltration of the rectal submucosal plane, they performed an endoanal mucosal proctectomy to a level of 35 cm above the sphincters, using the method of intussuscepting the bowel upon itself. Thereafter, the denuded colon was excised, leaving a length of colonic mucosa and the denuded rectal stump. These were then anastomosed with silk sutures (Figure 2.5). Four animals survived, three being fully continent from the

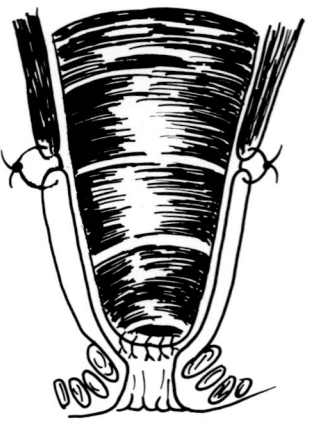

Figure 2.5 Colonic mucosal grafting (after Glotzer and Pihl, 1969)

outset. The fourth animal ultimately regained continence. Stools were semi-solid, and all animals had intact rectoanal inhibitory reflexes.

Encouraged by these results, they performed this procedure in two patients with ulcerative colitis. The first of these, a 48-year-old male, had an acceptable initial result. However, after 2 months he developed a stricture due to recurrent colitis in the retained mucosa and a proctectomy was performed. Their second patient was a 28-year-old male, who had previously undergone a subtotal colectomy with ileostomy formation. After initial urgency, he was fully continent by day passing 8–12 stools with good discriminatory function. There was a little nocturnal leakage. This group stressed the importance of careful patient selection, emphasizing that an emotionally stable and well motivated patient was required, and that evidence of 'granulomatous colitis' should be meticulously sought prior to performing any such procedures. These are sentiments which are equally as true today.

Throughout the 1960s, Peck and his co-workers had been working on the provision of an ileorectal mucosal graft to attempt to eliminate ileal peristalsis, and to alleviate fibrosis of the rectal muscular tube so preserving its muscular function (Peck and Hallenbeck, 1964; Peck, 1980). In 1968, this group performed its first such graft in a human patient, however profound frequency and nocturnal incontinence necessitated intestinal

diversion after 1 month. Further animal work was therefore undertaken to incorporate a reservoir, which culminated in their first patient receiving such a reservoir in 1971.

Peck's technique was to use a two-stage procedure. The initial procedure involved total colectomy, an abdominal and endoanal mucosal proctectomy and preparation of the mucosal graft. The latter underwent several modifications, ultimately being simplified to the technique used clinically (Figure 2.6). This method involves the grafting of ileal mucosa onto the denuded rectum. In this design, a conventional abdominoanal mucosal proctectomy is performed over a long rectal cuff. A 15-cm segment of terminal ileum is isolated on its blood supply. A 1-cm strip of the serosa and part of the muscular layer of the terminal ileum is excised from its antimesenteric border. The proximal end of the isolated terminal ileum is closed, and the segment is placed within the rectal muscular cuff. The upper rim of the rectum is anastomosed to the ileal segment. The distal open end of the grafted ileum is anastomosed endoanally to the dentate line. A temporary ileostomy is created in all patients (Peck, 1980).

After 6 weeks, if graft viability appears to be satisfactory, the neorectum is gently distended with retention enemas. Three months after the initial stage, the second phase takes place. The grafted rectum is mobilized, and is divided longitudinally on its ventral surface. After longitudinal division of the terminal ileum along its antimesenteric border, a two-layer anastomosis is created between the ileum and the grafted rectum.

Initial clinical experience with this technique was satisfactory. Bowel frequency per 24 hours was 5 for polyposis patients, and 6.7 for colitics. Ninety-two per cent of patients retained the ability to discriminate between flatus and fluids postoperatively. All patients could defer defaecation for anything up to 12 hours. Approximately 50% of patients evacuated at night. More than 90% were free from daytime leakage, and half were free from nocturnal leakage. Only four of 23 patients were required to wear pads. However, late complications including anastomotic stricture, intestinal obstruction, loss of the graft and fistulas occurred in 40% of patients. Hence, whilst complications were frequent and often serious, Peck had shown that acceptable results

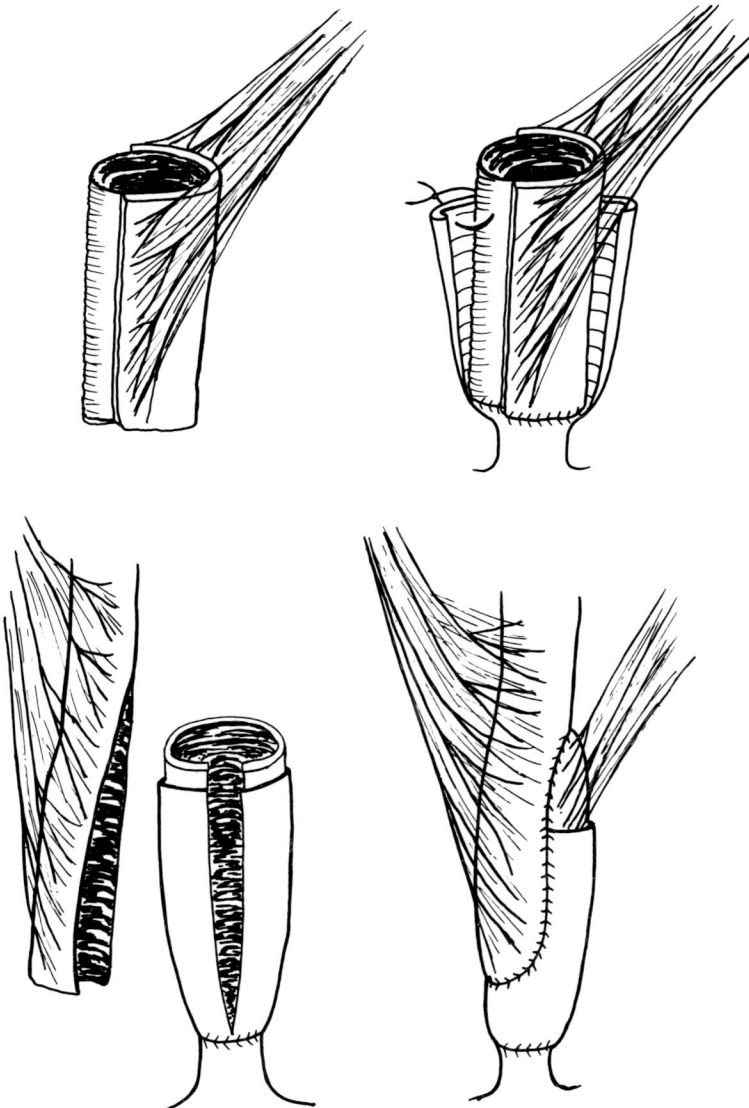

Figure 2.6 Ileal mucosal grafting (after Peck)

with excellent continence could be obtained after ileoanal anastomosis, and that a reservoir could be successfully utilized to decrease stool frequency.

An attempt has recently been made to revive the concept of grafting ileal mucosa onto the denuded rectal muscular cuff (Chaimoff *et al.*, 1989). Part of the incentive for such work is the continuing belief by some surgeons that there is little functional advantage conferred by the addition of a pelvic pouch, and that straight ileoanal anastomoses function equally well (Stoller *et al.*, 1987). In addition, complications such as pelvic sepsis and reservoir ileitis are much more common after pouch construction. Chaimoff *et al.* have therefore prepared a length of terminal ileum denuded of three-quarters of the antimesenteric seromuscular layers. The mucosal tube thus created is therefore well supplied through its mesenteric

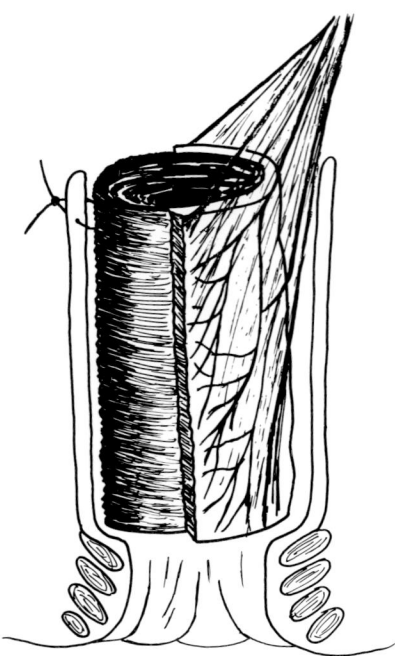

Figure 2.7 Ileal mucosal grafting (after Chaimoff *et al.*, 1989)

vasculature (Figure 2.7). An abdominal rectal mucosectomy is then performed, retaining a long rectal muscular cuff. The ileal mucosal tube is then placed within the rectal tube, where the proximal intact serosa of the ileum is loosely anastomosed to the superior edge of the rectal cuff. In this series of animal experiments, continence was satisfactory, and three or four bowel actions were passed per day. Macroscopically, the ileal mucosal graft was found to be adherent to the rectal wall. Interestingly, after only 6 weeks or so, the ileum showed areas of colonic metaplasia. As of yet there is no reported clinical experience with this model, which is similar to that previously described by Peck.

However, there has been little enthusiasm for any of these techniques in the clinical situation. Coincident with these developments of mucosal grafting and balloon dilatation, many workers had been assessing the potential of providing for such neorectums by constructing reservoirs from segments of small intestine.

Ileal pouch–anal anastomosis

It is now a little over 60 years since the first description of an ileal pelvic reservoir. This was constructed from an isolated segment of ileum fashioned into a doubly folded loop after rectal excision for malignancy (Figure 2.8). This was then analogous to the V-shaped ileal bladder substitute depicted in Figure 1.8. The postoperative course of this patient was complicated by a fatal bronchopneumonia, and hence the functional sequelae of adding an antiperistaltic segment to an ileocolorectoplasty are not clear (Dimitriu, 1928).

Encouraged by the efficacious use of isolated intestinal segments for 'pantaloon' gastric replacement, Valiente and Bacon (1955) studied the use of such reservoirs for rectal replacement in dogs. They constructed three configurations of reservoir (Figure 2.9). Doubly folded pouches were constructed with the apex of the pouch directed either caudad or cephalad. In addition, triplicated pouches were also assessed. These were clearly the forerunners of the reservoirs utilized today. Their technique involved transection of the rectum at the dentate line, and a two-layer ileoanal anastomosis. Unfortunately, five of the seven animals so treated died in the postoperative period. Three suffered leakage from the ileoanal anastomosis, succumbing to peritonitis. In one animal, the anastomosis failed to heal completely. The fifth animal died due to hypokalaemia. However, in both the other two animals, the functional results were satisfactory. They evacuated their pouches approximately three to five times per 24 hours. With time, their frequency of evacuation reduced as the consistency of the stool improved. Perianal skin excoriation was not significant. This now classic report documented the future potential of rectal replacement with ileal reservoirs, and prompted further research into their use.

Later that same decade, Karlan and his colleagues reported the results of their animal experiments, which were aimed at defining the relative importance of, and interactions between, sphincteric continence and reservoir continence (Karlan, McPherson and Watman, 1959).

Five groups of mongrel dogs were studied (Figure 2.10). In the first group the rectum and colon within the territory of the inferior mesenteric artery were resected to within 4 cm

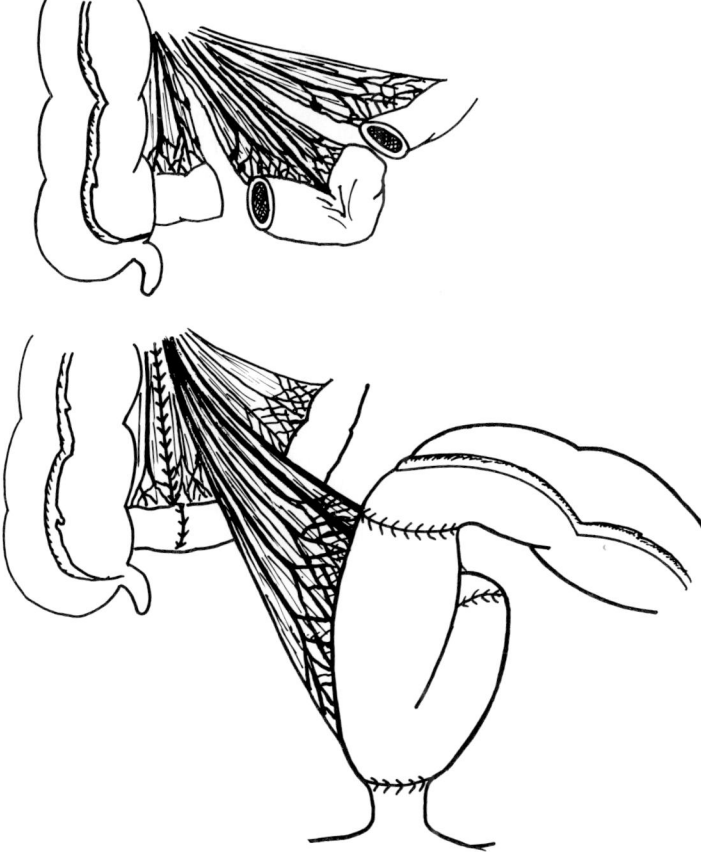

Figure 2.8 Ileocolorectoplasty (after Dimitriu, 1928)

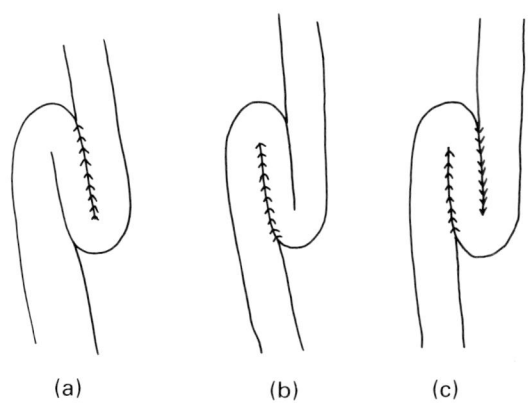

(a)   (b)   (c)

Figure 2.9 Ileal pouches (after Valiente and Bacon, 1955)

of the dentate line. A mucosal proctectomy was performed over the remaining rectum. A loop of ileum was isolated, its proximal end oversewn, and distal end anastomosed end to end with the rectal cuff. Small intestinal continuity was restored by ileoileostomy, and a terminal end colostomy fashioned. After a period of 10 days to allow healing of the ileorectal anastomosis, the colostomy was taken down and anastomosed to the previously fashioned ileal loop, thus restoring complete intestinal continuity. At 1 month postoperatively, continence was complete, the stool was improving in consistency, and frequency declined to three or four bowel actions per day.

In the second group, a similar procedure was performed, with the exception that a total coloproctectomy to the mucocutaneous junction was performed (Figure 2.10(b)). As no rectal cuff was left *in situ*, a direct pull-through ileoanal anastomosis restored continuity. All

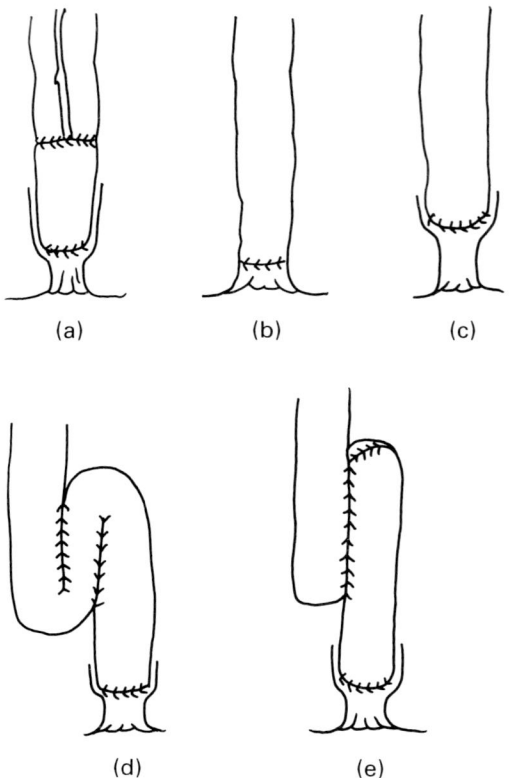

Figure 2.10 Ileal pouches (after Karlan, McPherson and Watman, 1959)

of these animals suffered complete anorectal incontinence with numerous fluid and electrolyte problems, and all died of progressive cachexia. The third group again underwent total colectomy, but the terminal ileum was anastomosed to a 4-cm rectal cuff after mucosal proctectomy (Figure 2.10(c)). All the surviving animals had severe frequency of defaecation, with up to 20 motions in a 10-hour period. However, all remained continent.

The fourth group of dogs was identical to the third, except that an S-shaped ileal reservoir was fashioned and anastomosed to the rectal cuff (Figure 2.10(d)). All survivors showed a tendency towards constipation, and it was frequently necessary to pass a rectal tube to evacuate the pouch. Fluoroscopy revealed the pouch to be large and atonic.

In the final group, the only difference from group (d) was that an isoperistaltic double-barrelled ileal pouch was constructed (Figure 2.10(e)). These animals passed stools which

progressively became more solid, with a frequency of between four and six bowel movements per day. All were fully continent with excellent control.

This important report concluded that the reflexes involved in sphincter function could be maintained by preservation of a short denuded rectal cuff. However, as witnessed in group (b), resection of the whole of the rectum to the mucocutaneous junction resulted in loss of sphincteric control in this animal model, in spite of an adequate reservoir for the stool consistency. The results from the group (c) animals show that even when sphincteric continence is provided, incontinence will result if the reservoir capacity is inadequate, particularly if the stool is liquid.

Whilst the results of these important experiments may not be completely applicable to man, the provision of a surgically created reservoir did result in full continence. However, the design of such reservoirs was important. These workers attributed the poor performance of the S-pouch to its having an antiperistaltic segment, presumably altering normal intestinal motility. Certainly, in their hands the isoperistaltic pouch provided very acceptable results, and they apparently applied such a technique in a 29-year-old female patient requiring a total proctocolectomy for polyposis coli. Few details were given other than the procedure was technically very difficult and that the results were equivocal. However, in their animal experiments both mortality and morbidity were extremely high, and so the idea of ileoanal reservoir formation was not pursued. This in part was the impetus for surgeons to focus their attention on the other methods for rectal replacement considered in this chapter. Generally, none of these other techniques proved to be any more easily performed or efficacious than the pelvic pouch procedure. Consequently, it was this latter technique which attracted most attention.

Throughout the 1970s, workers continued to examine the use of the ileal reservoir designs, as described by Valiente and Bacon in 1955. In July 1978 two papers were published which were to give new impetus and enthusiasm to the practicalities of sphincter preservation after total colectomy.

Fonkalsrud, a paediatric surgeon from the UCLA School of Medicine, had been continuing animal experimentation into the use of the S-shaped reservoir (Ferrari and Fonkals-rud, 1978). In seven dogs a total colectomy was performed, and an abdominal mucosal proctectomy commenced 2 cm above the peritoneal reflection, this being completed to within 1 cm of the dentate line after rectal eversion. The small bowel mesentery was mobilized, and the terminal ileal segment brought down and anastomosed to the divided rectal stump. The reservoir was then constructed by flexing the terminal ileum into an S-shaped loop with 6-cm limbs, the pouch being completed in two layers. Of the four dogs that survived more than 4 weeks, all were fully continent, passing a soft stool four to six times per day.

Such positive results with this technique prompted its undertaking in a 14-year-old boy with severe ulcerative colitis complicated by uncontrollable diabetes. An S-shaped reservoir was constructed and a defunctioning end-ileostomy brought out 8 cm proximal to the pouch. This was closed after three and a half months, with an initial frequency of defaecation of up to 20 stools per day. An elemental diet and antidiarrhoeal agents reduced this frequency, and one attack of ileitis distal to the reservoir was successfully managed with antibiotics and steroids. Subsequently, function improved, and both the ability to defer defaecation and to discriminate were good.

However, of perhaps greater importance was the report from the late Sir Alan Parks describing his initial experience with the S-shaped reservoir in eight patients (Parks and Nicholls, 1978). In this group of patients, a total colectomy was performed retaining an 8-cm rectal cuff. The reservoir was constructed from the terminal 30 cm of ileum, retaining the last 5 cm to act as a conduit. The 25-cm segment was opened along its antimesenteric border, and folded into three loops. A two-layer closure completes the pouch. An endoanal mucosal proctectomy is performed after infiltration with dilute adrenaline, and the ileoanal anastomosis completed with interrupted sutures. A large catheter was placed per anum and left on continuous drainage, and a loop ileostomy was fashioned above the pouch.

The results were encouraging, and there were no postoperative deaths. Five patients were available for assessment, two of whom had suffered with pelvic abscess. One of these had a partial anastomotic dehiscence, and

subsequent stenosis which responded to dilatation. There was one relaparotomy for small bowel obstruction, however two patients had an uncomplicated postoperative course.

With regard to function, at a follow-up of 1–9 months after ileostomy closure, only one patient evacuated the pouch spontaneously. Three other patients had to pass a catheter between four and eight times per day to evacuate a stool which varied between liquid and semi-solid. Nocturnal emptying and leakage were not witnessed in this group. In one patient, tenesmus, frequency and soiling presented difficulties, and a successful postanal repair was performed to restore the ano-pouch angle. Unfortunately, this patient developed an aversion to self-catheterization necessitating excision of the pouch, and conversion to a permanent ileostomy. Subsequent early follow-up revealed good results in two further patients after closure of the ileostomy, and encouraged the performance of this operation in a patient with familial polyposis associated with a carcinoma of the upper rectum, this patient having refused to accept a permanent ileostomy.

Updates on the initial results using S-pouches became available, and soon documented that spontaneous defaecation was more common if a shorter (i.e. less than 5 cm) efferent limb was used. The St Marks group also described that, in the first 21 operations, severe rectal disease did not preclude this procedure. Indeed, pouch–anal anastomosis had even been performed successfully in the presence of a rectovaginal fistula (Parks, Nicholls and Belliveau, 1980). This group continued to use a 6–8 cm rectal cuff, performing the dissection close to the rectum. Encouragingly, they did not describe any urinary or sexual complications, however other postoperative complications were common.

Later that same year, the next major development came from Utsunomiya working at the Polyposis Center of the Tokyo Medical and Dental University. He described his initial results in 11 patients who received one of three types of ileoanal anastomosis, two of which involved reservoir construction (Utsunomiya *et al.*, 1980). In all patients they performed a mucosal proctectomy to just above the dentate line, and utilized a long rectal cuff (from the level of the sacral promontory), believing this to be necessary for the maintenance of anorectal function. Patients received either a straight ileoanal anastomosis, a 20-cm isoperistaltic double-barrelled reservoir sited 20 cm above the ileoanal anastomosis, or a stapled pouch with a J configuration. More than 60% of patients suffered complications, usually septic and including cuff abscesses. The J-type reservoir reached a stable frequency of five to eight bowel actions per day in the shortest time, and compared with the other techniques, soiling was not a problem. Importantly, emptying was always spontaneous. This design of reservoir, as advocated by Valiente and Bacon some 25 years previously, was subsequently adopted by many surgeons working in this field. Many protagonists of restorative proctocolectomy have subsequently reported their use of the duplicated J-pouch (Taylor, 1986).

Johnston from Leeds reported his early experience with anal sphincter preservation, performing either a caecoanal, straight ileoanal, or ileoanal pouch anastomosis (Johnston *et al.*, 1981). Straight ileoanal anastomosis in eight patients resulted in good daytime continence, but nocturnal soiling was commonplace. Bowel frequency was usually between six and ten per day. Six patients underwent caecoanal or ascending coloanal anastomosis, however recurrent colitis was universal. Whilst responsive to steroids, its severity necessitated conversion to an ileal pouch–anal anastomosis in three cases. Ileal reservoirs (2 S- and 1 J-pouch) were performed in three patients with mixed results. Continence was excellent, but there was one early failure due to urgency and anal pain. The important conclusions of this early report were that incomplete colonic resections, involving retention of the caecum or ileocaecal valve, would probably not be met with success due to recurrent colitis. Also, with increasing experience ileal pouch–anal anastomosis should ultimately provide gratifying results. Subsequently, a few authors have documented occasional success with caecoanal anastomosis. However this procedure is not to be generally recommended.

Clearly, in selected cases ileal reservoir formation was beginning to produce very encouraging results. Debate was commencing upon the relative merits of various reservoir designs, and as such continues to the present. Over the last decade several further reservoir designs have been described, and each con-

tinues to receive the attention of its own advocates (see Chapter 5).

However, it was still to be shown that any long-term metabolic sequelae would not mar the success of this new procedure. Experience with the continent ileostomy suggested that several pathophysiological sequelae might develop in patients after restorative proctocolectomy, but that on the whole such complications should not be severe. The first major pathophysiological assessment of the latter procedure was reported by Nicholls *et al.* (1981). They studied 14 of their patients, all of whom were at least 6 months postoperation. Numerous metabolic investigations were carried out, including serum urea and electrolytes, full blood count, basic haematinics, a Schilling test, faecal fat estimation and pouch biopsy. Their results showed that metabolic sequelae of ileal pouch–anal anastomosis were few and generally not dramatic, features subsequently confirmed by most other workers (see Chapters 12 and 13).

Whilst early reports suggested that the pelvic pouch procedure was both metabolically safe, and functionally satisfactory, it did represent a more extensive procedure than the straight ileoanal anastomosis. The Mayo clinic group therefore compared the straight ileoanal anastomosis with the ileal reservoir in a nonrandomized fashion. Because of their increasing enthusiasm for the pelvic pouch, only the initial patients in the series had the straight form of anastomosis (Taylor *et al.*, 1983a). Over 30% of their straight anastomoses failed because of diarrhoea or sepsis, compared with only 1.3% of the pouch group. In the group of J-pouches, stool frequency was approximately seven per 24 hours after 3 months' follow-up, this being significantly less than in the patients without a pouch. Similarly, nocturnal incontinence was also significantly reduced.

These few early experiences with ileal pouch formation, particularly coupled with the endoanal sleeve technique devised by Parks for cancer operations, encouraged more colorectal surgeons to embark upon these procedures. Subsequently, there has developed an increasing enthusiasm for restorative proctocolectomy as an alternative to permanent ileostomy formation after colectomy for certain colorectal conditions, most notably ulcerative colitis and adenomatous polyposis.

However, even with the advent of the pelvic

pouch procedure, further experimental work into ways of avoiding ileoanal anastomosis for rectal replacement has continued. To some degree, this bears testimony to the relative complexity of the pelvic pouch procedure, and to the ingenuity of surgeons interested in this field.

Other techniques of rectal replacement

It has been reported that after a conventional mucosal proctectomy with adrenaline infiltration, the denuded rectum can be covered with skin grafts which may remain viable (Harrison, Oka and Owen, 1984). In this animal model, mongrel dogs underwent subtotal colectomy and abdominal mucosal proctectomy after submucosal infiltration with adrenaline. Skin grafts of 0.5 mm thickness were taken from the chest and applied to the balloon of a Sengstaken–Blakemore tube. This was placed within the denuded rectum, and an end-ileostomy constructed (Figure 2.11). After

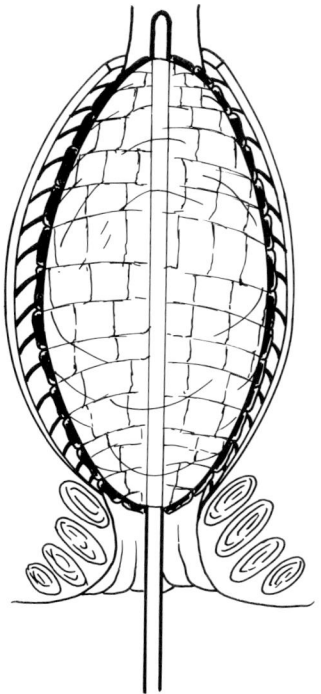

Figure 2.11 Skin-grafted rectum (after Harrison, Oka and Owen, 1984)

7–10 days the balloon was deflated and the tube expelled. Four weeks later the end-ileostomy was closed by ileorectal anastomosis to the grafted rectum. This was protected by a loop ileostomy. Again, the oesophageal tube was placed into the rectum, and the balloon inflated. After a further month the loop ileostomy was closed, the balloon was deflated and the tube finally removed. Frequency and diarrhoea were common within the first month after ileostomy closure. However, it was said that the stools were formed by the end of the second month, and that a 'normal' bowel habit was attained after 3 months. Follow-up to 1 year reinforced these satisfactory functional results. These workers felt that this procedure deserved further attention, as it represented an easier technical exercise than pouch–anal anastomosis.

Johnston has reported recently his early clinical experience with his 'Two-Sphincter' operation. This has been devised to retain the normal arrangement of the ileocaecal valve after colectomy (Johnston, Holdsworth and Smith, 1989). Johnston argues that excision of this specialized region, and manipulation of the terminal ileum into a folded pouch, may result in abnormalities of motility, intestinal transit and absorption. Twelve patients underwent his new technique, in which the ileocaecal junction and a 2-cm cuff of caecum are isolated from the remaining caecum, which is then excised with the colectomy specimen. In order to prevent recurrent colitis in the small amount of retained caecal mucosa, a 'conventional' mucosectomy is performed around the ileocaecal valve after infiltration with dilute adrenaline. In a manner analogous to that in the pelvic pouch operation, perirectal mobilization of the rectum is performed to the level of the pelvic floor. A linear stapling gun is used to transect the rectum, leaving a short rectal stump. Commencing some 60 cm proximal to the ileocaecal valve, a 50-cm segment of terminal ileum is isolated, leaving the last 10 cm incorporating the ileocaecal valve. After oversewing of the proximal end of this isolated loop (the future neorectum), an end-to-side anastomosis between the ileocaecal valve and the loop is created (Figure 2.12). The isolated neorectum is then anastomosed end to end to the anal stump using a circular stapling gun. An end-ileostomy is created, and the proximal end of the terminal ileal segment containing

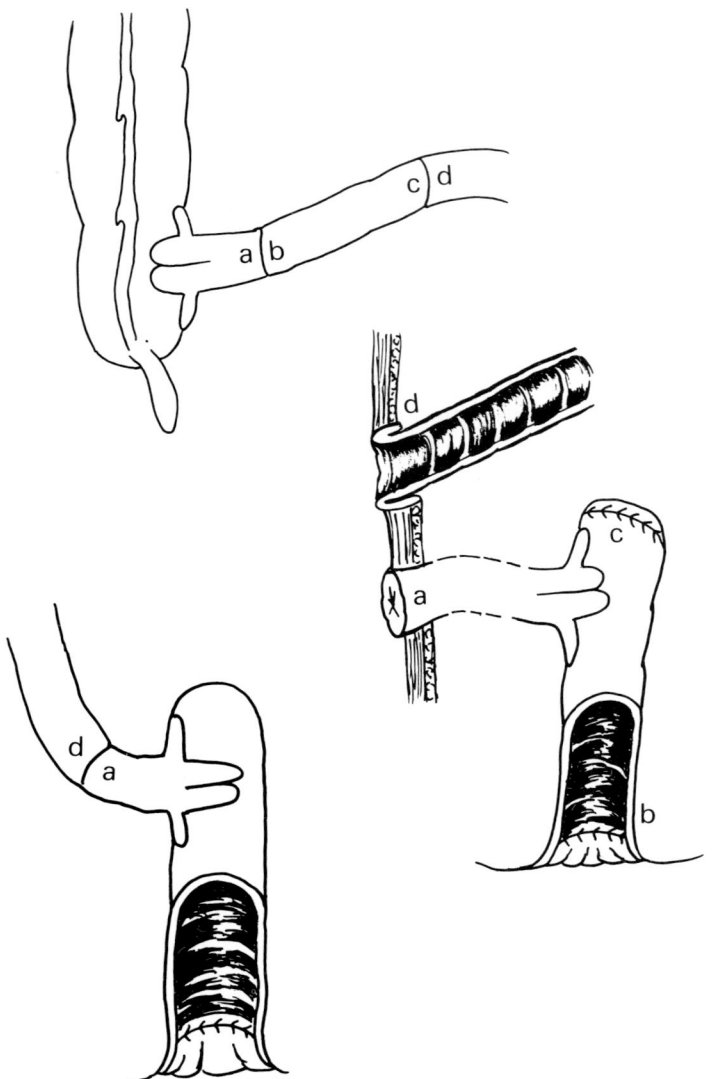

Figure 2.12 'Two-sphincter' operation (after Johnston, Holdsworth and Smith, 1989)

the ileocaecal valve is brought to the surface as a mucous fistula. After 2 months, continuity is restored by ileoileostomy.

Follow-up of these patients was for a median of 1 year. Functional outcome was satisfactory. Continence was virtually complete. One patient had minor leakage. Two patients had excessive frequency, necessitating reconstruction of their ileostomy. In the remaining patients in whom the ileostomy has been closed, frequency has declined to six per 24

hours. Neorectal functional capacity, maximal tolerated volume and compliance have all improved significantly. In spite of this improvement, the values obtained were still less than Johnston had achieved with his ileal pelvic pouches. Both procedures resulted in neorectums which emptied similarly. Bile acid absorption, as assessed by the SeHCAT test, was similar to that in Johnston's pouch patients. Excluding the 20% of patients requiring a return to ileostomy, functional results were very similar to those obtained with pelvic pouches. It remains to be determined whether this innovative procedure, retaining the ileocaecal valve above the neorectum, results in less bacterial overgrowth, less clinical pouchitis, and possibly less colonic metaplasia, than after 'conventional' pelvic pouch formation.

Fonkalsrud has also described another design of neorectum, constructed from a myotomized segment of ileum (Aly and Fonkalsrud, 1988). In this report, 15 dogs underwent colectomy followed by a straight ileosigmoid anastomosis. A 15-cm longitudinal myotomy was then created on the antimesenteric border of the ileum (Figure 2.13). The procedure was

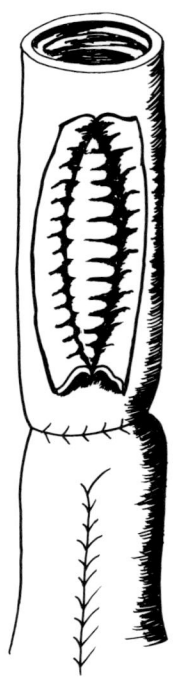

Figure 2.13 Ileal myotomy (after Aly and Fonkalsrud, 1988)

uncomplicated, and well tolerated. Unfortunately, peristalsis was unaltered, and the volume of this segment did not increase postoperatively. Indeed, a 50% occlusion of the sigmoid colon failed to result in any further dilatation of the 'pouch'. Whilst a much more simple technical procedure than the conventional ileal reservoir, it would appear that there is little role for this technique. However, what effects

differing patterns of myotomy might have are unclear. Others have reported that a straight ileoanal anastomosis with terminal ileal myotomy can provide for a neorectum with similar performance characteristics as the more accepted ileal pelvic pouch (O'Malley *et al.*, 1985; Sagar, 1990; Turnage, Coran and Drongowski, 1990).

Leite and his colleagues have attempted recently to define the role of an ileal valve sited at the afferent limb of either J-, S- or W-pouches. The presence of a valve did not affect intestinal transit time, and at this stage appears to have little foreseeable role in the pelvic pouch procedure. (Leite, Fausto-Pontes and Martins, 1990).

Conclusions

Thus far consideration has been given to the various surgical options available for patients with ulcerative colitis. In the following chapter the topic of surgery for adenomatous polyposis coli will be discussed. However, many of the facets discussed herein will be relevant to that discussion, and should be related to it.

Concerning first the formation of a permanent Brooke everted ileostomy. More than 95% of patients will conform to the following characteristics: are happy with their stoma, can manage their stoma adequately, are employed, and have few restrictions with regard to diet and daily activities. In addition, only approximately 10% will require ultimate stoma revision. Importantly, the majority of general surgeons both know and trust this operation. It gives reliable results in most surgeons' hands.

On the negative side, numerous 'minor' inconveniences may disrupt the patient's life; for example, skin irritation, occasional excessive ileostomy output, and rarely leakage. Persistent perineal wounds are relatively common, are inconvenient to the patient, and are both time and finance consuming in district nurse facilities. In addition, stoma care is extremely expensive often for both the patient and society. A minority of patients (perhaps one-quarter) experience some restriction on activity, be it sexual and/or social.

Importantly, and even when aware of alternatives, of all our patients who have an ileostomy, less than half are even remotely interested in such restorative operations. Only 25% or so express a more concrete interest, but very few seriously consider further surgery with a view to restoring more 'normal' anatomy. To date, we have not converted any such patients to ileal reservoirs, either abdominal or pelvic.

Prior to discussing the role for ileorectal anastomosis in colitis and polyposis, it should be re-emphasized that Crohn's disease is a condition which is not curable. Therefore, conservative 'palliative' procedures must be performed whenever possible. Colectomy with ileorectal anastomosis is the preferred treatment option for patients with extensive colonic involvement with this disease. Whilst ultimate proctectomy may be required in up to one-third of patients, this should not detract surgeons from the efficacy of ileorectal anastomosis, and at least the temporary deferment of a permanent stoma.

In the minority of colitics who have relative rectal sparing, ileorectal anastomosis will result in satisfactory results. Therefore, in such patients, and in those who refuse the other surgical options, ileorectal anastomosis may be considered. However, many surgeons do not feel able to offer this operation, mostly because of the risks of subsequent disease and malignancy. Whilst we do not subscribe to the efficacy of ileorectal anastomosis in ulcerative colitis, we do feel that it has a role in the management of patients in whom the diagnosis is in doubt.

Most surgeons, including ourselves, have little difficulty in recommending ileorectal anastomosis for the treatment of adenomatous polyposis coli, particularly if the rectum contains relatively few polyps. Whilst the risk of rectal preservation is relatively well documented, it has to be emphasized that the reduced risk of malignancy after ileorectal anastomosis is just that, a *relatively reduced risk*. No series has yet documented that this operation is as safe (with regard to cancer) as total proctocolectomy. One is therefore balancing between surgical expediency (and the functional results obtained), with the risk of subsequent malignancy.

Kock has documented that, with increasing experience, the success rate for the continent ileostomy (using Kock's own pouch design) is of the order of 95%. Such patients need only evacuate their pouches three or four times per day. Nipple valve desussception has been significantly reduced. However, it must be re-emphasized that few non-specialist surgeons have exhibited marked enthusiasm for this procedure. There can be little doubt that, in many cases, this is due to the long (and well-documented), turbulent history of Kock's operation. However, it must now be acknowledged that many of the operative details have been both standardized and simplified. Surgeons willing to embark upon pouch–anal anastomosis should be prepared to perform continent ileostomy in selected circumstances. In our view, there is a conceptual divergence between the advocacy of the ileal pelvic pouch, whilst admonishing the value of the intra-abdominal ileal pouch. It has been demonstrated repeatedly that the continent ileostomy is associated with a superior quality of life when compared with conventionl ileostomy.

The ileoanal pouch procedure has now come of age. The last decade has been associated with almost as many technical problems and modifications as that for the continent ileostomy. However, no doubt due to the maintenance of a normal route for defaecation, the pelvic pouch procedure has captured the imagination of the surgical fraternity in a way which the continent ileostomy has singularly failed to do. Whilst, to date, it has usually remained within the domain of the specialist, the technical details have become much simplified. In particular, changes with regard to the mucosal proctectomy, and the advent of improved stapling instruments have encouraged many other surgeons to attempt this procedure than ever performed continent ileostomy. Some now consider this procedure to be the treatment of choice in all patients requiring colectomy for colitis and polyposis. We certainly agree that there should be a good reason for *not* performing the procedure, rather than vice versa.

So what effects have resulted from the advent of these new procedures? Comparing the surgical preferences of two samples of gastroenterologists at world conferences separated by one decade, there appeared to be little effect on the emergency surgery for colitis (de Dombal and Prantera, 1989). In the urgent situation, there has been little reduction in the enthusiasm for proctocolectomy and ileostomy formation, with approximately one-third of all patients continuing to undergo this procedure.

Not surprisingly, neither ileostomy nor colostomy as isolated procedures were performed commonly. However, even in 1988 both were performed in some 5% of cases. Nevertheless, there was a significant reduction in enthusiasm for subtotal colectomy with ileostomy formation in the urgent situation. Perhaps surprisingly, this appeared to be almost totally because of an increase in the willingness to perform other varied procedures including presumably ileorectal anastomosis and ileal pouch–anal anastomosis.

In the elective situation, proctocolectomy with ileostomy formation retained its enthusiasts, being performed in approximately one-third of cases. Subtotal colectomy with ileostomy formation became significantly less popular, reducing from over 50% to some 27%. Interestingly, colectomy with ileorectal anastomosis became more popular, being performed in some 15% of elective cases in 1988. In the decade from 1978, procedures such as pouch–anal anastomosis increased 20-fold to 28% of elective cases operated upon.

It would therefore appear that, with increasing experience and an increasing literature, surgeons are becoming more prepared to perform sphincter-saving surgery, even in the urgent situation. How many of the proctocolectomies described above were of either the conservative or intersphincteric varieties is unclear. However, it is likely that there remains a core of surgeons who are well satisfied with proctocolectomy with ileostomy formation for both urgent and elective cases. It is interesting that many of the protagonists of sphincter-saving surgery appear to come predominantly from those surgeons who previously advocated subtotal colectomy with ileostomy formation.

Many reports of experience with ileal pouch–anal anastomosis have appeared from all over the world. Over the last decade, an increasing number of workers, including ourselves, have attempted to preserve the anal sphincters after colectomy. The results and experiences thus reported form the basis for the rest of this book.

3

Surgery for adenomatous polyposis

There can be few other conditions throughout the whole sphere of medicine which are so obviously premalignant as adenomatous polyposis coli. Untreated, there is a universal incidence of colorectal cancer. In approximately 80% of cases, the disease is familial, the other 20% being presumed to be spontaneous mutations.

At the time of writing, it is exactly 100 years since the first description of the association between cancer and multiple polyposis of the colon (Handford, 1890). Since then, increasing realization that many patients presenting with symptoms of polyposis already harboured at least one colorectal malignancy has encouraged the instigation of several registries of families with this disease. These have provided for screening of asymptomatic relatives of affected individuals, and allowed for scientific evaluation of the various treatment modalities, particularly their extent and timing.

There are basically four forms of surgical treatment for colonic polyposis syndromes, namely proctocolectomy with permanent ileostomy, subtotal colectomy with ileorectal anastomosis, and restorative proctocolectomy with or without ileal reservoir formation.

Many of the arguments regarding the relative merits of each procedure also pertain to ulcerative colitis, and have been discussed in the previous chapter. On a theoretical basis, proctocolectomy with formation of a permanent Brooke ileostomy has much to commend it. It certainly eradicates all the colorectal mucosa in which there is the field potential for development of both adenomas and carcinomas. However, the necessity for permanent ileostomy is a particularly major drawback in adenomatous polyposis.

Even when symptomatic, such patients frequently only have minor symptoms, such as slight frequency and occasional looseness of the motions. Hence, even at this stage they may not present clinically. More severe symptoms, such as severe diarrhoea, the passage of mucus and/or blood per rectum are often associated with malignant degeneration in one or more adenomas. These latter symptoms are common in colitics, and enable such patients to more readily accept a permanent stoma. In addition, apart from any psychological sequelae, such a procedure has little direct relevance to the family of a colitic.

Clearly, young patients with very minor presenting symptoms will be somewhat reluctant to accept a permanent stoma. Even more opposed are likely to be the totally asymptomatic patients found on subsequent screening. Indeed, knowing of the surgical trauma which their relative has undergone, there is a significant possibility that such individuals might not present for such screening.

Consequently, many surgeons managing such families have favoured the use of colectomy with ileorectal anastomosis. In order to improve function, many retain as much rectum as possible, often performing an ileosigmoid anastomosis. In such circumstances the retained rectal stump requires further management. It has been noted that, after colectomy, rectal polyps may regress spontaneously (Shepard, 1971). It may be that changes in stool chemistry, particularly a reduction in pH, may be at least partly responsible. Watne and colleagues have also suggested that oral vitamin C may aid such regression (Watne, Core and Carrier, 1975). Whatever its aetiology, such regression is not universal, and is frequently only transient. Hence, whilst some surgeons may postpone treatment of the retained rectum for some months in the hope of regression, many will treat rectal polyps perioperatively.

Subsequent to ileorectal anastomosis, regular patient review is required with sigmoidoscopy and fulguration of residual polyps. Such a policy is dependent upon the principle that carcinoma occurring in retained rectums will have arisen from malignant degeneration of a pre-existing adenoma. That this is a universal event is far from clear. It is certainly possible that a previously 'normal' area of mucosa may develop a malignancy *de novo*. In addition, the aggressive nature of such lesions may allow for adenoma-cancer progression within the space of only a few months, and hence 6-monthly surveillance may not be adequate in such circumstances.

So what of the experience with this procedure in adenomatous polyposis? Do such possibilities actually materialize in the clinical situation? Reported results vary considerably. Certainly, in the non-familial variant of adenomatous polyposis, where the rectum is often spared, ileorectal anastomosis is the treatment of choice. Such a distinction is not always possible, due to lack of information regarding relatives. Therefore, most reports assess the whole spectrum of adenomatous polyposis.

Since 1948, it has been the policy of surgeons at St Mark's Hospital to perform colectomy and ileorectal anastomosis (Bussey *et al.*, 1985). Reporting their first 216 patients, they were able to perform ileorectal anastomosis in 174 (80%). The majority of the rest had a rectal carcinoma at the time of diagnosis, and hence underwent rectal excision. They were however able to preserve the rectum in two such patients. In addition, a further 27 cancers were found in 18 patients at the time of operation. Four of these patients subsequently died of disseminated carcinoma. Their results certainly demonstrate that the operation is safe, in that there were very few postoperative complications. Ninety per cent of their patients had an uneventful postoperative course. Functional outcome was similarly very encouraging with the vast majority of patients having three to four bowel actions per 24 hours.

What of management of the retained rectums. This same group found 611 polyps in 115 patients. Diathermy fulguration proved generally to be safe, but had a small but significant risk of secondary haemorrhage. Eleven patients subsequently developed rectal carcinoma, three of whom died of this disease. Hence, whilst not eradicating the risk of malignancy, ileorectal anastomosis reduces this risk considerably. It is also hoped, and perhaps expected, that the majority of such lesions will be Dukes' A tumours. The St Mark's patients had a cumulative risk of cancer development of 13% at 25 years, and 30% at 35 years. The cumulative risk of dying of rectal cancer was some 4% at 15 years.

Whilst many workers have reported similarly encouraging results (Waugh, Harp and Spencer, 1964), others have had less satisfactory experience with ileorectal anastomosis (Flotte, O'Dell and Coller, 1956; Moertel, Hill and Adson, 1970). Moertel and colleagues found a cumulative cancer risk of 25% at 15 years, and more than 50% at over 20 years. It is likely that length of follow-up is important, as Waugh had previously demonstrated a 4% incidence of rectal cancer in patients from the same parent group (Waugh, Harp and Spencer, 1964). In addition, Moertel found that females are five times as likely to develop rectal cancers as are males. Patients with a malignancy in their resected colons were also particularly predisposed to cancers in the retained rectum, as were patients with 100 or more polyps in their rectum.

Consequently, the results from the Mayo clinic have cast doubts upon the safety of ileorectal anastomosis. There would appear to be no greater risk after ileosigmoid anastomosis (Bess, Adson and Elveback, 1980). However, most surgeons on both sides of the Atlantic continue to perform ileorectal anastomosis for adenomatous polyposis (Gingold, Jagelman and Turnbull, 1979; Beart, 1985).

Early reports with straight ileoanal anastomosis for adenomatous polyposis have varied (Safaie-Shirazi and Soper, 1973; Martin *et al.*, 1977; Beart, Dozois and Kelly, 1982; Heppell *et al.*, 1982; Hrabovsky, Watne and Carrier,

1984; Soave, 1985). Soave reported excellent results with eight patients, who had occasional nocturnal incontinence and only slight perianal soiling. Longer follow-up recorded that stool frequency was between three and five per 24 hours. Heppell and colleagues similarly demonstrated that this procedure could result in acceptable results in polyposis patients (Heppell *et al.*, 1982). This group however used the technique of balloon dilatation of the straight ileal segment in order to increase neorectal capacity (see Chapter 2). Not all reports have been so encouraging. Others have reported that excessive frequency may mar functional results. Indeed daily frequencies of ten or more have been described (Hrabovsky, Watne and Carrier, 1984).

The increasing enthusiasm for ileal pouch–anal anastomosis has led many surgeons favouring ileoanal anastomosis to abandon straight ileoanal anastomosis after colectomy for colonic polyposis. In an early report of their experience with all procedures, Heimann and colleagues described 77 patients, 21 of whom had undergone ileoanal anastomosis (Heimann, Bolnick and Aufses, 1986). The others had undergone ileorectal anastomosis (42 patients) or proctocolectomy with ileostomy (14 patients). In the ileoanal group, nine had undergone pouch–anal anastomosis. Stating that the surgical management of polyposis must be individualized, this group felt that ileorectal anastomosis represented a reasonable prophylactic procedure, especially in the young. This group of patients also appeared to poorly accept the formation of an ileostomy, even if continent. As has been found by others, the complication rate of mucosal proctectomy is less in polyposis patients than in colitics.

Describing his ten polyposis patients, Everett performed W pouch–anal anastomosis in patients whose rectal polyposis would preclude them from ileorectal anastomosis (Everett and Forty, 1989). Postoperative complications were few, and in particular septic complications were not witnessed in this group. Continence was absolute, and discrimination complete. Functional results were excellent, a fact witnessed by many workers using this procedure for adenomatous polyposis.

The Mayo clinic group have compared their results with pouch–anal anastomosis in 94 polyposis patients and 758 colitics (Dozois *et al.*, 1989). Whilst postoperative complications occurred with equal overall incidence, pelvic sepsis was not witnessed in the polyposis group. This group of patients also benefitted from a reduced stool frequency, less nocturnal soiling and less pouchitis. The use of antidiarrhoeal medications and bulk-forming agents was similar in both groups, as was the incidence of perianal irritation and sexual dysfunction. As surgeon-related differences are likely to have cancelled out in this large series, it can be proposed that some features of this procedure, especially pouchitis and pelvic sepsis, may be disease related. Only one polyposis patient required pouch excision, the indication being a mesenteric desmoid tumour. This compared with a total of 48 colitics who required pouch excision. The low incidence of mesenteric desmoids (see below) is interesting as it can be postulated that such lesions might become more common after such complex mesenteric manipulation performed as part of the pelvic pouch procedure. In addition, the Mayo clinic group have not found intestinal obstruction to be problematical in polyposis patients after pouch construction. Others have previously reported that postoperative small bowel obstruction is more common in polyposis patients (Sener, Miller and de Cosse, 1984). These workers therefore recommend ileoanal pouch construction for patients with polyposis coli in preference to ileorectal anastomosis. This group have recently described that whilst postoperative complication rates and functional outcome are similar in polyposis patients undergoing either ileorectal anastomosis or pouch–anal anastomosis, the former procedure may in fact preclude ultimate performance of the latter. In particular, shortening of the ileal mesentery and adhesions prevented pouch construction after proctectomy subsequent to a previous ileorectal anastomosis. Mesenteric desmoids may result in a similar inability to convert to a pouch–anal anastomosis (Ambrose *et al.*, 1990a; Ratelle *et al.*, 1990). However, it remains our practice to recommend ileorectal anastomosis for patients with colonic polyposis, so long as the rectum is relatively spared, and that the patient understands the necessity for and is willing to undergo prolonged endoscopic follow-up. In addition, it is important that the surgeon has a relatively low threshold for advising proctectomy in this group of patients (Skinner *et al.*, 1990).

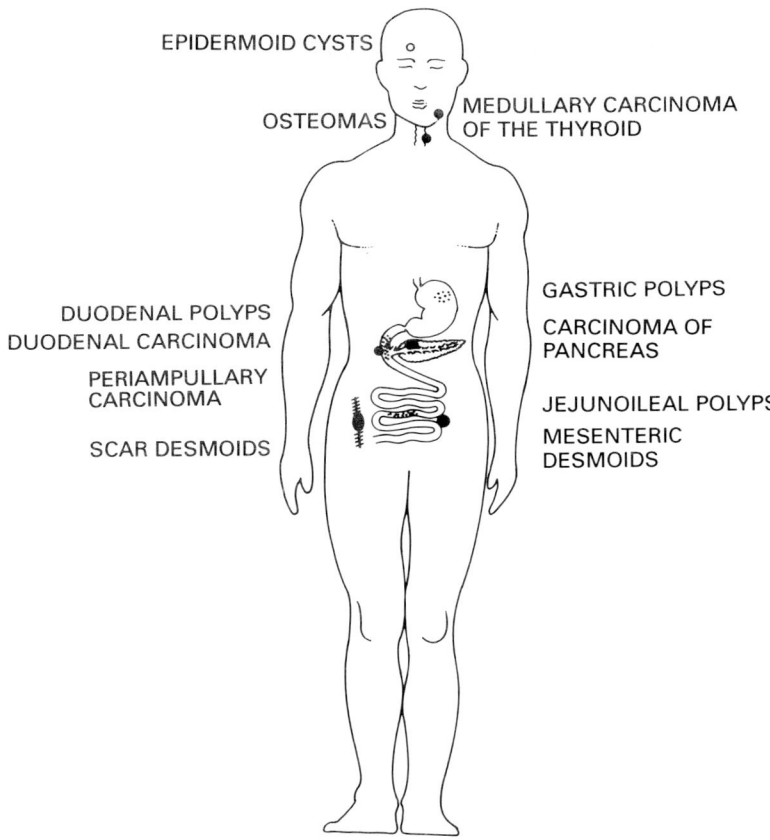

EPIDERMOID CYSTS

OSTEOMAS

MEDULLARY CARCINOMA
OF THE THYROID

DUODENAL POLYPS
DUODENAL CARCINOMA

PERIAMPULLARY
CARCINOMA

SCAR DESMOIDS

GASTRIC POLYPS

CARCINOMA OF
PANCREAS

JEJUNOILEAL POLYPS

MESENTERIC
DESMOIDS

Figure 3.1 Complications of familial adenomatous polyposis coli

Further to this discussion of the relative merits of ileorectal anastomosis versus ileoanal anastomosis for colonic polyposis is the problem of other extracolonic manifestations of this condition. These are depicted in Figure 3.1. Numerous extracolonic complications have been reported in patients with adenomatous polyposis coli. The majority of these are benign conditions. However, two such associations require further scrutiny.

Desmoid tumours

Desmoid tumours are locally invasive, usually non-metastasizing tumours of fibrous tissue. In the context of polyposis coli, they usually arise in the musculoaponeurotic structures of the abdominal wall, or from elsewhere within the abdomen. Within the general population, such lesions are extremely rare, accounting for less than one in three thousand of all neoplasms. In contradistinction, they occur with a frequency of up to 5.7% in Gardner's syndrome (Bussey, 1975). In those patients who have undergone a previous colectomy, the incidence of such lesions increases up to 29% (Naylor, Gardner and Richards, 1979). Whilst those lesions occurring within the abdominal wall may be resectable, only small mesenteric desmoids are amenable to resection. More often mesenteric and/or retroperitoneal desmoids are diffusely infiltrating, precluding surgical excision. In such cases, tumour may impinge upon vital structures, such as the ureters or small intestine, resulting in obstruction to these tracts and possibly in the ultimate demise of the patient. Naylor *et al.* reported such mortality in one-third of their patients with desmoids. Studying these patients more closely, half of those patients who formed postcolectomy desmoids did so within the abdominal cavity (i.e. 14% of all postcolectomy patients). All desmoid-associated deaths occurred within this subgroup. Therefore, up to three-quarters of polyposis patients with an intra-abdominal desmoid may ultimately die of this complication. Overall, postcolectomy desmoid formation resulted in death in approximately 10% of this group of polyposis patients (Naylor, Gardner and Richards, 1979).

In part, such a high patient mortality and morbidity associated with desmoid tumours may be explained by the fact that such lesions are frequently only diagnosed at a stage when they are advanced (Lopez *et al.*, 1990). It is also likely that these tumours may be underestimated in their extent, and consequently undertreated. Other treatment modalities have been assessed in this condition, particularly radiotherapy. Opinions vary, in that both reduced and enhanced local control of desmoids have been reported after radiotherapy.

Periampullary carcinoma

Bussey (1975) has reported previously that various periduodenal cancers, including periampullary carcinoma, duodenal carcinoma proper and pancreatic carcinoma, occur in approximately 12% of polyposis patients who survive for more than 5 years after colectomy. Whilst the majority occurred after this duration, a wide range was recorded (1–25 years postcolectomy). These lesions proved to be fatal in all cases. It remains uncertain as to whether these tumours have arisen in pre-existing benign adenomas, or have arisen *de novo*.

In addition, it is well recognized that such adenomas may be found within the stomach, duodenum or jejunoileum in polyposis patients (Spigelman, Talbot and Williams, 1989). Many of these are hyperplastic polyps, or represent areas of lymphoid hyperplasia, but there is no doubt that many are adenomatous, and as such may have malignant potential. However, few polyposis patients present with such small intestinal malignancies.

Therefore, even after colectomy for polyposis coli, there remains a significant chance of the patient developing an extracolonic lesion which might result in ultimate death. This should be compared against the cumulative risk of dying of rectal cancer, found to be 4% at 15 years after colectomy with ileorectal anastomosis (Bussey *et al.*, 1975).

Recurrent polyposis

In addition to the above potentially fatal complications of polyposis, recurrent polyposis and its possible significance to the patient should be considered. It was initially thought that the procedure of colectomy, mucosal proctectomy and ileal pouch–anal anastomosis would eliminate any risk of subsequent adenoma and carcinoma formation (Hrabovsky, Watne and Carrier, 1984). However, it is now realized that this is not in fact the case. Considering first those patients in whom a rectal cuff was retained as part of the pouch procedure, recurrent adenomas have been reported as occurring at the ileoanal anastomosis (O'Connell *et al.*, 1987b). In addition, in those patients in whom a sleeve of rectal mucosa was retained in the belief that discrimination would be improved, recurrent polyps have been recorded (Wolfstein, Bat and Neumann, 1982). Whilst these polyps recurred at the anastomotic line, retained rectal mucosa may have been the causal factor. However, multiple adenoma formation has occurred in areas of colonic metaplasia, both within conventional (Nakahara *et al.*, 1985; Johnson and White, 1988) and continent ileostomies (Stryker, Carney and Dozois, 1987). Carcinomas developing within conventional ileostomies have also been reported after colectomy (Ross and Mara, 1974; Roth and Logio, 1982; Primrose, Quirke and Johnston, 1988). In these case reports, the carcinomas were reported respectively 19, 14 and 28 years after colectomy.

Myrhoj and colleagues have reported recently the late development of multiple adenomas after straight ileoanal anastomosis (Myrhoj, Bulow and Mogensen, 1989). This patient had undergone colectomy, mucosal proctectomy to the dentate line and ileoanal anastomosis some 25 years prior to the development of recurrent polyps. These recurrences were found up to 12 cm from the ileoanal anastomosis, suggesting that retained rectal mucosa was not causal. We have also reported the occurrence of a juvenile polyp within a duplicated J-pouch in a patient who had undergone restorative procto-colectomy for very extensive juvenile polyposis coli (Sene *et al.*, 1989). Therefore, restorative proctocolectomy, with or without reservoir, should not be seen as completely removing the risk of subsequent adenoma and possibly carcinoma formation in polyposis patients. Regular endoscopic follow-up is therefore recommended in this group after pouch–anal anastomosis. Whether this necessity will attain the significance of surveillance after ileorectal anastomosis is unlikely. However, these recent findings at least partly negate one of the potential benefits of pelvic pouch construction over ileorectal anastomosis.

Iida and colleagues have described the appearances of recurrent polyps within the ileum after ileorectal anastomosis. Interesting-ly, multiple (more than 20) recurrences were found in all patients at a mean of 79.7 months after colectomy. Endoscopically, these lesions were whitish and sessile. Generally, there was little correlation between endoscopic appear-ance and histological diagnosis. In half of these polyps, the histological diagnosis was tubular adenoma; in the other half it was lymphoid hyperplasia alone. Of the patients with adeno-mas, 20% had adenomas containing numerous Paneth cells; one-third had adenomas in areas of colonic metaplasia; 44% had adenomas associated with lymphoid hyperplasia. Whilst the postoperative interval, the patient age, the extent of examination and the number of biopsies were statistically similar in those patients with and without adenomas, adeno-mas generally were found more frequently in patients followed up for longer periods (Iida *et al.*, 1989).

Conclusions

There is general agreement that if patients with adenomatous polyposis coli are left untreated, the vast majority will develop one or more colorectal cancers, and succumb to their disease. Future developments in our under-standing of the molecular biology of this condition may allow for diagnosis of asymp-tomatic individuals without recourse to endos-copic evaluation (Dunlop, Wyllie and Steel, 1990). In affected patients, colectomy remains a satisfactory procedure for avoiding the development of colonic tumours. However, it is only in those patients in whom the rectum is absolutely spared that ileorectal anastomosis is completely satisfactory. There is evidence that colectomy may reduce the incidence of malig-nancy developing within the retained rectum. The precise magnitude of this reduction is uncertain.

In those patients who have any rectal polyps, ileorectal anastomosis becomes a compromise between the surgical expediency of rectal preservation, and the attendant relative risk of such retention. With the advent of the ileoanal pouch procedure, it may be that, for many surgeons, these arguments have become irrele-vant. However, increasing understanding of, and expertise in the recognition of 'pre-cancers' of the rectum may allow for even earlier diagnosis of potentially malignant le-sions. This may subsequently rekindle interest in ileorectal anastomosis. For patients with adenomatous polyposis who have relative rectal sparing, we still consider that ileorectal anastomosis has a valuable role to play in their management.

4

Aspects of anorectal continence

Continence is that normal, mostly unconscious, process by which the contents of the rectum are maintained until sociably acceptable circumstances can be found for their controlled evacuation. In addition, there should be the ability to both discriminate between flatus and faeces, and to avoid nocturnal evacuation. Whilst this definition provides lip service to the extremes, it leaves a grey area in between. Few would have problems in ascribing terms to those who have complete anorectal control, or conversely to those who evacuate their rectal contents unconsciously. However, there is a wide spectrum betwixt these two, in which the perception of what constitutes normality depends upon numerous factors.

Various personal and social factors will dictate what, to any one individual, constitutes an unacceptable degree of lack of control. This has obvious implications for those assessments of continence performance relying completely upon the patient's perception. Hence, it is important that such studies should make patients document the presence or otherwise of certain features, rather than asking the patient merely whether they are continent or not.

Several factors make important contributions to anorectal continence, and numerous theories have been promulgated as to their interrelationship. As far as possible each individual factor will be discussed separately, prior to the description of theories interrelating them.

Sensory components

Rectal sensation

The rectum is largely insensitive to many of those noxious stimuli which may induce unpleasant sensations if applied to the skin or elsewhere. On the other hand, intraluminal distension is perceived, as it is elsewhere in the gut. However, this perceived sensation is somewhat different in its localization from other parts of the intestinal tract. Even distension of the terminal parts of the sigmoid colon are interpreted as 'wind', and felt suprapubically. This same stimulus within the rectum is referred to the perineum, and is associated with the call to stool.

In addition to these qualitative differences, it would appear that the normal rectum is also quantitatively more sensitive than the remainder of the colon. Smaller changes in intraluminal pressure are discernible within the rectum, particularly in the region of the ampulla. Whilst the precise mechanisms remain obscure (be they mechanical and/or chemical), the rectum also has more discriminatory abilities than the more proximal large intestine. Flatus cannot be distinguished from faeces within the colon, whereas it can within the rectum.

Whilst the above features are well recognized, much else regarding rectal sensation remains unanswered. Throughout the bowel, there is an absence of encapsulated organized nerve endings. Consequently, it has been assumed that the sensory afferent nerves from the bowel have their origins at free unencapsulated endings, identical to those of the intramural plexuses. The bowel mesentery is sensitive however, and much of what is perceived as gut pain may in fact be due to stretching of the mesentery.

Studying patients with Hirschsprung's disease after surgical correction, it was found that pelvic reservoir sensation and the desire to defaecate may be initiated from within the puborectalis muscle itself (Scharli and Kiesewetter, 1969). Similar conclusions have been drawn after coloanal anastomosis in adults (Lane and Parks, 1977).

Anal canal sensation

As will be discussed more fully in Chapter 7, the region of the anal canal between the perianal skin and the upper limit of the pecten is lined with a modified skin. It is therefore sensitive to all the common sensory modalities.

The anal mucosa above the pecten contains a varying number of both specialized encapsulated nerve endings, and unencapsulated endings. Painful stimuli can be perceived within the anal canal, particularly in the region around the anal valves and above, i.e. the transitional zone. This correlates with the anatomical distribution of the nerve endings within the anal canal (Figure 7.2). The precise role of such features in the maintenance of gross continence is debatable, however it remains likely that the transition zone is important in the ability to discriminate. Conflicting evidence for the latter has been provided from studies directly resulting from the development of restorative proctocolectomy (see Chapter 7).

Mechanical and motor components

The internal sphincter and anal canal resting pressure

Using the manometric techniques discussed in Chapter 7, at rest there is a definable high pressure zone within the anal canal. Generally, this is to be found some 2–3 cm from the anal verge, and is distal to the palpable sling of the puborectalis muscle. Anatomically it coincides with the region of overlap between the internal and external anal sphincters, and may be between 25 and 120 mmHg (3.32 cmH$_2$O and 16.0 kPa).

At rest, continuous electromyographic activity has been recorded from the internal sphincter (Kerremans, 1968), from the external sphincter (Kawakami, 1954), and from the pelvic floor musculature (Porter, 1962). Therefore, each could have a role in the genesis of the anal resting pressure. Bennett and Duthie (1964) calculated that the visceral internal sphincter contributed some 80% to this high pressure zone. That this zone is at a greater pressure than both the more proximal anal canal and the rectum, is suggestive that the high pressure zone makes a contribution to normal faecal continence.

In spite of its major contribution to the anal canal resting pressure, Bennett and Duthie (1964) have also demonstrated that division of the internal sphincter is associated merely with poor control of flatus. Similarly, the 20% contribution to resting pressure made by the striated external sphincter, results in little disability should it be lost (Milligan and Morgan, 1934). During provocative acts, such as straining and coughing, intraluminal rectal pressure exceeds that of the normal high pressure zone. Despite this supremacy, such acts are not normally associated with incontinence. Clearly, other factors must be important in maintaining continence.

The external sphincter and anal canal squeeze pressure

Division of the external sphincter results in a loss of some 20% of the resting tone of the anal canal. The external sphincter provides the major contribution towards the maximal anal canal squeeze pressure. As a mechanism of continence, the external sphincter is probably only of relevance when the stool is particularly fluid, especially if other facets of the system are in any way compromised.

Plainly, neither the internal nor the external anal sphincters are the prime movers in maintaining continence under normal conditions.

The puborectalis sling

The study of Milligan and Morgan found that division of the puborectalis muscle during surgery for fistula-in-ano universally resulted in gross faecal incontinence. The loop effect of the puborectalis around the rectum allows for the forward pulling of the region of the anorectal junction, resulting in an angle of 60–100°. As mentioned in the previous section, it can be demonstrated electromyographically that there is continuous activity in the pelvic floor musculature. A spinal reflex has been shown to be responsible for this continuous activity, which is present even during periods of sleep (Parks, Porter and Melzack, 1962). Only during defaecation, where electrical activity is abolished, or when the hips are flexed to greater than 90°, is there loss of the normal anorectal angle.

Valves of Houston

Indirect evidence of a possible role for the valves of Houston in the maintenance of continence has come from studies of rectal manometry (Hill *et al.*, 1960). When this group utilized a compliant balloon for manometric analysis within the rectum, discrete zones of high pressure were recorded. Further examination using slim open-tipped probes failed to confirm these high pressure zones, presumably due to failure of the slimmer catheter to meet any resistance from the mucosal 'valves'.

Anal canal resistance

Putative evidence for the importance of this factor has again come from manometric studies (Harris and Pope, 1964). These workers found that greater anal canal pressures were recorded when the anal probe was being inserted per anum, than were recorded when the same catheter was being pulled out of the anal canal. This suggests that there may be partial resistance to opening of the anal canal. Harris and Pope suggested that anal canal surface tension may be the mechanism for such resistance.

Neurological considerations

In addition to the sensory components within the anorectum discussed above, other neurolo-gical factors may be important in maintaining continence. The external sphincter is inner-vated by the pudendal nerve (see Chapter 7). It has recently been found that what had pre-viously been termed 'idiopathic' faecal inconti-nence, is related to delayed conduction within the pudendal nerves. Elevations in intra-abdominal pressure result in increased electric-al activity within the musculature of the pelvic floor and the external sphincter (Taverner and Smiddy, 1959). This reflex remains even after complete transection of the spinal cord, im-plying that it is mediated within that structure.

Characteristics of the stool

It is certain that the physical characteristics of the stool are important in maintaining normal continence. In particular, stool consistency appears to have special relevance, and may be of even greater importance after pouch–anal anastomosis (see Chapter 8). The volume and chemical composition of intestinal gas may also be important, particularly after restorative proctocolectomy. This latter topic is likely to undergo further scrutiny in the future.

Summary

Under normal conditions, the internal sphinc-ter ensures that the walls of the anal canal are apposed. Other than perhaps allowing for minor adjustments, it is likely that the internal sphincter has only limited importance in preventing inadvertent passage of liquid stool and/or gas. The external sphincter also has only limited importance by allowing for strong voluntary contraction. This may be beneficial under circumstances where other components are deficient, particularly if they are also stressed by liquid stool. Sensory components are probably of little importance in the maintenance of continence (Ferguson *et al.*, 1989).

The anorectal angle produced by the con-figuration of the puborectalis sling has received much attention regarding its importance in the maintenance of continence. Primarily, two mechanisms have been proposed for the effectiveness of this action. Debate continues as to the relative merits of both. However, they are not mutually exclusive, and it is likely that

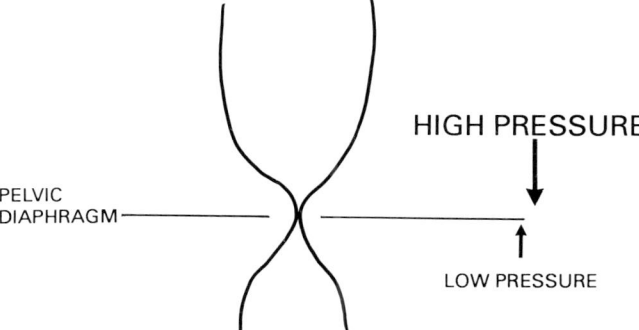

PELVIC
DIAPHRAGM

HIGH PRESSURE

LOW PRESSURE

Figure 4.1 Principle of the 'flutter' valve

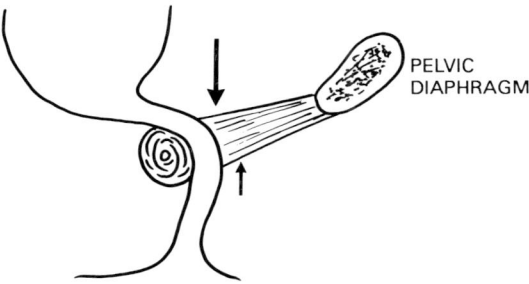

PELVIC
DIAPHRAGM

Figure 4.2 Principle of the 'flap' valve

both have a role in continence. It is generally accepted that the puborectalis muscle is of paramount importance in the maintenance of normal continence. The 'flutter valve' theory suggests that the anorectal segment assumes a slit-like configuration as it passes through the puborectalis muscle and other pelvic floor musculature (Figure 4.1). Therefore, elevations in intra-abdominal pressure might result in the forced apposition of the bowel wall. Both radiographic (Phillips and Edwards, 1965) and manometric evidence (Collins, 1967) have supported this theory. In addition, the slit-like configuration of the anal canal is probably of fundamental importance as it is in the shape of the urethra.

More recently, the 'flap valve' theory has attracted many advocates. It is well recognized that there is a pressure differential between the anal canal and abdomen. At rest, the abdominal pressure is some 100 cmH$_2$O greater than the anal canal. Under provocative acts, such as lifting, the pressure differential may increase to 250 cmH$_2$O. This differential may have the effect of compressing the anterior rectal wall onto the upper aspect of the anal canal lumen (Figure 4.2).

5

Restorative proctocolectomy – operative and technical aspects

Indications for surgery

Ileal pelvic reservoir construction is indicated in patients who have undergone proctocolectomy for diseases which predominantly affect the large bowel mucosa. Consequently, it is in the management of chronic mucosal ulcerative colitis and familial adenomatous polyposis that these procedures have been particularly useful.

Concerning ulcerative colitis, it is generally accepted that the enthusiasm for the new methods of sphincter preservation should, at least for the present, alter neither the indications nor the thresholds for surgery.

Failure of medical management over a prolonged period, results in a chronic state of morbidity for the patient, the degree of which is often not appreciated prior to colectomy. In younger patients, this may be particularly manifest as growth retardation. This is the indication for colectomy in the majority of our patients. The second major indication is an episode of acute fulminant colitis. Whether a toxic dilatation develops or not, emergency colectomy may be required. Generally, a subtotal colectomy with either a Hartmann's-type procedure or formation of a mucous fistula is best performed. We have had limited experience with creation of a pouch as a primary procedure in such circumstances. One such patient developed a pouch–vaginal fistula postoperatively.

The majority of other patients requiring colectomy for ulcerative colitis will be suffering either from some other local complication of their colitis, such as severe haemorrhage, perforation, colonic stricture, dysplasia or frank carcinoma, or from severe extracolonic manifestations of their disease.

What then are the effects of adding a mucosal proctectomy and ileal pouch–anal anastomosis on the indications for surgery in colitis? Generally, any patient requiring surgery for ulcerative colitis can be considered for sphincter preservation. However, certain exceptions should be stressed. Patients found to have a rectal carcinoma pre- or perioperatively have often been considered to be unsuitable for pelvic pouch construction. Nevertheless, as will be discussed in Chapter 14, so long as the principles of cancer surgery can be followed, a pelvic pouch need not be contraindicated. However, it is probably also important that the mid and/or lower rectum are not severely involved in the malignant process.

A low rectal stenosis, even if benign, is likely to make mucosectomy technically difficult. Consequently, some surgeons may recommend complete rectal excision in such circumstances. With the new stapling techniques, this need not preclude pouch–anal anastomosis. Similarly, other local complications of colitis, particularly rectovaginal fistula, have not been thought to contraindicate pouch construction (Parks and Nicholls, 1978; Harms, Hamilton and Starling, 1987). Indeed, such endoanal sleeve techniques have proved to be particularly efficacious in these circumstances. The pelvic pouch procedure is really only an extension of those techniques adapted for patients who require both treatment of their fistula and excision of their diseased large bowel.

With any procedure designed to preserve anorectal continence, it is important that the patient's anal sphincter complex is sufficiently efficient to withstand its new stress. Therefore, the presence of faecal incontinence preoperatively is a contraindication to pouch construction. Other assessments, either digital or manometric/electromyographic, may be used in borderline cases. It is our practice to perform preoperative anorectal manometric studies in all of our patients.

Patients who have previously undergone proctocolectomy for colitis may also be considered for ileoanal pouch construction, so long as at least part of their anal sphincter musculature remains intact. Therefore patients after either conservative proctectomy, intersphincteric proctectomy, or subtotal proctectomy with an extended distal mucosal proctectomy may be considered. As discussed in Chapter 1, a pelvic pouch can be anastomosed to the retained internal and external sphincters after conservative proctectomy (Fasth *et al.*, 1986). Such conversion has taken place 24 years after conservative proctocolectomy (Pearl *et al.*, 1985). Intestinal continuity has also been restored 5 years after mucosal proctectomy and Kock continent ileostomy formation (Hulten *et al.*, 1988). Similarly, patients who have previously undergone construction of a straight ileoanal anastomosis may be converted to a pelvic pouch should their straight anastomosis be unsatisfactory (Bulow and Kirkegaard, 1987; Fonkalsrud, Stelzner and McDonald, 1988a). Interestingly, conversion of a conventional 'sphincter ablating' panproctocolectomy to a pelvic pouch has also been reported (Ryan and Fink, 1988). In this case, continence was provided merely by the pelvic floor musculature, the anal sphincters previously having been excised (see Chapter 15).

Finally, any patient accepted for pelvic pouch construction must be fully aware of the potential risks and benefits of the procedure. Patient selection continues to be important. Patient motivation must be high. Even though results have improved considerably, complications often ensue, and may frequently require further surgery. Even in suitable patients, psychological preparation might be necessary. We frequently encourage our patients to discuss the operation with patients who have

had variable outcomes after pouch formation. It is certainly to be recommended that some degree of patient contact should occur preoperatively.

In the past, surgeons were understandably cautious about advising this procedure in older patients. More recently, accepting the above parameters with respect to preoperative continence, providing that the patient does not have seriously debilitating coexisting medical conditions, most surgeons are extending the upper limit of acceptance of patients for pouch construction. Indeed, some would now consider that, as such, there is no upper age limit for restorative proctocolectomy; biological age being more important than chronological age. However, it must be remembered that this is a prolonged surgical procedure, and patients must be fit enough to withstand it.

Total proctocolectomy with a Brooke everted end-ileostomy remains a satisfactory procedure for most cases of inflammatory bowel disease, including Crohn's colitis. However pelvic pouch formation is not. We have had one patient, subsequently shown to have Crohn's disease, who continues to have an excellent result 6 years after pouch formation. Our other two patients with Crohn's colitis have subsequently undergone pouch excision. The experience of all major series is that patients with Crohn's disease generally do very badly after ileal pouch–anal anastomosis (Deutsch *et al.*, 1990). In cases where the diagnosis is in doubt, it is prudent to perform a subtotal colectomy, and await definitive histological diagnosis from the colectomy specimen. Workers, particularly in the USA, often seek the intraoperative advice of a pathologist on the resected colonic specimen, prior to deciding upon the best course of action. Frequently, an experienced pathologist will be able to give sound advice based upon the gross appearence of the colectomy specimen. Should an ileoanal pouch be constructed in a patient subsequently shown to have Crohn's disease, there is an increased likelihood of developing local complications such as fistulas and abscesses. However, an alternative argument should be presented. There is evidence that, in the absence of clinical features suggestive of Crohn's disease, a histological diagnosis of this disorder may not be the harbinger of disaster. Interestingly, perhaps only 10% of patients with both clinical and histological evidence of

Crohn's disease will retain their pouch in the long term. Conversely, the vast majority (perhaps more than 80%) of patients with only histological evidence of Crohn's disease may have a satisfactory outcome after restorative proctocolectomy. This has led one group recently to suggest that such patients with Crohn's colitis may still be considered as candidates for pouch–anal anastomosis (Hyman *et al.*, 1990). Others have reported that, in the absence of postoperative complications requiring pouch excision, patients with Crohn's disease and pelvic pouches may have extremely satisfactory results (Johnson and Wolff, 1990).

Whilst the major indications for restorative proctocolectomy remain ulcerative colitis and adenomatous polyposis, the operation has also been performed for functional disorders of the large bowel, including constipation associated with megarectum (Hosie, Kmiot and Keighley, 1990). In this series of 13 patients, functional outcome was satisfactory.

Staging of the ileal pouch procedure

Ileal pouch–anal anastomosis can be performed in one, two or three stages. The three-stage procedure involves a preliminary colectomy with rectal stump preservation as either a mucous fistula, or as a Hartmann's-type operation. Alternatively, the rectum can be resected using the intersphincteric approach. The next stage of this three-stage operation involves resection of most of the remaining rectum; mucosal proctectomy over the most distal rectal segment; creation of the ileal reservoir and pouch–anal anastomosis protected by a loop ileostomy. The final stage of this method is to close the loop ileostomy sometime thereafter. The two-stage procedure involves proctocolectomy, mucosal proctectomy and pouch construction with its anastomosis to the anal canal performed at one sitting. A loop ileostomy is utilized, to be closed at a later date. A single phase operation is identical to the two-stage procedure, except that a loop ileostomy is not created.

Obviously, the major advantages of reducing the number of stages in restorative proctocolectomy are: to reduce the hospital stay; to reduce patient exposure to anaesthesia; and to reduce the expense of the procedure.

Three- or two-stage procedure?

A preliminary colectomy might make subsequent laparotomy more difficult and possibly hazardous. In particular, the thickening and possibly foreshortening of the mesentery associated with previous surgery can make intestinal mobilization and pouch construction somewhat more difficult. Thus in certain patients a two- or even one-stage procedure might be safer in the long term. So long as its safety can be proven, the single-stage procedure would appear to have greater advantages (Galandiuk *et al.*, 1990). As yet, no randomized, prospective trial has been performed to answer these questions.

It is generally agreed that in severe cases of ulcerative colitis, with the patient receiving high doses of systemic steroids, a three-stage procedure is in the patient's best interests. Nicholls has compared his results with both two- and three-stage procedures in 152 patients (Nicholls, Holt and Lubowski, 1989). Ninety-five patients underwent a three-stage procedure (67 of the colectomies having been performed at other institutions); 57 patients underwent two-stage operations. Assessing these patients prospectively, patients' details were similar for the two groups. Major complications (pelvic abscess and intestinal obstruction) were comparable in both groups. Overall, complications were similar between both patient cohorts. Functional results were the same in both groups. Patients with Crohn's disease or malignancy suffered higher complication rates. Therefore, if the diagnosis is in doubt, it is probably wiser to undertake a preliminary colectomy, allowing for more definitive histological examination. Neither low albumin levels nor the taking of corticosteroids were, in isolation, predictors of increased complication rates. However, in conjunction they were powerful predictors of a poor outcome. In such circumstances, Nicholls recommends a three-stage procedure.

Two- or one-stage procedure?

Recent evidence suggests that in polyposis patients, and in colitics who have already undergone colectomy or are not receiving oral corticosteroids, then stapling of the ileoanal anastomosis may enable the surgeon to avoid the use of a diverting loop ileostomy (Kmiot and Keighley, 1989b). Some surgeons have advocated single-stage procedures throughout their series (Thow, 1985). However, it should be stated that in Thow's series, patients had a full length intestinal tube in-situ in the early postoperative period. Such one-stage procedures have rarely been reported after hand-sewn anastomoses, but often with very satisfactory results (Everett and Pollard, 1990).

Preoperative preparation

There is little specific preparation for this procedure, most elements being similar to those for any other major colorectal operation. Any metabolic abnormalities should be corrected and the patient well hydrated. Preoperative anaemia, if less than 10 g/dl, should be corrected. Transfusion if required should preferably be undertaken at least 24 hours prior to surgery. Between 4 and 6 units of blood are cross-matched, and should transfusion be required, a blood warmer is recommended.

If the patient is malnourished, a period of alimentation may be required. In a few cases, resort may have to be made to parenteral hyperalimentation.

Even though a decision regarding the necessity for colectomy has been made, it is well worth continuing an intensive course of corticosteroid enemas. This may limit rectal inflammation, and aid in the performance of the mucosal proctectomy. This same advice applies to patients who have had a previous subtotal colectomy. Telander has questioned the necessity for either parenteral nutrition or steroid enemas in younger patients (Telander and Perrault, 1981).

If a staged procedure is contemplated, the site for the proposed loop ileostomy should be marked preoperatively. Standard guidelines used in the siting of a permanent ileostomy should be used. Ideally, the patient should be seen by a stomatherapist.

We have found aggressive preoperative bowel preparation to be not only unnecessary, but also to be poorly tolerated. The vast majority of these patients have severe diarrhoea, so intensive mechanical preparation brings little objective benefit. Indeed, a case can be made for the avoidance of any mechanical bowel preparation in selected patients. It is our policy to administer one sachet of sodium picosulphate orally the day prior to surgery, and to follow this by one phosphate enema on the morning of the procedure. Other workers have reported the use of almost all of the other recognized forms of colonic preparation prior to ileal pouch–anal anastomosis.

In our experience, the majority of patients will be receiving high dose steroids preoperatively, and so will require parenteral steroids in the perioperative period.

At induction of anaesthesia, a urethral catheter and a nasogastric tube are inserted, and both an aminoglycoside and metronidazole are administered parenterally. If the procedure is uncomplicated, two further doses of these antimicrobials will be given at 8-hourly intervals thereafter. Pneumoflators are fitted to both calves as prophylaxis against deep venous thrombosis.

Even the most uncomplicated of procedures results in a prolonged period of anaesthesia. Standard techniques of temperature monitoring and control must be carried out. Care with pressure points must be taken. We have had one case of transient peroneal nerve palsy postoperatively. Other surgeons have reported similar occurrences. The corneas must be covered.

Logistics of the pelvic pouch procedure

We favour the initial performance of a complete laparotomy. After colectomy, the ileum is divided. At this stage we fully mobilize the small intestinal mesentery, and ensure that sufficient length is available for a pouch–anal anastomosis without tension. Whilst such an occasion has never arisen, should insufficient length be available and the pouch procedure have to be abandoned, no irrevocable damage has been done elsewhere. After constructing the pouch, we then move onto the perineal phase of the operation. After completion of the mucosectomy and ileal pouch–anal anastomosis, the site for the loop ileostomy is chosen, and the abdomen closed. After closure and dressing of the abdominal wound, the loop ileostomy is fashioned.

Other surgeons perform the endoanal mucosectomy prior to opening the abdomen (Thow, 1985). There would appear to be potential advantages to this policy (Sullivan and Garnjobst, 1982). In such cases, the mucosectomy is usually performed under light sedation, with adequate local anaesthesia.

We have used the Lloyd-Davies position, with a Trendelenburg tilt of 15°, to allow for adequate access both to the abdomen and to the perineum throughout the whole procedure. Whilst most surgeons utilize foot stirrups to attain the Lloyd-Davies position, Coran (1985) has found that popliteal rests provide for improved access during these procedures. Many other surgeons, particularly in the USA, have found the prone jack-knife position to be useful for both the mucosectomy and the subsequent ileoanal anastomosis. By necessity, this requires repositioning of the patient during the operation.

Total colectomy for inflammatory bowel disease

The whole abdomen and perineum are prepared and draped as for abdominoperineal resection of the rectum. We perform a long midline incision, although a long left paramedian incision is also adequate. A full laparotomy is performed. The colon is closely inspected for signs of Crohn's disease and carcinoma. Should a carcinoma be present, it is fully evaluated at this time. Similarly, the entire small intestine is inspected for signs of Crohn's disease. Other lesions associated with ulcerative colitis are sought.

Total colectomy is performed as in a standard panproctocolectomy for inflammatory bowel disease. A close perirectal dissection is performed (Figure 5.1). Whilst somewhat tedious, it has been associated with less complications attributable to division of the pelvic autonomic nerves (see Chapter 6). It is important to dissect as close to the rectosigmoid segment as is possible, particularly in the midline posteriorly. Similarly, the lateral attachments of the rectum, including the lateral ligaments, must be divided close to the rectal wall.

The remainder of the colon is mobilized, remaining close to the bowel wall (Figure 5.2). This process has been termed 'coring' of the large bowel. Thereafter, the terminal ileum is divided as near to the caecum as is possible

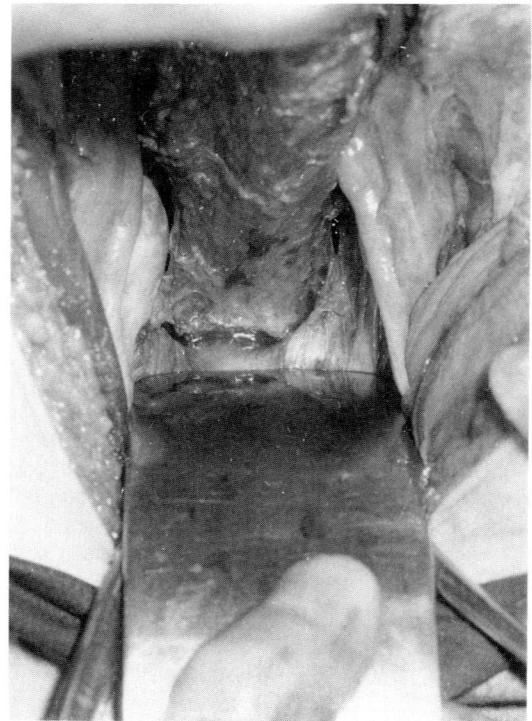

Figure 5.1 Perirectal dissection

(Figure 5.3). A right-angled clamp is placed across the rectum as low as is possible. The rectum is divided, and the specimen removed (Figures 5.4, 5.5). The terminal ileum is oversewn in two layers (Figure 5.6). Alternatively a transverse stapling instrument may be used, such as the TA55. The small bowel mesentery is mobilized completely at this stage (Figure 5.7).

General principles of pouch construction

After oversewing of the terminal ileum, the ileum is folded into the general configuration of the pouch to be constructed (Figure 5.8).

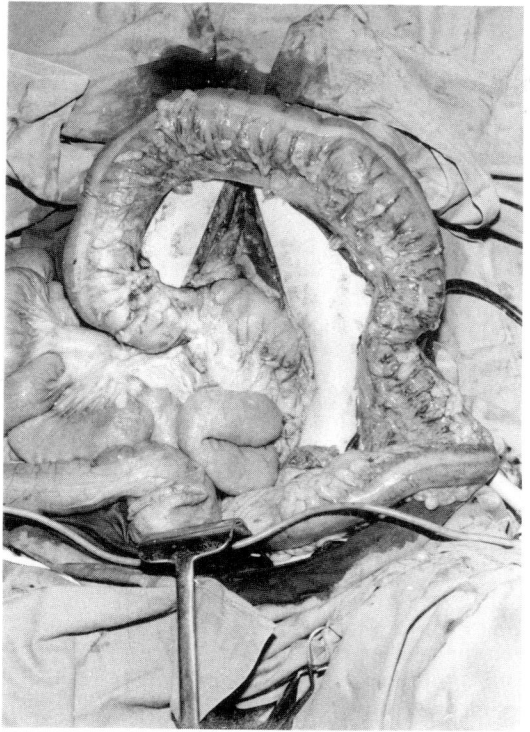

Figure 5.2 'Coring' of the colon

Whilst limbs of 15 cm are generally used for J-pouches, it is important to use the most inferiorly reaching point around this region as the apex of the pouch (see later). Babcocks forceps are placed both proximally and distally to aid subsequent anastomosis. We use a hand-held straight needle to facilitate placement of a continuous seromuscular layer of catgut (Figure 5.9). The pouch is then opened, keeping close to the previously placed suture line (Figure 5.10). Various modifications have been described to facilitate longitudinal opening of the ileum, including the use of a plastic rod (Go *et al.*, 1986). A full thickness layer of continuous catgut is then placed, hence forming the pouch, which is completed by an anterior line of seromuscular catgut (Figure 5.11). We perform the pouch–anal anastomosis to a defect left in the anterior suture line (Figure 5.12). However, many surgeons close the pouch completely, and create a new enterostomy at the apex of the pouch. Most other suture techniques that are described for intestinal anastomoses have also been described for the construction of ileal reservoirs.

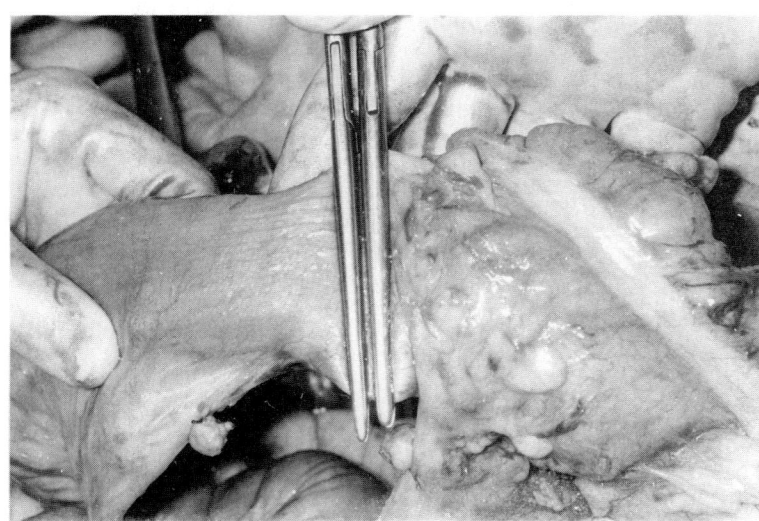

Figure 5.3 Division of terminal ileum

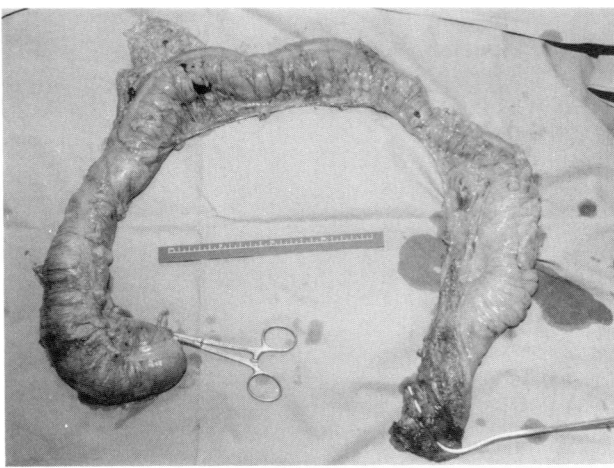

Figure 5.4 Proctocolectomy specimen

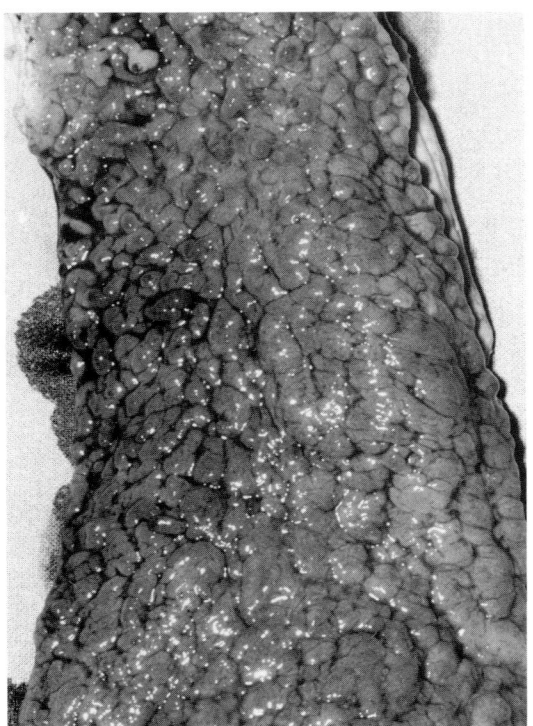

Figure 5.5 Ulcerative colitis

Like all such anastomoses, surgical technique and attention to detail are probably of greater importance than the precise suture technique used.

Which pouch?

That many designs of ileal pelvic reservoir have been popularized, to some degree bears testimony not only to surgical preference, but also relates to the fact that there is considerable overlap between the functional results obtained with all such designs. Modifications have been applied to these basic designs so as to improve various parameters of reservoir function; most notably volume and compliance characteristics. In Chapter 1, mention was made of the progression through which the continent ileostomy passed. In this chapter, this theme will be continued with particular reference to the ileal pelvic reservoir.

As described in the previous chapter, the first clinical experience with the pelvic pouch was obtained using the hand-sewn triplicated or S-configuration pouch. That this reservoir dramatically decreased stool frequency was without question, and subsequent reports fuelled the optimism in this reservoir type (Taylor *et al.*, 1983a). Many workers have favoured this design of reservoir. Whilst accepting the efficacy of the S-pouch (Figure 5.13), several technical modifications to the basic designs have been reported.

Stern and colleagues have described, in both animals and humans, a modified stapled form of S-pouch construction (Stern *et al.*, 1987). The rationale for this technique was to avoid the potential complication of ischaemic necrosis of the central bridge of reservoir tissue

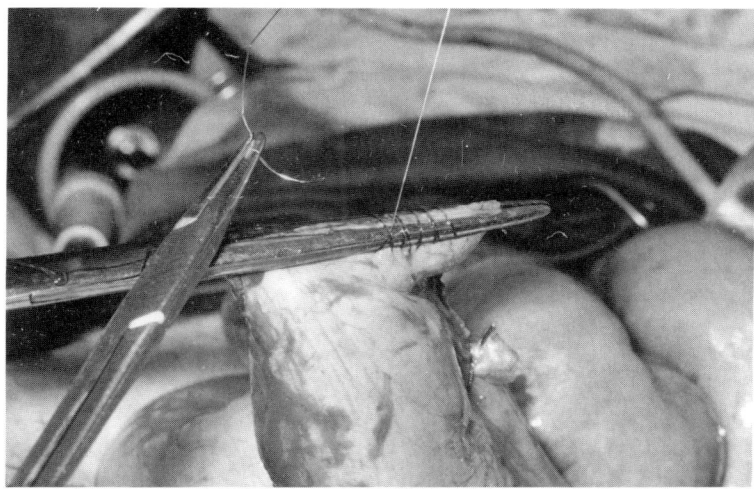

Figure 5.6 Oversewing terminal ileum

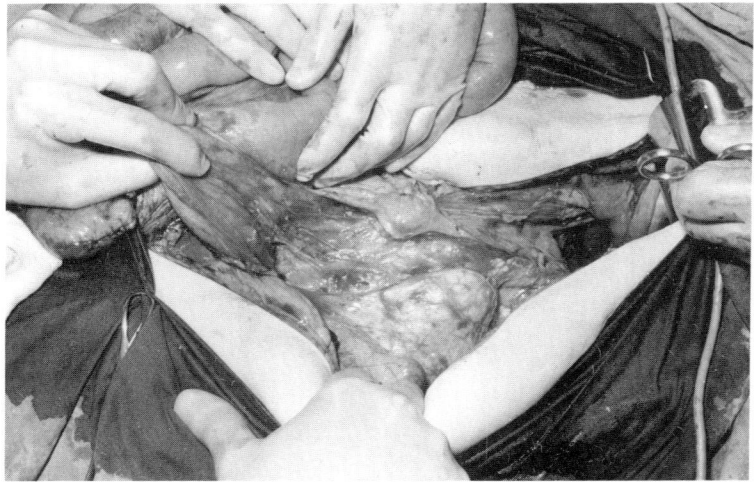

Figure 5.7 Mobilization of root of mesentery

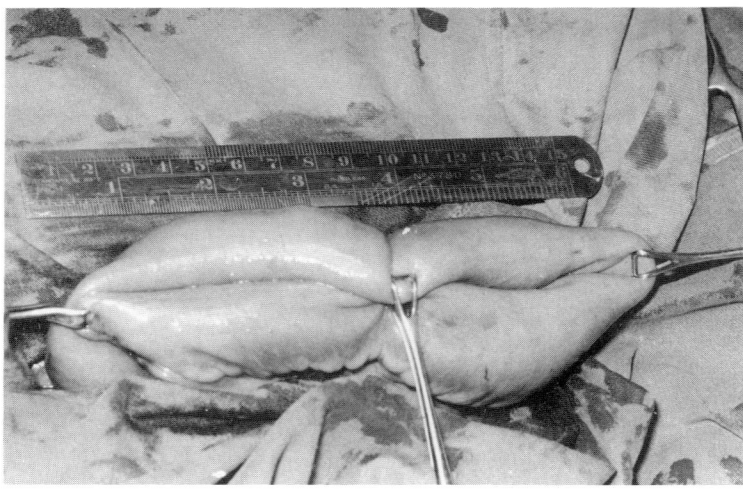

Figure 5.8 Folding of ileum

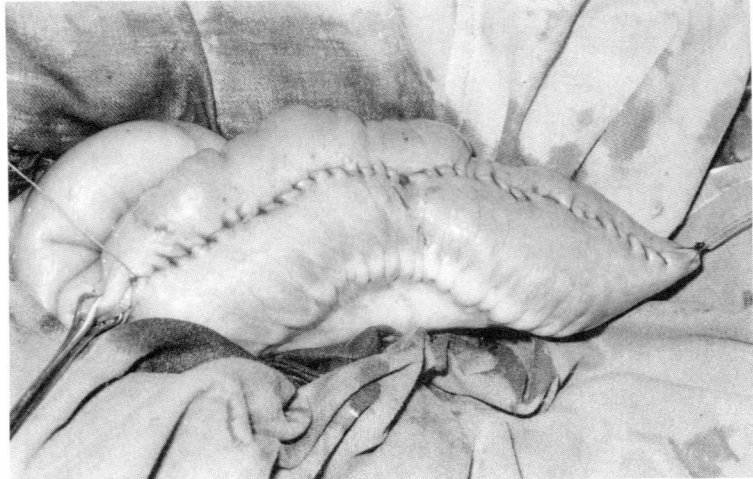

Figure 5.9 Seromuscular layer

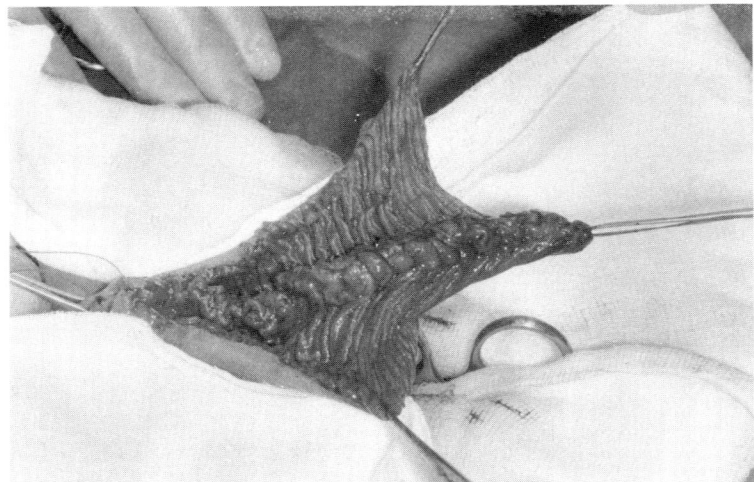

Figure 5.10 Opening of pouch

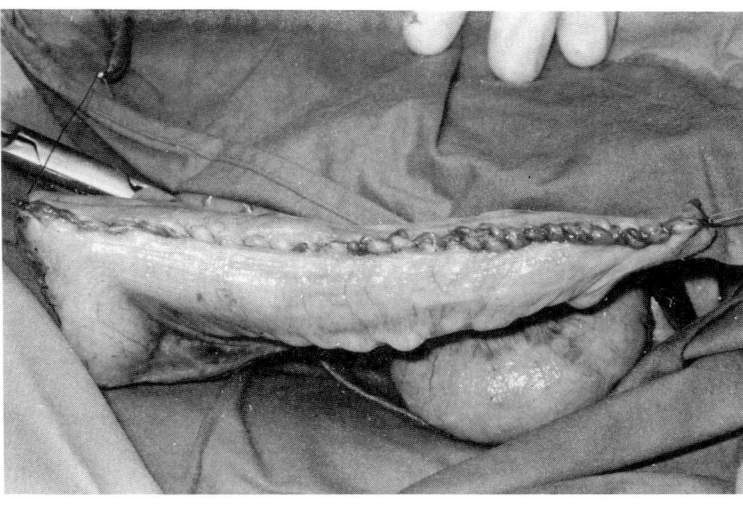

Figure 5.11 Full-thickness layer

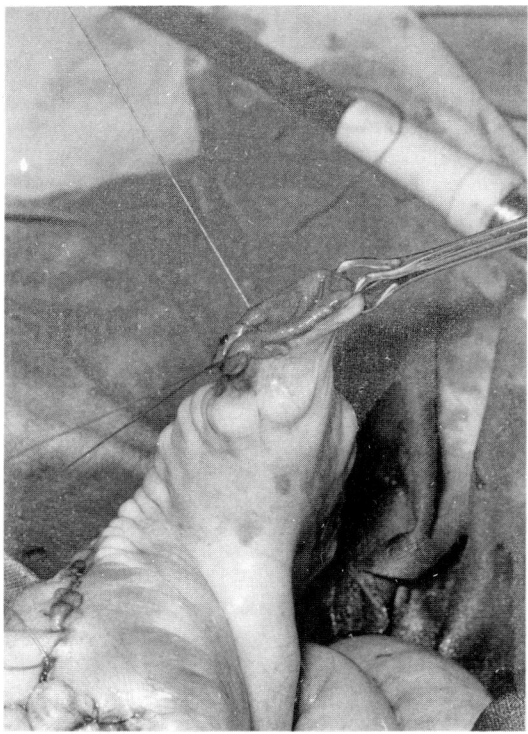

Figure 5.12 Apical defect

between the two longitudinal staple lines. Theoretically, this complication could ensue if the pouch was fashioned in a manner directly analogous to that for a duplicated J-pouch. This technique results in there being no such completely isolated segments.

The inability to evacuate the S-pouch spontaneously has always been the Achilles heel of the triplicated reservoir. With the realization that long efferent limbs were the major reason for poor evacuation (see later), this problem has been much improved with the use of shorter pouch outlets (Figure 5.13(a),(b)). However, even with such modifications, there is still a small but significant incidence of catheterization. In order completely to avoid this complication, whilst maintaining the volume and compliance characteristics of the S-pouch, Pescatori described a design in which an end-to-side pouch–anal anastomosis is constructed in a manner analogous to that performed for J- and W-pouches (Figure 5.13(c)) (Pescatori, 1988). Clinical assessments of six standard S- and four modified S-pouches concluded that the modified design resulted in improved clinical and functional outcomes (Pescatori *et al.*, 1989).

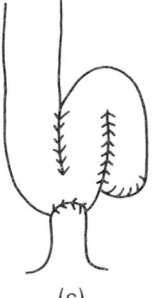

(a)   (b)   (c)   **Figure 5.13** Triplicated S-pouches

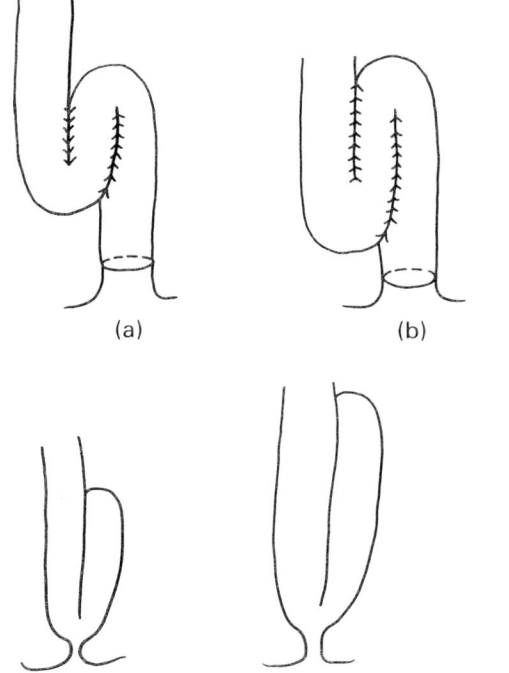

(a)   (b)   **Figure 5.14** Duplicated J-pouches

After Parks' initial description of this procedure, the next significant change in reservoir design was described by Utsunomiya. His group originally described the use of three forms of ileoanal anastomosis, two of which involved the construction of a reservoir (Utsunomiya *et al.*, 1980). Whilst modest experience was gained with the isoperistaltic double-barrelled reservoir, it was the J-configuration pouch which aroused the most interest from Utsunomiya's group and other workers (Figure 5.14). With this form of reservoir, functional stability was attained in the shortest period of time compared to their other designs, soiling did not prove to be problematical, and evacuation was always spontaneous. These results encouraged others to adopt this design, most notably the Mayo clinic group (Taylor *et al.*, 1983a). A modified J-pouch (termed the B-pouch) has recently been used in experimental animals to assess peptide YY and enteroglucagon levels after pouch construction (Mariani *et al.*, 1989). As yet, there is no report of its clinical use.

Further innovation was to come from St Mark's Hospital, in the form of the quadruple or W-pouch (Nicholls and Pezim, 1985; Nicholls and Lubowski, 1987). Initially, such reservoirs were hand-sewn in two layers using four 12-cm lengths of terminal ileum (Figure 5.15(a)). This enabled an end-to-side ileoanal anastomosis, in the manner of that utilized for duplicated pouches. In the first clinical reports of its use, 23 patients had undergone such a procedure (Nicholls and Pezim, 1985). Encouragingly, 17 of these patients had no complications whatsoever. After allowing for a learning curve, postoperative complications probably did not differ from the S- and J-pouches also considered in this report. All patients evacuated spontaneously, with a bowel frequency of 4.1 per 24 hours. Some 22% had to evacuate at night. These figures compare very favourably with those for the other pouch designs, in that almost 60% of patients with J-pouches described nocturnal evacuation, with a bowel frequency of 5.5 per 24 hours. Interestingly, intraoperative volumes of the reservoirs were 325 ml (W), 177 ml (S) and 172 ml (J). This compared with 322 ml, 416 ml and 197 ml respectively when measured after closure of the ileostomy. However, time-corrected figures for pouch distension are difficult to assess. Such discrepancies between the S- and W-pouches are probably related to obstruction of the efferent limb of these pouches, as only 41% of the latter could evacuate spontaneously.

This same group described their combined experience with the W-reservoir in 64 patients (Nicholls and Lubowski, 1987). This report included a modification to their initial design, in which the four-loop reservoir was somewhat staggered (Figure 5.15(b)). As can be seen, the pouch is made up of two J-type intestinal loops, with the cephalad loop lying 2 cm proximal to the caudal loop. This modification permitted an easier ileoanal anastomosis, by avoiding the bulk of the pouch having to lie within the rectal cuff.

Harms has similarly reported a modification to the originally described W-pouch (Harms, Pellett and Starling, 1987). In this, the apex of the pouch is intended to be some 12 cm from

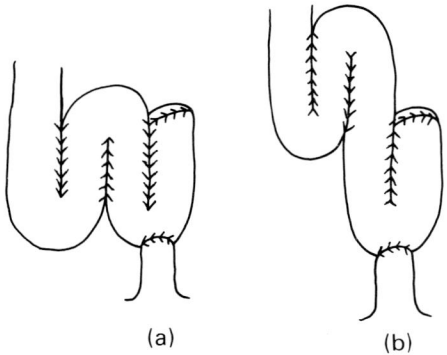
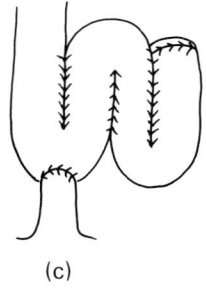

(a)   (b)

(c)

Figure 5.15 Quadruple W-pouches

the oversewn end of the terminal ileum. This point is tagged in order to ascertain that it will in fact reach the site for the ileoanal anastomosis. A standard J-type loop with 12-cm limbs is created, to which is added two further limbs of length 9 cm, staggered from the former by 3–4 cm. This allows an easy ileoanal anastomosis as for a J-pouch, whilst providing for an increased capacity. In ten patients so treated, the mean intraoperative volume was 220 ml. All patients had good to excellent continence control, with no patients having anything more than minimal nocturnal leakage. At 6 months, bowel frequency was approximately six per 24 hours. This reservoir therefore resulted in quite acceptable performance characteristics, but requires some 8 cm more of small intestine for its construction than does a standard S-pouch. However, because of the nature of its construction, should excision be necessary, this configuration allows that no more bowel need be excised than for an S- or J-pouch.

It therefore appears that increasing the volume of the ileoanal reservoir results in an improved functional performance, particularly with regard to frequency and nocturnal evacuation. Might not a similar result be witnessed merely by doubling the length of the J-pouch (Figure 5.14(b))? Nicholls argues that for a given set of dimensions, i.e. the length of terminal ileum to be utilized in reservoir construction, that a spheroid will theoretically result in the greatest volume. He continues that the W-pouch is the configuration which most resembles a spheroid. However, he concedes that there is insufficient data to answer the question of whether a J-pouch of double length would prove to be equally effective.

In addition to these three major forms of folded reservoirs, several other forms of neorectum have been described. Perhaps the most frequently used of the rest is the lateral isoperistaltic reservoir (Figure 5.16) (Fonkalsrud, 1981). Utsunomiya terms this reservoir the 'H-pouch'. Again, this procedure can be performed in stages or at one sitting. After colectomy and mucosal proctectomy, a straight ileoanal anastomosis is performed and the ileum divided 30 cm above the anastomosis. An end-ileostomy is created, and the proximal end of the distal ileal segment is brought to the skin as a mucous fistula. After healing of the ileoanal anastomosis the ileostomy is mobil-

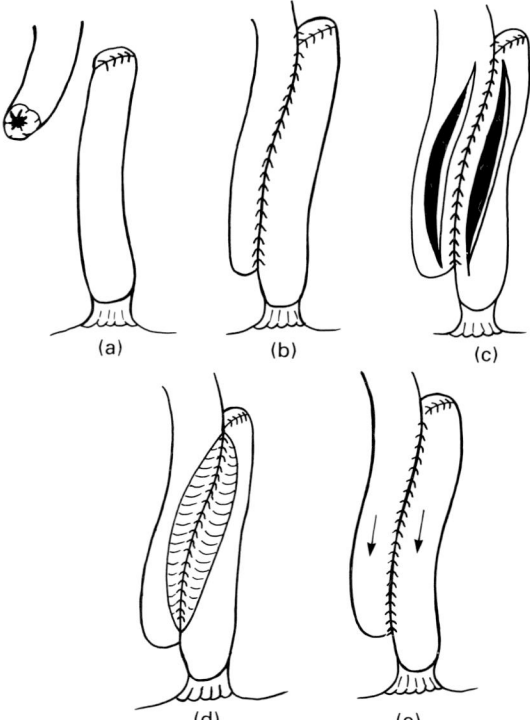

Figure 5.16 Lateral isoperistaltic reservoir (after Fonkalsrud, 1981)

ized. The distal 20 cm of this segment is anastomosed side to side isoperistaltically with the ileoanal segment. Consequently, Fonkalsrud left a 10-cm efferent limb from the pouch, but this has been reduced in later patients.

Excepting Fonkalsrud, clinical experience with this design has been limited, and not always favourable (Canty, Self and Bonaldi, 1983). However, in the latter report the results obtained were with the initial patients in the series, and were probably on the steepest part of the learning curve. Several surgeons have created lateral reservoirs on occasions, but few have used them extensively.

A similar reservoir construction, but incorporating an antiperistaltic segment, has also been described. In this lateral antiperistaltic reservoir, the terminal ileum is folded upon itself, in a manner analagous to the J-pouch. The apex of the pouch is subsequently divided. The distal antiperistaltic limb is anastomosed side to side with the proximal isoperistaltic segment. The latter is left protruding distal to

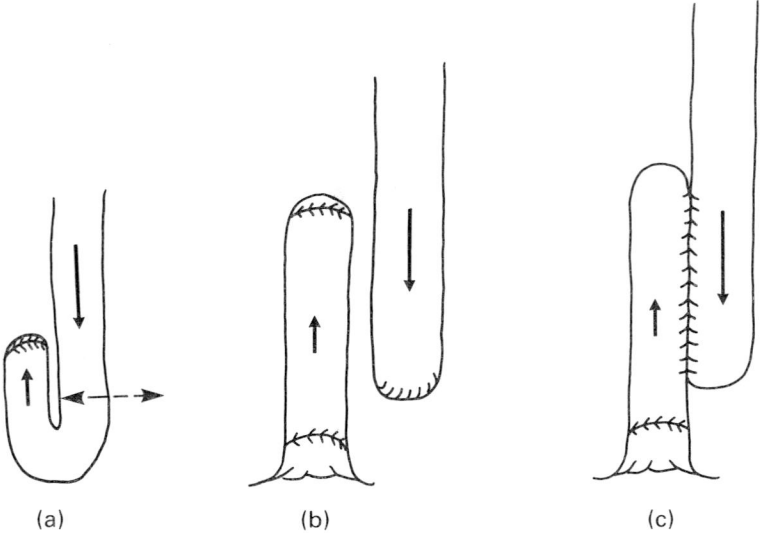

(a)   (b)   (c)

Figure 5.17 Lateral antiperistaltic reservoir (after Thow, 1985)

the former by 2–5 cm as an antiperistaltic efferent spout, which is anastomosed to the anal canal (Figure 5.17). Clinical experience with this pouch design has been provided by Thow, who utilized a full length intestinal tube to obviate the necessity for a defunctioning stoma (Thow, 1985). Describing his results in 21 patients, stool frequency averaged five per 24 hours after 3 months. Nocturnal leakage was infrequent, and continence was complete.

In Chapter 1, the fundamental principles of pouch mechanics were briefly discussed. The major contributor to this subject has been Professor Nils Kock. He described the filling-pressure profiles of several reservoirs culminating in his design of the doubly folded Kock pouch. With excellent filling characteristics, the use of the Kock pouch as both bladder substitute and continent ileostomy has met with considerable success. It is perhaps surprising that this configuration has received little enthusiasm for its use as a pelvic pouch (Myrvold and Thoresen, 1989). Early clinical experience with this design came from a patient in whom a Kock continent ileostomy was converted to a pelvic pouch. This patient requested the restoration of intestinal continuity some 5 years after a conservative proctocolectomy with endoanal mucosectomy and construction of a Kock continent ileostomy. Clinical results with this conversion were

extremely satisfactory, probably due in part to the fact that the pouch had already become dilated. This prior dilatation was emphasized as the key to this procedure, as the intra-abdominal reservoir reached the pelvis with very little mobilization. This therefore represents a treatment option should insufficient length be available for primary pouch–anal anastomosis. After a period to allow for dilatation, the pouch can be moved to the pelvis as a secondary procedure (Hulten *et al.*, 1988).

Kock's own experience with this design used as a pelvic conduit has been limited (Kock, Hulten and Myrvold, 1989). After conventional colectomy and mucosal proctectomy over a 5-cm rectal cuff, the terminal ileum is divided flush with the caecum. The site for ileoanal anastomosis is chosen some 15 cm proximal to the terminal ileum. A 30-cm segment of terminal ileum is opened on its antimesenteric border. Importantly, the opened bowel is placed so as to lie in the U-shape, with the efferent end pointed cranially and with the base of the U pointing to the patient's left (Figure 5.18). The limbs of the U are anastomosed leaving a small defect. This will be the ultimate site for the ileoanal anastomosis. Folding of the intestine allows for formation of the pouch. After suturing of the pouch, the corners of the pouch are passed between

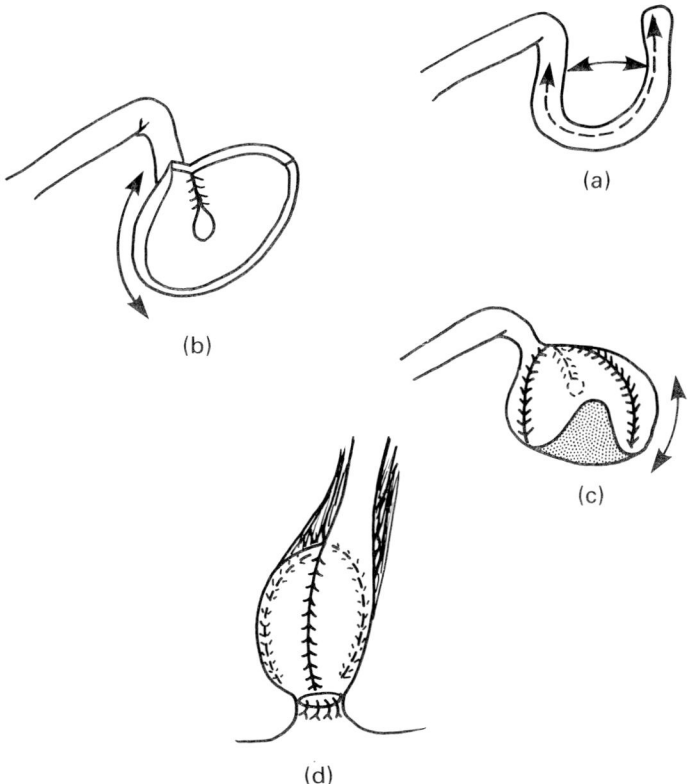

Figure 5.18 Kock pouch–anal anastomosis

the leaves of the mesentery. As a consequence, the posterior wall of the pouch comes to anteriorly. This manoeuvre facilitates positioning of the enterotomy site for ileoanal anastomosis. A temporary loop ileostomy was employed in all six patients. Very acceptable functional and physiological results were obtained with this reservoir design.

Few clinical studies have attempted to compare different reservoir designs. Randomized prospective trials have not been performed generally. Most such studies have compared one surgeon's early results with one reservoir design with his later experience with a differing design. Alternatively, several different surgeons' experiences with their own preferred pouch design have been compared (see Chapter 8).

Generally, the greater the pouch volume and compliance, the better the functional outcome. In particular, reduced frequency and nocturnal frequency are seen (Nicholls and Pezim, 1985;

Nasmyth, Williams and Johnston, 1986; McHugh *et al.*, 1987).

Hand-sewn or stapled pouches?

With all reservoir forms, stapling devices were soon utilized to aid pouch construction (Hughes, Bauer and Bauer, 1988; Ramos and Bode, 1988; Soper, Kestenberg and Becker, 1988; Brough and Schofield, 1989). Generally, two methods have been used in the stapling of pelvic pouches; either telescoping the pouch, or using multiple enterotomies.

Hughes described construction of a 15-cm J-pouch using a linear stapling gun inserted through an apical enterome and purse-string. After firing, the pouch was telescoped over the gun, which was refired up to four times. Similar techniques have been described by others (Ramos and Bode, 1988). Upon removal of the gun, the purse-string suture is tied, thus preventing contamination. The same apical site is also used for the ileoanal anastomosis. As there are no formal enterotomies within the pouch, there are no repair lines which might subsequently leak. Also, this technique avoids the formation of a septum within the pouch, as occurs in the Utsunomiya design. Finally it has the additional advantage of most stapled anastomoses, in that it is faster to construct than a hand-sewn anastomosis.

Brough and Schofield described a modification for stapled J-pouch construction. After colectomy, a 40-cm loop of terminal ileum is fully mobilized. Three stay sutures are placed in the antimesenteric border of the bowel. After insertion of an apical purse-string, an enterotomy is placed within the latter. Through the enterotomy a long linear stapling gun is passed and fired. A small enterotomy is made in the junction of the afferent limb with the pouch and the same gun similarly placed into the pouch and fired. The divided end of the terminal ileum is then anastomosed end to side with the afferent limb (Figure 5.19) in order to avoid stenosis of the pouch entrance.

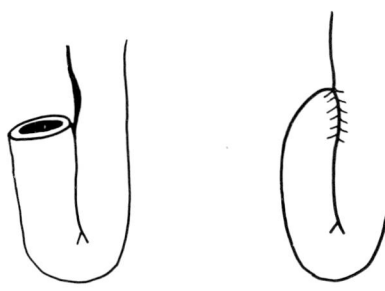

Figure 5.19

The purse-string facilitates a stapled ileoanal anastomosis.

Further support for the use of stapling instruments has been provided by experimental reports (Soper, Kestenberg and Becker, 1988). The former group assessed a group of six mongrel dogs, in each of which they created three J-pouches with 15-cm limbs. The first pouch was situated 10 cm proximal to the ileocaecal valve, with 10 cm between each subsequent pouch. Reservoirs were constructed in a random fashion, and each intestinal segment was isolated by transverse

stapling. Three pouch designs were assessed, including a hand-sewn pouch in two layers of continuous Dexon, and two forms of stapled pouch. The first stapled pouch entailed the forming of enterotomies in each limb of the pouch at the junction of the proximal and middle thirds. A stapling gun was inserted both proximally and distally into the pouch and fired. The enterotomies were closed in two layers with Dexon. The final group of pouches was formed by performing an apical enterotomy through a Prolene purse-string suture, and inserting the linear gun. Construction was facilitated by telescoping the pouch, as described above.

After occlusion of the afferent limb of the pouch, saline was infused into the reservoir to a pressure of $30 \, \text{cmH}_2\text{O}$. Any leaks were noted. The volume infused to reach this pressure was recorded as the 'crude volume'. The mean ileal circumference (C) was recorded at three sites, allowing for the calculation of a 'corrected volume' of the pouch from the equation:

$$\frac{\text{crude volume}}{\text{corrected volume}} = \frac{C^2}{2\pi}$$

In addition to these calculations, the time for each anastomosis was noted, and the ease of the procedure graded on a scale of 1 to 5, with 5 implying an easy anastomosis. The hand-sewn pouch had a corrected volume of approximately 50% as compared to the stapled pouches, which were approximately equal. How relevant such figures are, taken as they were at the time of construction, is open to debate. Whether such relationships continue to hold with time is presently unclear. The apically stapled pouch was the easiest to construct (score 4.2), with the laterally stapled pouch being intermediate, followed by the hand-sewn pouch (3.1 and 2.4 respectively). As for the time to construct the pouch, both stapled techniques took approximately 5 minutes, whilst the hand-sewn pouch took 30 minutes to construct. There were no leaks associated with any of the pouches.

Keighley randomized his patients into those who would receive either a stapled J-pouch or a hand-sewn W-pouch (Keighley, Yoshioka and Kmiot, 1988). The duplicated reservoirs were constructed from 20-cm limbs, whereas the W-pouches had 10-cm limbs. Hence, equivalent lengths of small intestine were utilized. The operative capacity of the designs was 190 ml and 230 ml respectively. Generally, complication rates were equivalent, and bowel frequency was found to be the same in both groups. Keighley found that whilst stapled reservoirs were quicker to construct, functional results were more related to postoperative pelvic sepsis rather than to pouch design.

Reservoir length

Whilst differing forms of reservoir designs have received much attention, little attention has been given to the subject of reservoir length and its relationship to ultimate functional outcome after restorative proctocolectomy. As many workers have shown reservoir capacity to be a statistically important discriminator of ultimate function, it would not be surprising if doubly folded reservoirs of twice the length of a standard J-pouch provided similar results to W-pouches (Nicholls and Lubowski, 1987). Such a series has not, to our knowledge, been reported. Keighley found that longer J-pouches were easier to place in the pelvis than W-pouches (Keighley, Yoshioka and Kmiot, 1988). In the authors' series, all except one of the J-pouches had 15-cm limbs. In the other patient a 30-cm pouch was constructed. In this

patient, functional outcome was not initially satisfactory, with a clinical history of incomplete and repeated evacuation of the pouch. Complete bowel evacuation often took more than 1 hour, but interestingly these episodes only occurred in the morning and early evening. Cinepouchography revealed evidence of folding of this reservoir on defaecation, leading to a sump effect in the cephalad half of the pouch (Figure 5.20(a)). Pouchopexy of this reservoir to the left psoas muscle has resulted in resolution of these symptoms (Figure 5.20(b)), with two or three complete bowel evacuations per day. There is no nocturnal evacuation.

Only one report has specifically examined this aspect of pouch construction (Stelzner, Fonkalsrud and Lichtenstein, 1988). In this series, all 153 patients had undergone formation of an isoperistaltic lateral reservoir. The majority had pouches of between 14 and 20 cm in length, however 14 patients had pouches of 30 cm in length. Considering the complications and results in both groups, it was found that postoperative complications requiring further surgery were five times more common in the group with longer reservoirs. Recurrent pouchitis was also found much more frequently in this group. Significantly, almost total improvement was noted in all patients in whom a conversion from a long to a short pouch was undertaken.

The rectal cuff

Initial descriptions of the pelvic pouch procedure incorporated long rectal cuffs (Figure 5.21(a)) (Utsunomiya *et al.*, 1980). The rationale for such cuffs was to lead to improved continence compared to that achieved with more complete rectal incision. It was thought that receptors were present in the perirectal tissues which were important in registering rectal distension and that these might in part contribute to the ability to discriminate between fluid and flatus. Certain authors soon began to utilize shorter rectal cuffs (Figure 5.21(b)) (Parks and Nicholls, 1978; Taylor *et al.*, 1983a), in particular as this more limited cuff resulted in the need for less dissection and anal retraction when the whole of the mucosectomy was performed from below. Longer cuffs

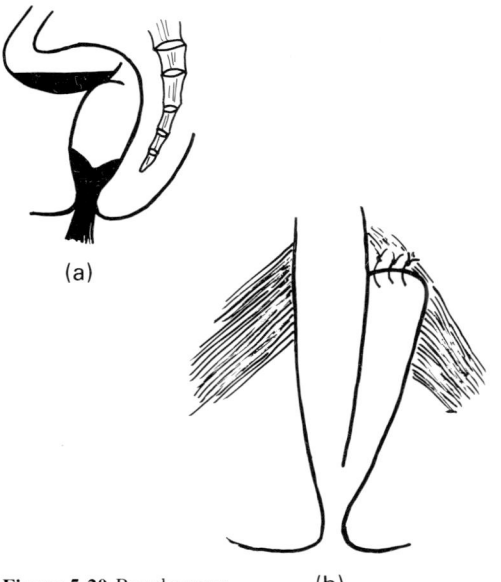

(a)

Figure 5.20 Pouchopexy   (b)

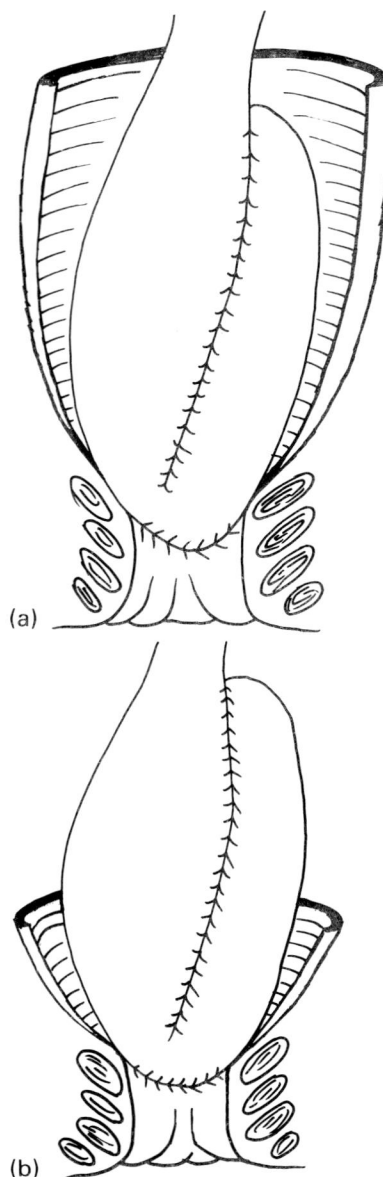

Figure 5.21 Long (a) and short (b) rectal cuffs

had often necessitated an abdominal mucosectomy (see below).

Clinical experience soon made it apparent that very acceptable functional results could be achieved with the adoption of short rectal cuffs (McHugh *et al.*, 1987). Certainly, these shorter cuffs resulted in a considerable reduction in operating time. There is now anecdotal evidence that the complication of cuff abscess is

less frequent when shorter rectal cuffs are used. However, this finding is not universal (Lindquist, Nilsell and Liljequist, 1987). Mucosectomy is facilitated by a shorter cuff, and hence any particular risk of leaving islands of mucosa should be reduced.

In an attempt to determine the necessity for the retention of any rectal cuff whatsoever, Chaussade *et al* have compared 18 patients after J-pouch–anal anastomosis to the dentate line with controls (Chaussade *et al.*, 1989c). After eversion of a short rectal stump, the remaining rectum was transected at the dentate line, and a hand-sewn ileoanal anastomosis performed. Several tests of ano-pouch function were performed, including two forms of anal manometry (see Chapter 7). Seventeen of the 18 patients had normal continence and defaecation. As with other groups, anal canal resting pressure was approximately halved postoperatively. The anorectal inhibitory reflex was absent in 17 patients. Squeeze pressures were not reduced compared with controls. The maximal tolerated pouch volume was similar in both groups, although the threshold volume at which sensation was first felt was significantly higher in the pouch group.

Other functional parameters were similar to those reported by other units constructing J-pouches. Therefore, sacrifice of the complete rectum was found to be compatible with satisfactory results after restorative protocolectomy. Chaussade describes that such resection might be useful when mucosectomy proves difficult, or when the rectum is found to be small.

Over the last decade, there has been a trend towards shorter rectal cuffs, most surgeons now utilizing a 2–3 cm cuff, and some of them have abandoned the preservation of a cuff altogether.

The efferent limb

Parks' initial description of the pelvic reservoir utilized a 5–6 cm efferent spout from his triplicated 'S' pouch (Figure 5.13) (Parks and Nicholls, 1978). Of the first 21 patients so treated, only 10 were able to void spontaneously (Parks, Nicholls and Belliveau, 1980). Since this time, two further reservoir designs have incorporated efferent limbs. Both of these are of the 'lateral' configuration, one iso- the other antiperistaltic (see above). Early experience with duplicated so-called J-reservoirs revealed that this design was associated with spontaneous evacuation in all cases. Both duplicated and triplicated designs incorporate antiperistaltic segments, and so it appeared that the efferent limb was responsible for the failure to evacuate spontaneously.

The St Mark's group assessed the pressure-filling characteristics at several sites within S-pouches, including the efferent limb (Rabau, Percy and Parks, 1982). Using a double-lumen water-filled system, to which a balloon was attached, single, phasic-type waves were recorded in the efferent limbs, with a duration of 3–9 seconds (similar to those in the pouch themselves), and an amplitude of 10–60 cmH$_2$O (approximately twice that of those seen in the pouches). In addition, tonic waves were seen in the efferent limbs, with an amplitude of 35 cmH$_2$O (compared to 10 cmH$_2$O in the pouches). These tonic waves tended to occur in a sequential manner between the pouch and the efferent limb. In the fasting state, phasic waves were the predominant form (31.3% of the time in the reservoir and 51% in the efferent limb). Very little time was occupied by tonic wave forms. Eating increased the total time occupied by activity to 57.1%, with a modest increase in tonic activity, both in the efferent limb and the pouch. Reservoir distension during fasting resulted in a marked increase in both total activity and, to a greater degree, tonic wave duration. This was witnessed in the pouch and efferent limb. Tonic waves resulted in the desire to defaecate in the pouch patients. These waves are propulsive as shown by the fact that if external sphincter contraction was voluntarily resisted, their presence resulted in faecal leakage.

Further physiological studies of the efferent limb have compared the effects of long and short efferent limbs on pouch function in experimental animals (Rosemurgy, Schraut and Block, 1983). Twenty-five dogs, six with straight ileoanal anastomoses, and 19 after ileal reservoir construction, were studied. Nine animals had S-pouches (six with long and three with short efferent limbs), and ten had antiperistaltic double-barrelled reservoirs (seven with long and three with short efferent limbs). Reservoir motility patterns were studied by using a compliant latex balloon introduced into the pouch or distal ileum under light anaesthesia. Water was instilled into the balloon to a pressure of 20–25 cmH$_2$O. The balloon was connected to a strain gauge transducer allowing continuous pressure recording. Such records were obtained synchronously with electromyographic recordings. Filling of the reservoirs to a pressure of 25 cmH$_2$O, resulted in bursts of synchronous spike activity, with an associated increase in both amplitude and frequency of the recorded pressure waves. The presence of a long efferent limb resulted in a decrease in such activity, which in the case of the triplicated reservoir caused it to become an atonic bag by 4 months. The double-barrelled reservoir tended to retain both its contractile and electrical properties, particularly when it was placed proximal to a 2-cm efferent spout (2–8 waves per hour, amplitude 15–45 cmH$_2$O).

Clearly a long efferent limb frequently results in at least partial obstruction to the pouch. It has also been associated with an increased incidence of cuff abscess in the postoperative period (Lindquist, Nilsell and Liljequist, 1987).

S-pouch volumes have been seen to increase dramatically postoperatively, being greater than those found in W-pouches (Nicholls and Pezim, 1985). That kinking of a long efferent limb may be partly responsible for the inability to defaecate spontaneously was provided from the experience of the effects of pregnancy (Pezim, 1984). Enlargement of the gravid uterus may result in straightening of the efferent limb, and the ability to defaecate spontaneously. This process may be reversed after delivery.

Almost 25% of the early isoperistaltic reservoir developed outlet obstruction, attributable to a long rectal cuff and efferent limb in half of these (Stone, Lewin and Fonkalsrud. 1986). Clinically this was manifest by pouch distension, faecal stasis, pouchitis and diarrhoea. Division of the upper rectal muscle resulted in improvement in all patients. Reduction in efferent limb lengths has resulted in great improvement with regard to the necessity for self-catheterization (Vasilevsky, Rothenberger and Goldberg, 1987). Catheterization can be reduced to less than 5% by the adoption of efferent limbs of 3 cm or less.

Other defaecation disorders are often seen in patients with long efferent limbs; these include faecal incontinence and excessive straining at defaecation. In addition, efferent limb stenosis may occur, possibly resulting from repeated trauma due to self-catheterization.

Efferent limb outlet obstruction is well recognized in the clinical situation (Schoetz, Coller and Veidenheimer, 1986). This complication has been managed by endoanal posterior transmucosal myotomy. The technique involved submucosal infiltration of a dilute adrenaline solution, following which a 5-mm incision is made down to and including part of the longitudinal muscle of the efferent limb. This relatively minor procedure relieved outlet obstruction (Pescatori and Parks, 1984b). However, it is important to perform the procedure in the posterior midline, as the small bowel mesentery lies anteriorly.

In patients where obligative self-catheterization is associated with other problems, such as faecal incontinence, Nicholls has recommended reconstructive surgery (Nicholls and Gilbert, 1990). In six patients so treated, the efferent limb was excised. Initial attempts to perform the resection endoanally were inadequate. Transabdominal resection of the efferent limb proved to be more successful, but difficult technically. After endoanal reanastomosis, a temporary loop ileostomy was created. Symptoms were improved in all patients, but only four evacuated spontaneously. Whether improved results would be witnessed after conversion of such S-pouch–anal anastomoses to one as described by Pescatori, with closure of the efferent limb, has not been reported (Figure 5.13c).

The superior mesenteric artery

The anatomical disposition of the superior mesenteric artery is depicted diagrammatically in Figure 5.22. This vessel is of great importance with regard to the pelvic pouch procedure, as confirmed by reports of complications attributable to it. Adequate length of the artery is the limiting factor in permitting delivery of the pouch apex to the upper anal canal for anastomosis. At the end of the operation, the vessel often may be found to be stretched quite tight.

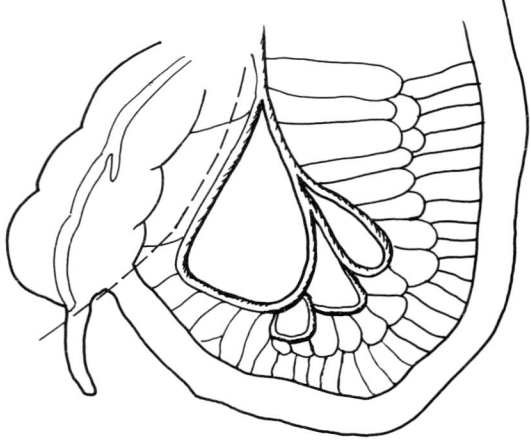

Figure 5.22 The superior mesenteric artery

The first report of complications attributable to the superior mesenteric artery came from Ballantyne and colleagues. In this case, the patient developed upper intestinal obstruction postoperatively. This settled on conservative management (Ballantyne *et al.*, 1987).

Subsequently, there followed further reports of the so-called 'superior mesenteric artery syndrome' after ileoanal anastomosis (Hines, Gore and Ballantyne, 1984; Christie, Schroeder and Hill, 1988). This latter group reported a 21-year-old male, who underwent semi-urgent construction of a stapled J-type reservoir. Transverse incisions in the ileal mesentery ensured that both the ileoanal anastomosis and the defunctioning loop ileostomy were easily placed without tension. After 6 days of uncomplicated recovery, vomiting of copious amounts of bile-stained fluid necessitated replacement of the nasogastric tube, and recommencement of parenteral nutrition. Contrast radiography demonstrated a band obstruction of the fourth part of the duodenum. Conservative therapy failed to relieve the high gastric aspirates, and after 6 weeks a further laparotomy was performed. A high duodenojejunal flexure was found, tethered by a particularly strong ligament of Treitz. Consequently, the superior mesenteric artery was tightly bow-stringed across the duodenum producing constriction. After complete mobilization of the duodenojejunal flexure and division of the ligament of Treitz, the duodenum was divided and reanastomosed anterior to the superior mesenteric artery. The loop ileostomy was also closed. The patient made an uncomplicated recovery with good pouch control.

Several subsequent reports have evaluated the relationship of the superior mesenteric artery and its branches to the ileoanal pouch procedure (Smith, Friend and Medwell, 1984; Burnstein *et al.*, 1987; Cherqui *et al.*, 1987).

A study performed in cadavers assessed tension in the pouch–anal anastomosis (Smith, Friend and Medwell, 1984). First, 12 cadavers were studied to assess the length of the ileocaecal artery. In addition, the two longest branches of the superior mesenteric artery were also measured. The length of the ileocaecal junction to the longest branch of the superior mesenteric artery was also noted. The length of the ileocaecal artery was 22 cm (range 19–28 cm), the longest branch was 30 cm (27–35 cm), and the second longest branch was 27 cm (24–29 cm). The distance from the ileocaecal region to the longest branch was 19 cm (15–20 cm).

In 12 post-mortem specimens, the same group constructed J-pouches so as to evaluate the potential gain in length after section of the longest branch of the superior mesenteric artery. Such division resulted in a gain in length of 2.5 cm (2–4 cm). Their third study assessed the relationship between the origin of the superior mesenteric artery and both the dentate line and the inferior margin of the symphysis pubis (Figure 5.23). This was studied in 25 eviscerated cadavers. The distance between the origin of the artery and the dentate line was found to be 33.7 cm (29–38 cm), whilst its distance from the symphysis pubis was 28.2 cm (24–36 cm). Importantly, there was a consistent discrepancy of 5.5 cm (2–8 cm) between the two.

A similar study was also performed in nine other post-mortem specimens in whom pouches were also constructed, giving corresponding values of 34.5 cm (28–36.5 cm) to the dentate line, and 31.2 cm (26–33 cm) to the inferior margin of the symphysis pubis; the mean discrepancy was 3.3 cm (2–5 cm). In this group, a J-pouch with 18-cm limbs was created and its overall length measured from the origin of the superior mesenteric artery. This was followed in the same group by construction of an S-pouch with 15-cm limbs and a 6-cm efferent limb. Finally, similar pouches and

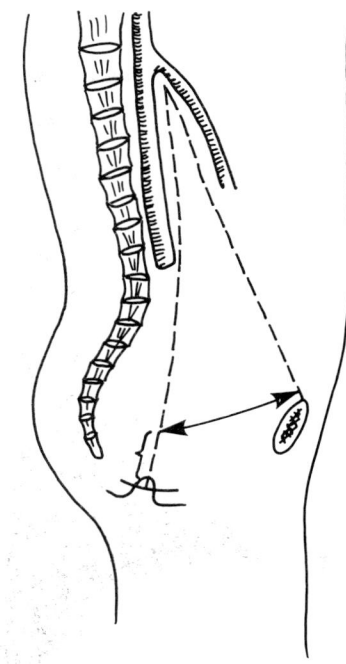

Figure 5.23

examinations were performed after resection of the last 20 cm of ileum. The S-pouches consistently reached a mean of 2.7 cm farther than the J-configurations; J-pouches reached a mean of 34.7 cm compared with 37.5 cm for the S-pouches. S-pouches reached 6.3 cm below the symphysis pubis compared with 3.6 cm for the J-pouches. After ileal resection, J-pouches reached a mean of 33.7 cm, and the S-pouches 35.7 cm. Therefore, if a 20-cm segment of terminal ileum has been resected, it will result in a mean loss in overall length of 1 cm for the J-pouch and 2 cm for the S-pouch.

Further experimental studies in cadavers have been performed in France (Cherqui *et al.*, 1987). In 13 cadavers, a right hemicolectomy was carried out after division of the ileal and caecal vessels flush with the caecum. The root of the mesentery was completely dissected. As in the previous study, the distances between the termination of the ileum and its most inferiorly reaching point, and between the antimesenteric border of this point and the inferior margin of the symphysis pubis, were recorded. The small bowel and its mesentery were then removed after division of the superior mesenteric artery at the lower border of the pancreas. Angiography was performed using a dilute solution of barium sulphate via a catheter in the superior mesenteric artery. Measurements of mesenteric length were made and angiograms were taken both before and after division of the ileocaecal artery. S-pouches of 15-cm limbs with a 3-cm distal efferent limb were created, and compared to J-pouches formed around the most inferior point of the ileum. The gain in length after vessel division was assessed in each case. In two cases the ileocaecal artery was spared, whilst the terminal branch of the superior mesenteric artery was divided at its point of greatest tension, as described by Utsunomiya (Utsunomiya *et al.*, 1980).

The most inferior reach of the ileum was 22.3 cm from the terminal ileum. In almost 50% of cases, this point reached between 1 and 2.5 cm distal to the inferior margin of the symphysis pubis. However, in the other half, it either reached exactly to this latter point or failed to reach it by some 1–2 cm. In all cases the limiting factor was tension in the superior mesenteric artery. Complete dissection of the root of the mesentery resulted in up to 1 cm gain in length in half of the specimens. There was no benefit in the other half.

Angiography revealed the terminal ileum to be supplied by terminal branches of both the ileocaecal and superior mesenteric arteries, which in all cases formed an arterial anastomotic loop. Clamping of either of these main vessels did not alter this vascularization. Importantly, however, in almost 40% of cases caecal vessels contributed markedly to the supply of the last few centimetres of the terminal ileum via recurrent branches. In 25% of studies, such recurrent vessels provided the sole supply to the terminal ileum.

Division of the ileocaecal artery resulted in movement of the most inferior portion of the ileum to within 18.5 cm (16–21 cm) of the terminal ileum. Irrespective of pouch design, such division resulted in an increase in distal reach (5.5 cm for S-pouches; 4.8 cm in J-pouches). In more than 80% of cases, this manoeuvre resulted in lengthening of 5 cm or more. In the two cases where the terminal superior mesenteric artery was divided, the mean extra reach was 4.5 cm. This resulted in the use of J-pouches with limb lengths of 21 and 22 cm respectively.

Clinical experience with methods to lengthen the mesenteric attachments to ileoanal reservoirs has been provided from the Lahey clinic (Burnstein *et al.*, 1987). In this series, 159 consecutive J-pouches were constructed and various techniques applied in order to generate satisfactory mesenteric length. The objective was to extend the inferior margin of the reservoir to 6 cm beyond the pubic symphysis. As they state, this level may occasionally be reached without recourse to further lengthening manoeuvres. However, in the majority of cases an additional 2–5 cm was required. Their method of lengthening consists of division of the terminal ileum flush with the caecum, and subsequent division of the mesentery immediately adjacent to the colonic wall. This method spares the ileocolic artery. All adhesions from the ligament of Treitz to the terminal ileum are released. Thereafter, the posterior attachments of the entire small bowel mesentery are mobilized, thus exposing the third part of the duodenum and the inferior portion of the head of the pancreas (Figure 5.24(b)).

A J-pouch was constructed with limbs of approximately 20 cm, however the apex of the pouch is chosen to be the most distal limit of the terminal ileum. Hence, the apex may be moved a few centimetres proximally or distally from the arbitrary 20-cm point. They note that distal shift is rarely required, so that limb length is usually between 20 and 25 cm. Serial incisions in the anterior and posterior aspects of the ileal mesentery along the superior mesenteric artery are said each to confer about 1 cm of additional length (Figure 5.24(d)). They are especially useful if a previous laparotomy has resulted in adhesions and mesenteric thickening. Subsequently, if mobilization is still inadequate, the mesentery is transilluminated. Traction on the mesentery allows identification of those vessels with greatest tension within the anastomotic loop between the ileocolic artery and the terminal branch of the superior mesenteric artery. These vessels are divided, usually providing an additional 2–5 cm of length (Figure 5.24(c)).

Rarely, in the experience of the Lahey clinic group, will further additional length be required. When it is, more proximal division of the superior mesenteric artery can be performed (Figure 5.24(a)). This should be proceeded by assessment of the adequacy of collateral flow by temporary occlusion of the

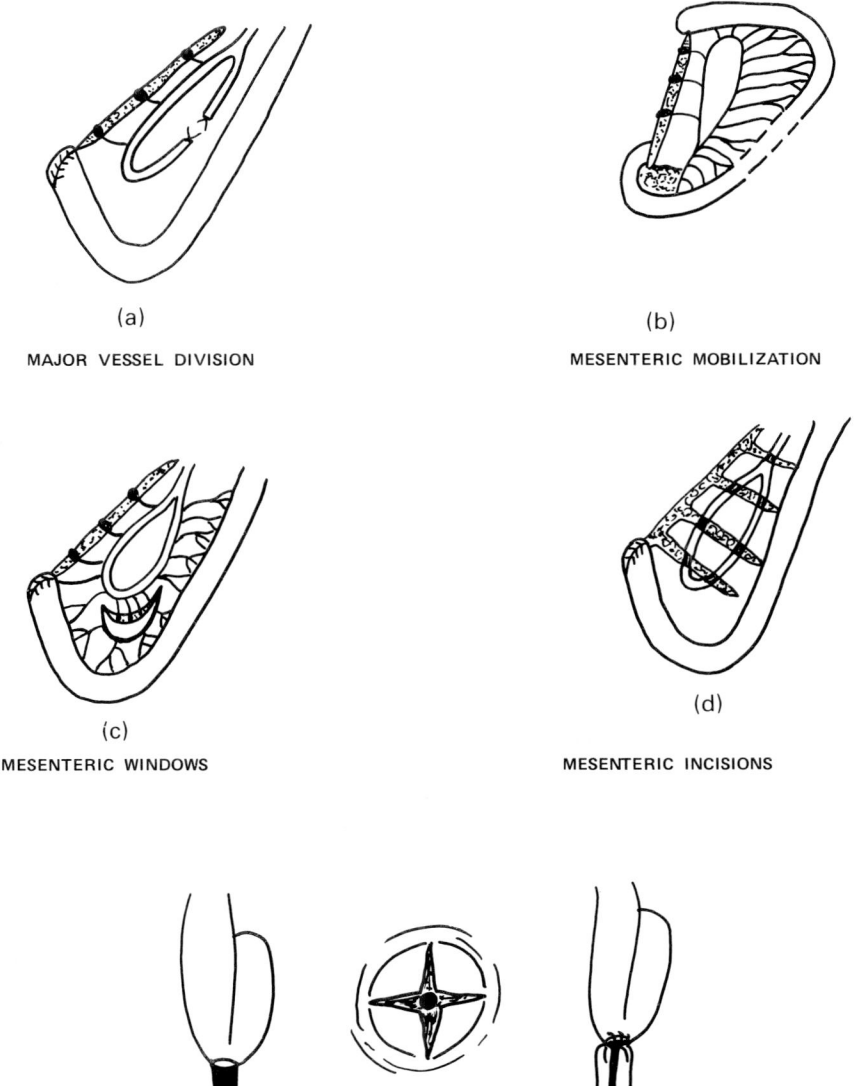

(a)

MAJOR VESSEL DIVISION

(b)

MESENTERIC MOBILIZATION

(c)

MESENTERIC WINDOWS

(d)

MESENTERIC INCISIONS

(e)

ANOPLASTY

Figure 5.24 Techniques used to gain length during IPAA

vessel and attention to pouch perfusion. Other techniques to reduce tension at the ileoanal anastomosis have been described, including anoplasty (Figure 5.24(e)). Microvascular reconstruction of a devascularized 'pouch', in the form of mesenteric vessel lengthening, has also been reported (Chick, Brown and Walton, 1988).

In conclusion, it would appear that the different designs of pouch constructed from terminal ileum depend, at least partly, upon different arterial configurations (Figure 5.25).

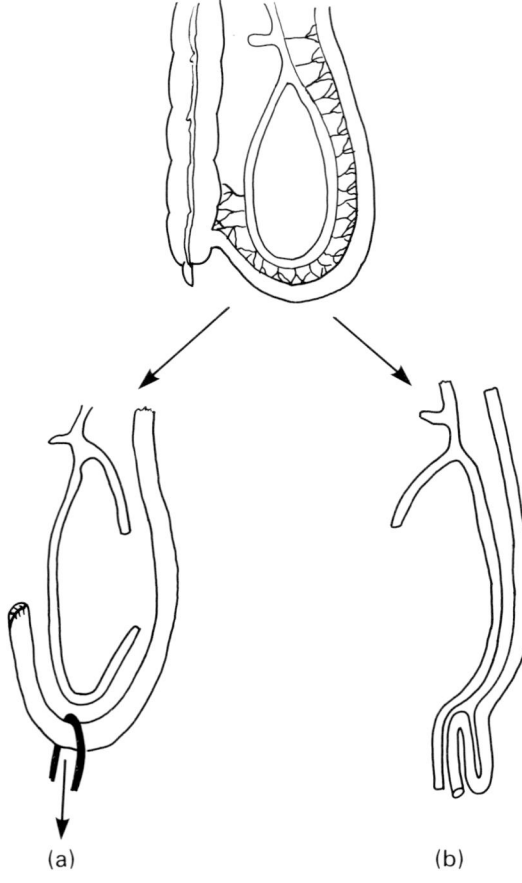

(a)   (b)

Figure 5.25

the apex of the pouch reaches 6 cm below the symphysis, it will always reach to the dentate line. Should the overlap be 4 cm, the pouch will reach in 50% of cases. This is reduced to one-third if there is only 2 cm of overlap. It is rarely necessary to divide more proximal vessels.

Angiography confirms constant anastomotic branches and a loop between the ileocaecal artery and the terminal branches of the superior mesenteric artery. One or other of these vessels can be divided safely, but should be test clamped prior to division. Recurrent ileal branches from the ileocaecal artery are more important than may have been first thought. It is therefore important to divide the ileal and caecal vessels as close as is possible to the bowel wall.

The mucosal proctectomy

The question of mucosal proctectomy and cancer is discussed in Chapter 14. Various techniques have been described for the stripping of rectal mucosa, including local hyperthermia (Ger *et al.*, 1986), chemical debridement (Kawarasaki, Fujiwara and Fonkalsrud, 1982; Kojima, Sanada and Fonkalsrud, 1982a), ultrasound fragmentation (Heimann *et al.*, 1985), and conventional surgical excision using various operative techniques.

There are three basic approaches to the performance of mucosal proctectomy (Figure 5.26). The stripping of the rectal mucosa can be performed from above in the abdomen, or from below via the perineum. From below, the mucosectomy can be performed either endoanally within the anal canal, or outwith that structure after eversion of the rectal stump.

Abdominal mucosal proctectomy (Figure 5.26(a))

At or just above the rectal peritoneal reflection, the anterior rectal wall is incised through its seromuscular layer with a scalpel or needle diathermy. A dilute solution of adrenaline (such as 1 in 200 000) is injected into the submucosal plane. This facilitates definition of this plane, easier dissection and aids in haemostasis. Using a mounted pledget, the mucosa is stripped away from the underlying muscular cylinder. Various methods have been

Duplicated J-pouches tend to be dependent upon the terminal branches of the superior mesenteric artery or the ileocaecal artery, depending on the longest loop of ileum. However, S-pouches rely mostly upon the ileocaecal artery. For any pouch design, the longest distal reach is obtained by transecting the ileum flush with the caecum. The extra few centimetres gained by this action are most likely to be lost, or at least unavailable to the surgeon, if the operation is performed in three stages.

Clearly, that the pouch will reach to the lower margin of the symphysis pubis is not a reliable indicator that it will reach to the dentate line. There is a consistent discrepancy between the two landmarks, with the distance to the dentate line always being the longer. If

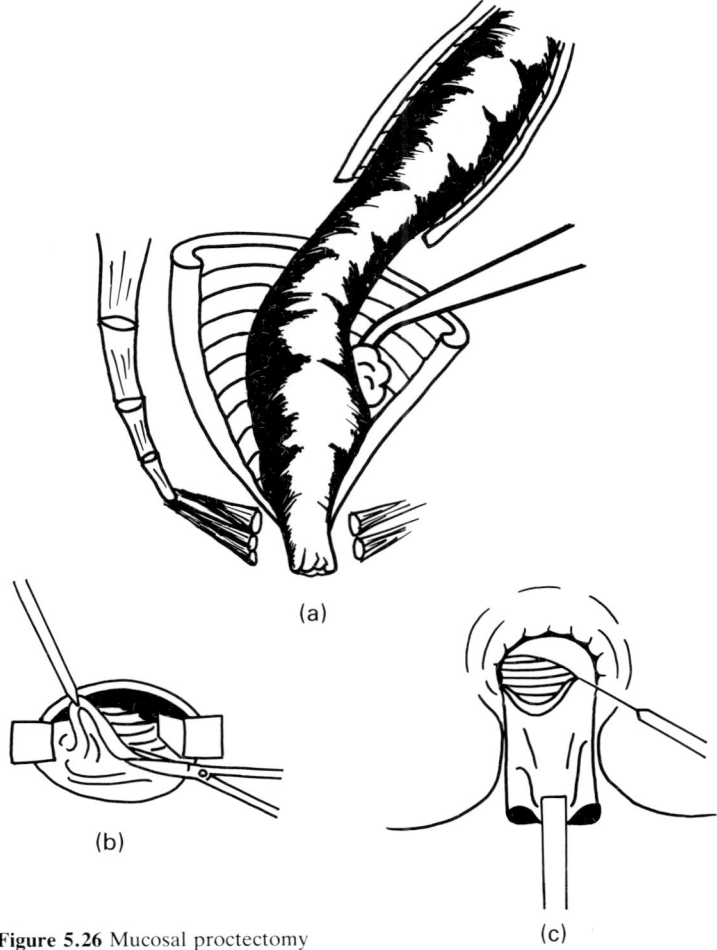

(a)

(b)

(c)

Figure 5.26 Mucosal proctectomy

described to provide stability to the mucosal tube during stripping. Utsunomiya has described the use of a balloon urinary catheter inserted per anum prior to either colectomy or mucosectomy. The catheter, with the balloon inflated, is advanced into the sigmoid colon, and a ligature is tied around the colon distal to the balloon. The catheter remains in place throughout the abdominal mucosectomy, and helps to prevent tearing of the mucosa during the procedure (Utsunomiya *et al.*, 1980).

Most surgeons utilizing an abdominal mucosectomy tend to add a perineal component to ensure complete stripping to the desired point (Utsunomiya *et al.*, 1980). Using this combined approach, Keighley (1987) reduced anal retraction time from 72 minutes

for a purely endoanal mucosectomy, to 18 minutes. In addition, cuff abscesses were avoided after abdominal mucosectomy, and resting anal pressure was maintained. In Keighley's experience, soiling was significantly more common after an endoanal procedure.

Endoanal mucosal proctectomy (Figure 5.26(b))

After preparation and draping, the anus is manually dilated with up to four fingers. We favour the use of the Parks' three-blade retractor, although many have reported the advantageous use of paired Gelpi retractors (Keighley, 1987). The latter avoid the use of intra-anal retraction, but may be associated with minor (and probably clinically insignificant) tearing of the anal skin.

Commencing at the dentate line (or 1–2 cm above depending upon preference), a dilute solution of adrenaline is again injected in the submucosal plane, in order to elevate this from the mucosa. An incision is made at the dentate line, and the plane opened up with sharp scissor dissection. Initially, it may be found useful to mark the dentate line around its full circumference with diathermy, as landmarks may become less obvious after commencement of mucosectomy. Due to the distal inflammation, the dissection is frequently bloody at this early stage. Bleeding points must be secured early and meticulously by diathermy. Any haematoma occurring between the rectal cuff and the pouch may be a cause of prolonged postoperative sepsis, and result in a poor functional outcome. Rotation of the Parks' retractor facilitates removal of the rectal mucosa as a confluent cylinder. This reduces the risk of leaving behind any islands of mucosa. Some surgeons excise the mucosa in sheets, but we feel that this may contribute to the retention of such islands.

Mucosal proctectomy after rectal eversion (Figure 5.26(c))

After preparing the rectum as for endoanal mucosectomy, a pair of tissue forceps is passed transanally and grasps the divided end of the rectum. Withdrawal of the forceps everts the rectal cuff. Commencing at the divided end, the submucosal plane is again infiltrated with dilute adrenaline solution. Progressing towards the anus, the now outer sleeve of mucosa is dissected from the submucosa. It is often possible to remove the mucosa as a confluent sheet. The dissection is stopped at the dentate line, and the denuded rectal stump, if necessary shortened to the required length, is replaced into the pelvis. Alternatively, the mucosectomy can be performed commencing at the dentate line and progressing to the divided edge of the rectal stump.

The ileoanal anastomosis

After construction of the pouch, its passage through to the perineum is required. There are several ways in which this can be facilitated.

The apex of the pouch can be grasped with tissue forceps, or can be pulled through to the perineum with stay sutures inserted into the pouch. Difficulty may be encountered in some patients, and various technical modifications have been described to facilitate the pull-through. Included amongst these have been the enterotractor (Barraza, 1988), a polythene sleeve inserted per anum (Rabinovici and Krausz, 1988). We often insert a de Pezzer catheter into the apex of the J-pouch, holding it in place with four sutures (Thomas and Taylor, 1990). However the pull-through is performed, it is extremely important to avoid twisting of, or tension on, the pouch.

If the pouch has been constructed without an apical enterotomy, this must first be created. Either a simple slit, a cruciate incision, or excision of a small ellipse have all been performed. Most surgeons create the enterotomy prior to inserting any ileoanal sutures. However, it may aid the procedure to insert four quadrant anchoring sutures between the anal canal and the pouch, so that the enterotomy can be made between these sutures. We perform a hand-sewn anastomosis using interrupted absorbable sutures (such as 2/0 Vicryl). A series of 10–15 sutures is usually required. Full thickness bites of the pouch are taken from within out, followed by taking a deep bite of the internal sphincter and the anal mucosa from its deep surface out to the anal canal. Initially, it is often easier to insert sutures in each of the four quadrants in order to aid with orientation. Special instruments have been described for such endoanal procedures, such as those invented by the late Sir Alan Parks, and the so-called 'fish-hook' needle (Glass and Mann, 1988).

Utsunomiya has described his method for obviating the need for anal retraction. He inserts six or so traction sutures between the perianal skin and the skin of the anal verge. These open up the anal canal and facilitate pouch–anal anastomosis (Figure 5.27).

As with the pouch itself, numerous surgeons have described the use of stapling instruments to facilitate the ileoanal anastomosis (Heald and Allen, 1986; Hughes, Bauer and Bauer, 1988; Brough and Schofield, 1989; Kmiot and Keighley, 1989b; Williams, 1989). Varying methodologies have been described for these anastomoses. Briefly, surgeons have performed a hand-sewn pouch construction, using

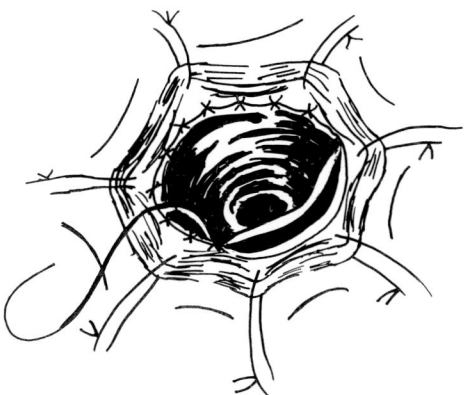

Figure 5.27 Anal canal retraction (after Utsunomiya)

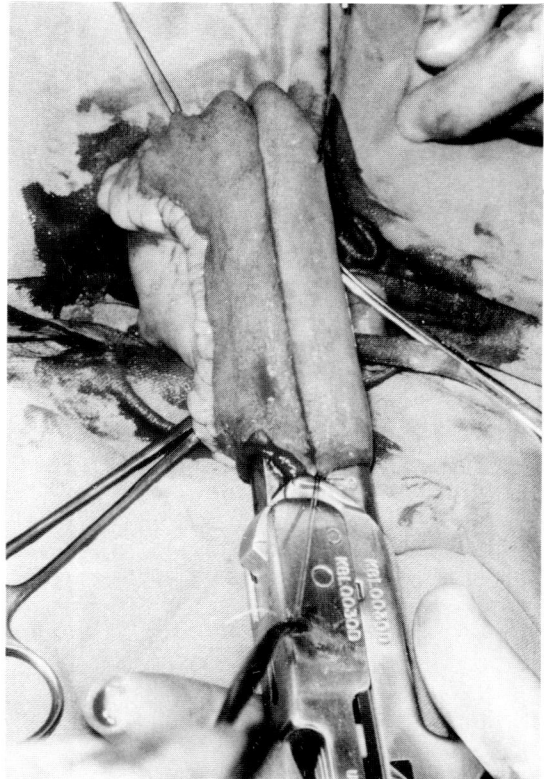

Figure 5.28 Stapled construction of a J-pouch

a circular stapling gun for the ileoanal anastomosis. Others perform a totally stapled procedure (Kmiot and Keighley, 1989b) (Figures 5.28, 5.29). A stapled ileoanal anastomosis also may be performed after a conventional mucosal proctectomy (Brough and Schofield, 1989). Alternatively, a mucosal proctectomy may not be deemed necessary, and a stapled anastomosis performed at the anorectal ring (Kmiot and Keighley, 1989b). A standard purse-string suture may be inserted into the denuded rectal stump. This may be performed from above, or from below. From below, it can be performed endoanally, or after rectal eversion (Brough and Schofield, 1989).

Alternatively, the new Premium E.E.A. circular stapling gun can be used to avoid the need for a purse-string (Kmiot and Keighley, 1989b; Williams, 1989). In the latter case, a transverse stapling gun is used to transect the rectum. The new Roticulator gun may also be useful for this manoeuvre. The shaft of the circular stapling gun is passed per anum through the closed rectal stump and into the pelvis. This can be performed either through the previously created staple line, or away from it. The shaft is then passed into the lumen of the pouch, where it is attached to the head of the gun (Figure 5.29). Closure of the gun approximates the pouch and rectal stump, and firing completes the ileoanal anastomosis.

Hughes and his colleagues have described a novel way of using a circular stapling gun to aid both mucosectomy and ileoanal anastomosis. A transverse stapling instrument was used to

transect the rectal cuff. An E.E.A. stapling instrument is then inserted per anum, and a purse-string suture applied around the rectal cuff and stapling gun. The gun is then gently retracted from the anus, thus everting the rectum and facilitating mucosectomy. After excision of excess rectal cuff, the latter was again purse-stringed over the gun, which was readvanced into the rectum. The J-pouch was manoeuvred over the anvil of the gun, and the anastomosis performed (Hughes, Bauer and Bauer, 1988).

Heald has described a method of performing the entire pelvic pouch procedure from within the abdomen (Heald and Allen, 1986). The key to Heald's technique is to mobilize the rectum down to the anorectal ring, extending even within the upper limit of the external sphincter (Figure 5.30). Strong upward traction on the rectum will draw at least part of the anal canal mucosa out of the anal canal.

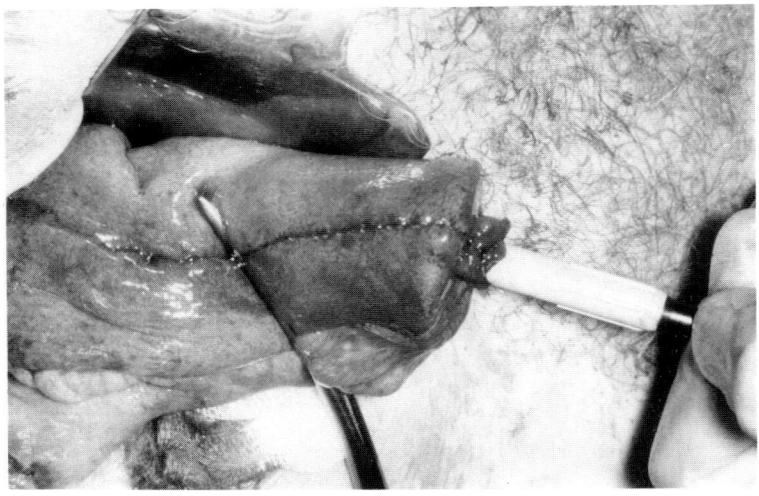

Figure 5.29 Stapled ileoanal anastomosis using the Premium E.E.A. stapling gun

Transverse division of the rectum at the level of the superior margin of the external sphincter will result in some degree of anal mucosectomy. A circular stapling gun is used for pouch–anal anastomosis, and hence approximately 1 cm more of anal canal lining will be resected. Consequently, the final ileoanal staple line should be very close to, if not at, the dentate line.

Drains

As in other major surgical techniques, particularly those within the field of colorectal surgery, the necessity for the use of drains will remain one of personal preference. Similarly, the type of drain utilized in such circumstances will vary between surgeons. Those which have been popular after pouch–anal anastomosis are depicted in Figure 5.31. In addition to these standard forms of drain, both a full length intestinal tube (Thow, 1985), and an intraluminal anastomosis bypass tube have been reported after pouch–anal anastomosis (Sackier and Wood, 1988).

The loop ileostomy

The temporary ileostomy used by most surgeons in performing the ileal pouch proce-

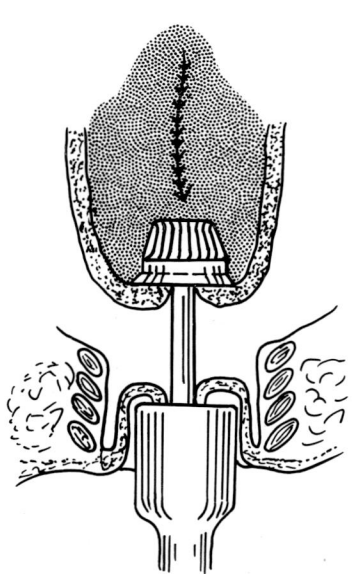

Figure 5.30

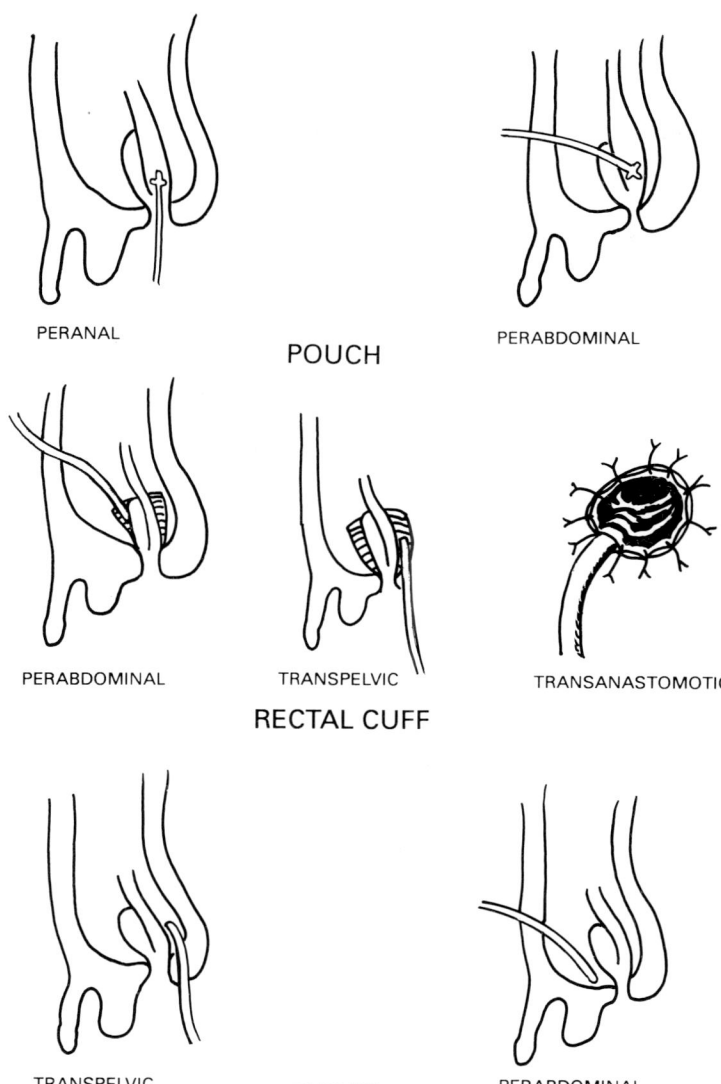

PERANAL POUCH PERABDOMINAL

PERABDOMINAL TRANSPELVIC TRANSANASTOMOTIC

RECTAL CUFF

TRANSPELVIC PELVIS PERABDOMINAL

Figure 5.31 Drains used in pouch construction

dure is the Turnbull asymmetrical loop ileostomy (Figure 5.32). Initially, the loop ileostomy had a poor reputation because of unreliable appliance fitting. Turnbull described the modification of protruding the proximal end, whilst making the inactive end flush with the skin; this represented a useful advance. Prior to closure of the abdomen after pouch–anal anastomosis, the ileum proximal to the pouch is assessed for the optimal site for the proposed ileostomy. This site must be relatively free from tension when brought through the ileostomy trephine. For metabolic reasons, it has been suggested that the most distal segment of ileum as is practicable should be used (see Chapter 13). The proximal portion of the proposed ileostomy should be marked prior to closure of the abdomen. We place a marker tie around a tissue forceps placed proximally. Another, unmarked, tissue

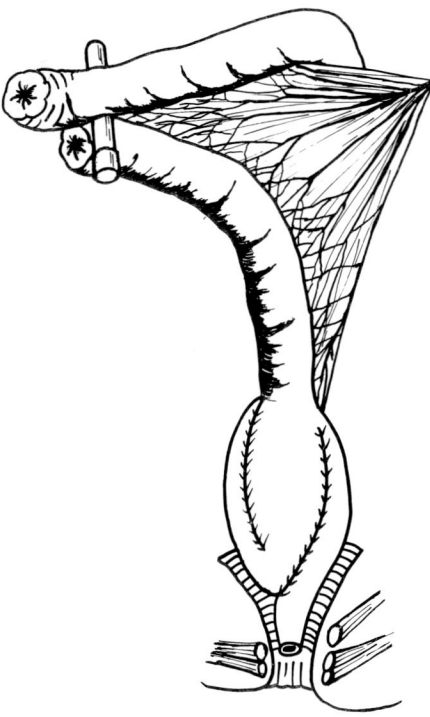

Figure 5.32 Loop ileostomy

forceps is placed distally. A skin trephine is made at the site determined preoperatively for the ileostomy. After extension of the trephine through the abdominal wall, the proximal end of the chosen ileal segment is grasped from without the abdomen, via the trephine, by the marked forceps. Similarly, the unmarked forceps are placed distally. This placement helps to prevent twisting of the ileum during closure of the abdomen. After dressing of the abdominal wound the ileostomy is fashioned, ensuring that the proximal limb is as prominent as is possible. The efferent limb is sutured flush with the skin. We tend to favour the use of a rodless technique for ileostomy formation, and have occasionally fashioned a modified 'split' stoma as described by Prasad (Prasad *et al.*, 1984).

All early reports of the ileoanal anastomosis, particularly when some form of capacitance reservoir was added to the procedure, described the utilization of a temporary loop ileostomy as a means of providing faecal diversion. Whilst it is well accepted that this

would not prevent anastomotic dehiscence, it is likely that any clinical effects of such an eventuality might be minimized. Hence, many surgeons embarking upon this form of therapy have incorporated loop ileostomy into their technique of restorative proctocolectomy. However, not all advocate such diversion. Several surgeons have reported the occasional omission of a diversionary ileostomy (Metcalf, Dozois, Kelly *et al.*, 1986; Brough and Schofield, 1989; Galandiuk, Wolff, Dozois *et al.*, 1990b); others have reported that this is now their usual practice (Thow, 1985; Matikainen, Santavirta and Hiltunen, 1990). It is worth analysing the merits of such a practice.

The Mayo clinic group have emphasized the importance of a meticulous technique, both in the construction and in the closure of these stomas (Metcalf *et al.*, 1986a). In their group of 180 patients who had undergone restorative proctocolectomy, 157 patients had been given a loop ileostomy, whilst 23 had received a Brooke ileostomy. Complications related to faulty technique occurred in 18% of the loop and 13% of the Brooke ileostomies. Peristomal irritation was twice as common in the loop ileostomy group (54% versus 26% respectively).

The commonest technical complication was retraction, often resulting in incomplete diversion of ileal effluent. This is associated with the passage of flatus and/or liquid faeces per anum. Such incomplete diversion is associated with a 44% incidence of pouch–anal anastomosis complications, compared to 14% if diversion is complete. This group also described that 13 cases of intestinal obstruction occurred in these patients prior to closure of the ileostomy. Twelve of these occurred in patients with loop ileostomies (seven due to lateral space herniation, three due to stomal retraction and two due to adhesions). One case of adhesive obstruction resulted from a Brooke ileostomy. Furthermore, 10 loop ileostomies required revision or closure at a date earlier than had been planned previously, whilst none of the Brooke-type stomas required such modification.

After closure of these stomas, small intestinal obstruction occurred in 13% of cases, whilst peritonitis was witnessed in 7% and wound infection in 1%. Interestingly, once the stoma has been taken down, there ceases to be any difference in the incidence of postoperative complications. The causes of peritonitis were anastomotic leaks, and tears sited either proximal or distal to the closure site itself.

Further evidence of the complication rate associated with the temporary loop ileostomy has come from Feinberg and colleagues. In a 4-year period they performed 117 pelvic pouch procedures. In 41 of these patients a previous subtotal colectomy with Brooke ileostomy formation had been carried out. In these patients the same stoma site was utilized for the loop ileostomy (Feinberg, McLeod and Cohen, 1987). Throughout this series, 59% of patients developed a complication attributable to their ileostomy. Excluding patients who developed either cholelithiasis or renal stones, 20% became dehydrated at some stage after ileostomy construction, 15% had some form of skin breakdown around the stoma, and 11% developed intestinal obstruction. Subsequently, 110 patients had their loop ileostomy closed, 15% of whom developed small intestinal obstruction. These workers concluded that obstruction was less likely to occur if the stoma was formally resected and a stapled anastomosis performed. A further 3% each suffered either an anastomotic leak or a wound infection. Others have reported highly satisfactory results with simple transverse suture closure of the loop ileostomy (van de Pavoordt *et al.*, 1987).

Various technical modifications, including a rodless technique (Prasad *et al.*, 1984), and one utilizing a Penrose drain through the mesentery to prevent loop retraction (Krausz, 1988), have been described. It is likely that such attention to detail, adopting modifications where necessary, will improve the functional results of the loop ileostomy.

Postoperative care

Postoperative care after pelvic pouch construction follows the format for any other major procedure in which a low pelvic anastomosis has been performed. Prophylaxis against deep venous thrombosis is essential. The authors use pneumoflators in the perioperative period. Careful observations of vital signs are continued throughout the postoperative course with 4-hourly recordings being made for 48 hours. Checks of haemoglobin and electrolyte concentrations are made, and abnormalities

are corrected when necessary. It is our practice to remove the urinary catheter after 3–5 days. If retained, the pouch catheter is removed after 5 days or so. At this time the anastomosis is examined digitally. In those uncomplicated cases where a pouch catheter was not retained, no such formal examination is undertaken in the early postoperative period. Other surgeons have reported the routine examination of all their pouch–anal anastomoses after 1 week (Williams and Johnston, 1985).

Patients are given instruction in the management of their temporary stoma. Changes of appliance type are not infrequent, depending upon the configuration of the stoma, and the patient's ability and preference. The loop ileostomy usually functions on or about the third postoperative day, and a light diet is allowed after the fifth postoperative day. We have found that a blood-stained mucous anal discharge is common in the early postoperative period. Patients are usually discharged from hospital after 12 days, after which a mucous discharge may persist. We encourage patients to perform anal sphincter exercises in the postoperative period, often accompanying this with manometric evaluation as a form of biofeedback (see Chapter 6).

Several surgeons advocate intubation of the distal limb of the loop ileostomy, allowing for irrigation of the defunctioned reservoir. This also encourages patients to retain intraluminal contents. During consultations with the stomatherapist, advice is given with regard to diet. This is an important facet of after-care (Faller, Welling and Lambert, 1986; Raymond and Becker, 1986). In particular, those foods which might thicken the ileostomy effluent (such as rice and bananas) are encouraged. Patients are advised that food should be chewed very well, that they should drink plenty of fluid every day, and admonished that they should avoid excessive weight gains.

Patients are reviewed routinely in the outpatient clinic after 1 month or earlier if necessary, when particular emphasis is placed upon the loop ileostomy. The patients' haemoglobin and electrolyte status are checked. A gentle examination is made of the ileoanal anastomosis. A degree of stenosis is not uncommon at this stage, and responds well to gentle digital dilatation, which can be performed in the outpatient clinic. Further review is made at 3–4 months postoperatively, when the pouch is again assessed digitally. Should all be well, endoscopic examination is usually performed at this stage and a defaecating cinepouchogram is performed, allowing for assessment of anastomosis integrity and initial pouch function (see Chapter 12). If there are no leaks, the loop ileostomy is closed, a procedure which should be associated with minimal morbidity (Lewis and Bartolo, 1990).

In the immediate postclosure period, patients are encouraged to hold onto their stools for as long as possible. Anal sphincter exercises are similarly to be encouraged. Patients may return to work as soon as they feel able, and we recommend early return whenever possible. Anecdotally, we feel that this may encourage the process of deferment of defaecation and improved function.

Perianal skin care is extremely important after closure of the ileostomy. When circumstances permit, patients should wash the perianal region after each evacuation. Soaps are best avoided; warm water is satisfactory. The area must be kept dry at all times. With this in mind, and should early postoperative leakage occur, cotton wool balls may be placed within the anal canal. With such conservative methods the vast majority of patients will maintain a healthy perineum. In more severe cases, a water-repellant based cream may be used to advantage. Others have recommended the occasional use of antifungal agents (Hanson, 1990). However, we have no personal experience with the application of such preparations to the perineum.

It is of vital importance that patients should have easy access to the surgical team and/or stomatherapist, so that problems can be assessed early. Frequently, these will be of a psychological nature, especially a lack of confidence. Therefore, the clinical attendants must demonstrate marked enthusiasm for this procedure, so that patient motivation can be maintained to a high level.

6

Clinical experience with the ileal pelvic pouch

The clinical series reported in the literature are illustrated in Table 6.1. These reports document the outcomes of approximately 3000 cases of restorative proctocolectomy. These series have been collated to provide an overall review of the clinical experience with ileal pouch—anal anastomosis.

Indications for surgery

A full discussion of the indications for restorative proctocolectomy was given in the previous chapter. Overall, 87.5% of the pouch procedures reported in the above series have been performed for ulcerative colitis. This figure includes all the cases of inflammatory bowel disease for which this procedure has been performed. Most series report an incidence of indeterminate colitis of between 3% and 8%. Of those patients thought to have ulcerative colitis peroperatively, again most series report a re-evaluation of the diagnosis to that of Crohn's disease in approximately 3% of cases. Approximately 12% of operations have been performed for colonic polyposis syndromes; the vast majority of these being familial adenomatous polyposis. Occasional reports of non-adenomatous polyposis coli requiring colectomy and pouch construction have been reported (Sene *et al.*, 1989). As already stated, most series include only a minority of polyposis patients. The series of Utsunomiya however differs in that 62% of the pouches which he has constructed have been for adenomatous polyposis, which reflects his practice at the Polyposis Centre at the Tokyo Medical and Dental University.

The miscellaneous indications for colectomy in the remaining 0.5% of cases include

Table 6.1 Reported clinical series on experience with the ileal pelvic pouch

Bodzin *et al.*, 1987
Bubrick, Jacobs and Levy, 1985
Chaussade *et al.*, 1989a
Damgaard and Kirkegaard, 1990
Davidson and Thornton-Holmes, 1990
Dozois *et al.*, 1989
Everett and Forty, 1989
Fleshman *et al.*, 1988a
Fonkalsrud, Stelzner and McDonald, 1988b
Harms *et al.*, 1987
Hatakeyama, Yamai and Muto, 1989
Hill, 1987
Keighley, Yoshioka and Kmiot, 1988
Keller, Salky and Gelernt, 1989
McGowan, Postier and Williams, 1987
Nicholls, 1990
Oresland *et al.*, 1989
Pescatori, Mattana and Castagneto, 1988
Ribotta *et al.*, 1988
Saeger *et al.*, 1985
Schoetz, Coller and Veidenheimer, 1986
Skarsgard *et al.*, 1989
Slors, Taat and Brummelkamp, 1990
Smith and Sircus, 1987
Thomas and Taylor, 1990a
Utsunomiya *et al.*, 1988
Wexner *et al.*, 1990
Williams *et al.*, 1989b

intractable constipation (Nicholls and Kamm, 1988; Pescatori, Mattana and Castagneto, 1988), and megarectum after previous colectomy and ileorectal anastomosis for constipation (Keighley, Yoshioka and Kmiot, 1988; Hosie, Kmiot and Keighley, 1990).

Age and sex

As is to be expected, the sex distribution of patients undergoing restorative proctocolectomy is approximately equal. Overall, some 53% of all reported patients are males, with 47% being females. Taking account of the reported mean ages, and the number of patients in each series, the overall mean age at which pelvic pouches have been constructed is approximately 28.3 years (range for mean ages 23–34 years). The reported age ranges for patients undergoing pouch construction are from 7 to almost 70 years. As stated elsewhere, many would not now have an upper age limit for pouch construction, accepting that the patient's anal sphincter function and 'physiological age' are perhaps of greater importance.

Pouch construction

In the series listed above, 55% of the pouches constructed were of the duplicated J-configuration. Figures for the other pouch designs were 25% for the triplicated S-pouch; 12% for the quadruple W-pouch; and 8% for the lateral reservoir.

Complications occurring after pouch construction

Creditably, the mortality after pouch–anal anastomosis has been extremely low throughout its history. Taking all the reported series, the operative mortality is approximately 0.5%. The majority of such mortalities have been caused by metastatic spread from previously present colorectal malignancies (see Chapter 14). In addition, adrenal insufficiency, pelvic sepsis, massive pulmonary embolus, abdominal sepsis after ileostomy closure, and perforated steroid-induced gastric ulcer have each been reported as the cause of isolated postoperative deaths.

The major complications of pouch construction are depicted diagrammatically in Figure 6.1. Where necessary, these will now be considered independently.

Complications related to the pelvic dissection

Autonomic dysfunction

Proctocolectomy with permanent ileostomy formation for colitis and colonic polyposis is associated with few complications, is reproducible in the hands of the majority of general surgeons and, perhaps most importantly, it is trusted by these workers. However, proctocolectomy is well recognized to be associated with certain complications, including a persistent perineal sinus. In addition, autonomic dysfunction may occur, resulting in impotence and bladder dysfunction (Neal, Parker and Williams, 1982). It is likely that rectal dissection at the time of the proctectomy is predominant in the aetiology of such complications, however by keeping the rectal dissection close to the rectal wall, damage to the autonomic nerve supply to the pelvis should be avoided.

In a prospective study of mucosal proctectomy and ileoanal anastomosis, both with and without formation of an ileal reservoir, evidence of pelvic nerve damage was sought (Neal, Williams and Johnston, 1982). In this study 33 patients were investigated by questionnaire both before and after mucosal proctectomy, two-thirds of them also underwent cystometry and measurement of urethral closing pressure. Six patients had undergone mucosal proctectomy alone, whilst 21 patients had an ileoanal anastomosis, in 11 of which a reservoir was also constructed. Six patients had a caecoanal anastomosis with poor results due to a recurrence of their colitis, often necessitating further surgery. They were therefore eliminated from the series. At cystometry, numerous parameters were assessed, including residual volume, maximum bladder capacity, bladder compliance, detrusor contraction pressure and maximum flow rate. Both the clinical and urodynamic assessments failed to demonstrate either sexual or bladder impairment after mucosal proctectomy, and similar but less detailed results have been described by others (Parks, Nicholls and Belliveau, 1980).

Many other series have documented that there is an infrequent occurrence of at most only very transient urinary or sexual complications postoperatively. Urinary complications such as a slight reduction in urinary stream are recorded in less than 5% of patients, usually males. Autonomic sexual complications are similarly reported in approximately 5% of males (Skarsgard *et al.*, 1989; Wexner *et al.*, 1990).

Complications related to the rectal cuff

Cuff abscess

In a study to assess possible aetiological factors in the development of cuff abscesses, 20 mostly duplicated reservoirs were described. Half of these patients had separation of the ileoanal anastomosis with development of a cuff abscess. Ten patients had uncomplicated procedures (Lindquist, Nilsell and Liljequist, 1987). It was found that the major determinant of cuff abscess was the presence of severe colitis, especially if it was associated with a difficult mucosal proctectomy.

Efferent cuff length from the pouch was also positively correlated with this complication. Indeed, no cuff abscesses were seen in patients with short efferent limbs from S-pouches, or who had J-pouches.

The use of a loop ileostomy relieves the symptoms of ileoanal anastomosis dehiscence, but does not offer any protection against this occurrence. Four out of ten patients who had intact colons developed cuff abscesses, compared with four of the ten patients who had previously undergone a subtotal colectomy. Of these ten anastomotic dehiscences, only one healed by secondary intention. In the others, recourse was made to further operative intervention.

Over the last decade the vast majority of surgeons with experience of this procedure have shortened their rectal cuffs. Indeed, some have abandoned the use of them altogether (see Chapter 5).

Carcinoma of the rectal cuff

Rectal cuff carcinoma has been recently reported in a patient who had undergone restorative proctocolectomy with a 10–12 cm rectal cuff 4 years prior to presentation of the

malignancy (Cohen, 1989; Stern *et al.*, 1990). This neoplasm presumably originated within retained mucosa after mucosectomy. It is perhaps surprising after more than a decade of experience with this procedure that the complication of malignancy developing within the retained cuff of rectum has not become a more recognized complication. Clearly, surgeons must be vigilant in the pursuit of this complication.

Complications related to the pouch

Pouch leak

Leakage from the ileal reservoir itself is generally uncommon, with an incidence of less than 5%. Such leaks may present as either abdominal sepsis or as an enterocutaneous fistula. Whilst pouch excision may ultimately be required in such circumstances, we would err on the cautious side, hoping that the fistula may spontaneously close. To ensure that there is no distal obstruction, we would perform a contrast study, and place a catheter into the pouch per anum. This has been successful in our one case of enterocutaneous fistula, which occurred after pouch damage during mobilization as part of the performance of 'pouchopexy' (Thomas *et al.*, 1990).

Pouch haemorrhage

Haemorrhage from the ileal pouch is uncommon after pouch construction. We ourselves have not witnessed this complication. Most patients with this complication have required laparotomy to stop the bleeding, but pouches can be generally salvaged.

Pouch necrosis

Fortunately, pouch necrosis is a rare complication of restorative proctocolectomy. Whilst many surgeons have not witnessed this complication, others have seen it in up to 4% of their cases (Pescatori, Mattana and Castagneto, 1988). Pouch excision has often been required in such circumstances.

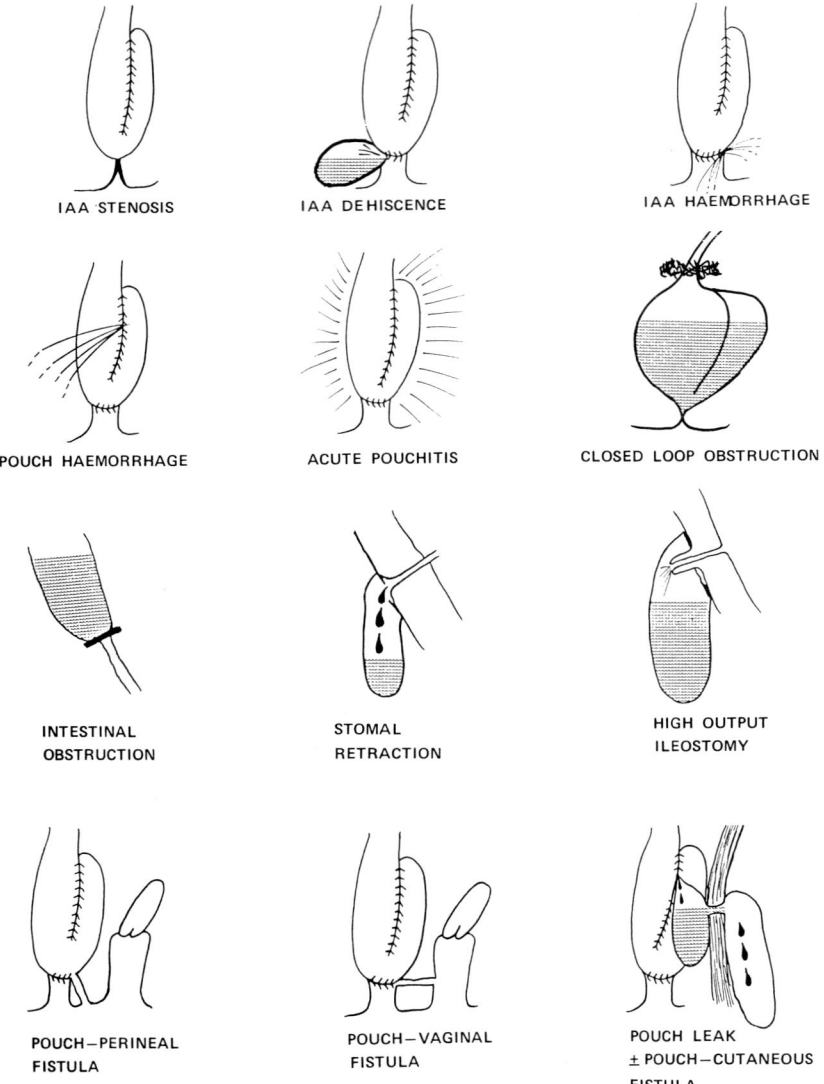

IAA STENOSIS

IAA DEHISCENCE

IAA HAEMORRHAGE

POUCH HAEMORRHAGE

ACUTE POUCHITIS

CLOSED LOOP OBSTRUCTION

INTESTINAL OBSTRUCTION

STOMAL RETRACTION

HIGH OUTPUT ILEOSTOMY

POUCH—PERINEAL FISTULA

POUCH—VAGINAL FISTULA

POUCH LEAK ± POUCH—CUTANEOUS FISTULA

Figure 6.1 Complications of ileal pouch formation

Pouchitis (see Chapter 9)

Superior mesenteric artery syndrome (see Chapter 5)

Closed loop obstruction

We have witnessed one case of closed loop obstruction of a pelvic pouch (Thomas, Hobbis and Taylor, 1990). This female patient had a generally uncomplicated postoperative course, except for numerous repeated episodes of poor pouch function, diarrhoea, severe abdominal pain, and electrolyte disturbances. Periods of pouch catheterization partially relieved the symptoms, but the pouch rarely functioned satisfactorily. Metronidazole was of no benefit. A cinepouchogram revealed a grossly dilated pouch, with virtually no retrograde filling of the afferent limb. At laparotomy, extremely

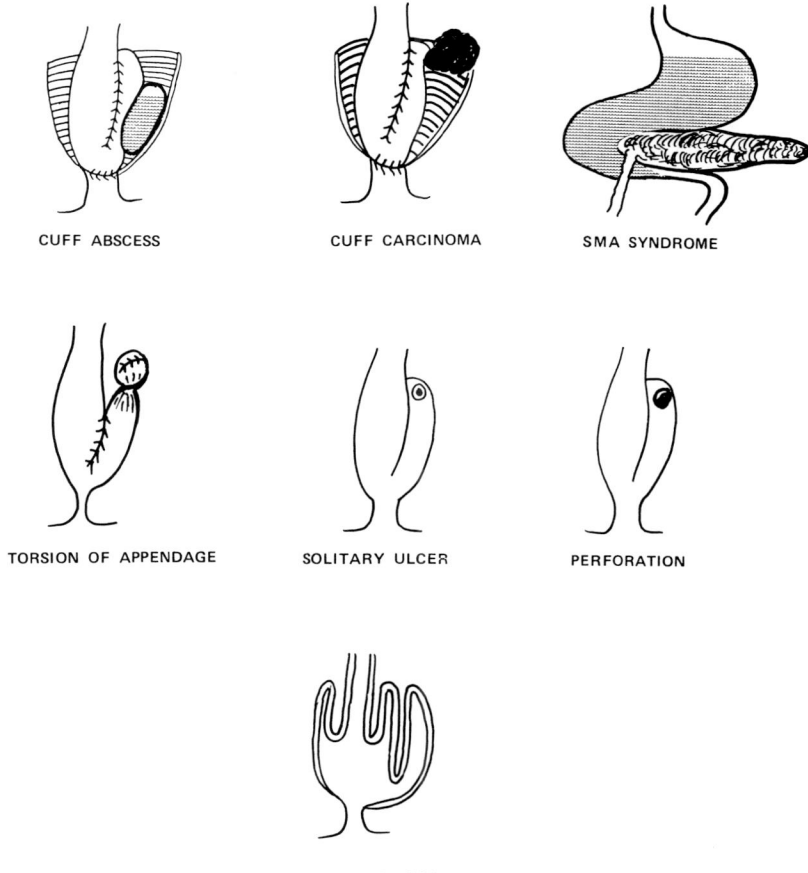

CUFF ABSCESS   CUFF CARCINOMA   SMA SYNDROME

TORSION OF APPENDAGE   SOLITARY ULCER   PERFORATION

AFFERENT LOOP
INTUSSUSCEPTION

Figure 6.1 Complications of ileal pouch formation (*Continued*)

dense adhesions were found around the pouch, which was grossly inflamed on its serosal aspect. Surprisingly, the proximal small intestine was collapsed and empty. It was thought that the diagnosis was likely to be Crohn's disease, and the pouch was excised. Subsequent histological examination demonstrated gross chronic inflammatory changes, but no specific evidence of Crohn's disease.

In this case, it appeared that the afferent limb of the pouch was partially obstructed, presumably by an adhesion. However, proximal bowel contents were generally able to pass this obstruction, which acted like a valve. The patient's efficient anal sphincter mechanism converted the pouch into a closed loop.

Complications related to the ileoanal anastomosis

Anastomic leakage and pelvic sepsis

Pelvic sepsis is a feared complication of the pouch–anal anastomosis. It has been reported as the most significant prognostic factor influencing the ultimate functional outcome after restorative proctocolectomy (Keighley *et al.*, 1989). Others have found it to be of less importance (Pemberton *et al.*, 1987). Almost all recent clinical series have documented an incidence of some degree of anastomotic dehiscence of between 1% (Wexner *et al.*, 1990) and 8% (Skarsgard *et al.*, 1989). Perhaps surprisingly, there would appear to be little evidence that an increased incidence of leakage is associated with an increased frequency of emergency procedures, or with the performance of more complicated reservoir designs.

This complication decreases with increasing surgical experience, as many early reports of this procedure documented incidences of up to 20% (Dozois *et al.*, 1986). The Mayo clinic group has reported that pelvic sepsis is more common in those patients who are underweight, or are suffering with malignancy or systemic toxicity preoperatively. Surprisingly, sepsis appears to be more serious in female patients (Scott *et al.*, 1988b).

Consistently, it has been shown that patients with ulcerative colitis form the major group in which pelvic sepsis occurs. Indeed, it has been shown that patients with polyposis rarely suffer with problems related to poor anastomatic healing (Scott *et al.*, 1988b). The use of long-term corticosteroids is not thought to be the causal factor in this increased incidence in colitics. It is more likely that the severe pelvic disease itself is the aetiological agent in this complication. Similarly, the use of prophylactic antibiotics does not appear to mitigate the effects of poor anastomotic healing.

Most reports document that some 50% of patients suffering a degree of anastomotic leak will require further surgery. In the majority, the loop ileostomy is retained, allowing for a period of time to elapse for the anastomosis to heal and for any pelvic sepsis to subside. Widening of the anastomotic defect allowing for free drainage may also be required. Should the anastomosis be found to heal, the ileostomy is then closed once again. Fleshman and colleagues have reported their favourable experience with the use of the technique of endoanal advancement of the pouch outlet with resuturing of the ileoanal anastomosis. Fifty per cent of such patients had their pouches salvaged, with satisfactory long-term functional results (Fleshman *et al.*, 1988b). The experience of most workers is that a very significant proportion of patients requiring further abdominal surgery for sepsis, perhaps up to 50%, will ultimately require excision of their reservoirs.

What factors can be taken into account in order to potentially avoid this complication? As stated above, many of the factors which might have proved to be important will often have little effect on the severity of pelvic sepsis. Clearly, surgical technique must be meticulous. Should there be any doubt regarding a stapled anastomosis, a loop ileostomy must be employed. Acceptable results can be obtained in selected patients after both a hand-sewn pouch and ileoanal anastomosis without recourse to temporary ileostomy formation (Everett and Pollard, 1990). However, most surgeons performing a hand-sewn ileoanal anastomosis would continue to utilize loop ileostomy in all circumstances. Adequate bowel preparation, rectal irrigation prior to laparotomy, early exclusion of the rectosigmoid, irrigation of the terminal ileum prior to pouch construction and irrigation of the efferent limb of the loop ileostomy at completion of the operation have all been advocated. At the time of writing, the potential benefits individually attributable to these manoeuvres is unclear. However, once cleared, it appears that pelvic sepsis no longer effects ultimate functional outcome adversely.

Anastomotic haemorrhage

Bleeding from the ileoanal anastomosis has been reported less frequently than the previous complication. Less than 5% of patients will develop this complication, but most will require endoanal suture of the suture line.

Anastomotic stricture

Anastomotic strictures are reported with varying incidences after pouch–anal anastomosis. To some degree, incidences varying between 5% (Pemberton *et al.*, 1987) and 22% (Skarsgard *et al.*, 1989) may be dependent upon different definitions of what constitutes this complication.

We have found a minor degree of stenosis to be extremely common during the defunctioned period. Most of these respond to digital dilatation in the outpatient department. Of our patients, approximately one-quarter have required further dilatation at the time of ileostomy closure. Only 6% of our patients have had recurrent problems with anastomotic strictures; none have required treatment other than intermittent dilatation. We have not felt that these patients' symptoms have warranted the performance of anoplasty.

Others have reported the use of instrumentation as the preferred method of treatment for anastomatic strictures. Caution must be voiced, as small bowel perforation has been reported after the use of this technique (Skarsgard *et al.*, 1989). It is important to exclude Crohn's disease as a cause for the stenosis. Occasionally, formal revision of the ileoanal anastomosis may be required, and again it is important that a diverting ileostomy is used to cover this.

Pouch–vaginal fistula

Since the first description of pouch–vaginal fistula after pouch–anal anastomosis in 1985, it has been recognized as a relatively uncommon, but often very difficult to manage complication. Most series document only occasional isolated fistulas (Wong, Rothenberger and Goldberg, 1985; Thomas and Taylor, 1990). As any one surgeon has but a limited experience of this complication, therapeutic strategies have been difficult to formulate. In order to provide such a consensus, a multicentre assessment of this complication has been undertaken (Wexner *et al.*, 1989b). Eleven colorectal practices throughout North America provided information regarding pouch–vaginal fistula; its aetiology and its management.

In this series, 304 pelvic pouch procedures had been performed in female patients. In this group 21 patients developed 22 pouch–vaginal fistulas, resulting in an overall incidence of this complication of 6.9%. Five other patients with such fistulas were incorporated into this study, being secondary referrals from the institution at which their pouch had been constructed. Of these 26 patients, 88.5% had ulcerative colitis, 7.5% had 'indeterminate colitis', and 4% had familial adenomatous polyposis. Therefore, it would appear that patients with inflammatory bowel disease (96%) are probably slightly more predisposed to fistula formation. Twenty-two of the patients had never undergone any previous anorectal surgery. One patient had undergone formal closed haemorrhoidectomy just 2 weeks prior to pouch construction.

Five patients had previously undergone a midline episiotomy; four of which had been performed within a year of ileoanal anastomosis. Thirty-eight per cent of patients had undergone an urgent or emergency subtotal colectomy; 16% had undergone a routine subtotal colectomy, and 46% underwent pouch construction at the same time as colectomy. Of the latter, half were elective procedures, 42% were urgent, and 8% were emergency procedures. Regarding pouch design, 46% were S-pouches, 50% were J-pouches or modifications thereof, and 4% were of the lateral configuration. Eighty-five per cent of patients had had a temporary loop ileostomy constructed, and 88% had pelvic drainage. One further patient had drainage of the rectal cuff.

Only 20% of patients had intraoperative complications, 80% of which were tension at the ileoanal anastomosis (16% overall). Seventeen complications ensued postoperatively: cuff abscess (five), pelvic abscess (three), partial anastomotic dehiscence (one), ileoanal stenosis (two), and other miscellaneous complications (six). Only 8% of fistulas failed to present clinically, and were discovered on routine pouchography. Thirty per cent presented prior to ileostomy closure. Only 12% of patients were subsequently shown to have Crohn's disease. Two of the cuff abscesses were converted to pouch–vaginal fistulas iatrogenically. In addition, drainage of both a 'Bartholin cyst' and a low vaginal abscess resulted in the development of a fistula.

Thirteen forms of treatment were utilized in this cohort of 27 fistulas. Seven of these involved local treatment, and six involved more aggressive non-local treatment (Figure 6.2). One patient had conservative medical treatment only. In total, these 26 patients with 27 pouch–vaginal fistulas underwent 73 surgical procedures. Pouch excision (Figure 6.2(l)) was ultimately required in five patients.

Of the local treatments, sphincteroplasty (Figure 6.2(g)) and endoanal ileal flap advancement (Figure 6.2(e)) were the most successful when performed as the sole procedure (cure rates of 75% and 60% respectively). Closure via either the transanal or transvaginal routes (Figure 6.2(a)) were moderately successful (29% and 27% respectively). Of note, debridement and fistulectomy was rarely successful (6%) (Figure 6.2(b)). This has certainly been our experience after five attempts at fistulectomy and primary closure in two patients, both of whom now have permanent ileostomies. High fistulas have successfully been closed transabdominally (Figure 6.2(c)). Several other techniques were used in isolated

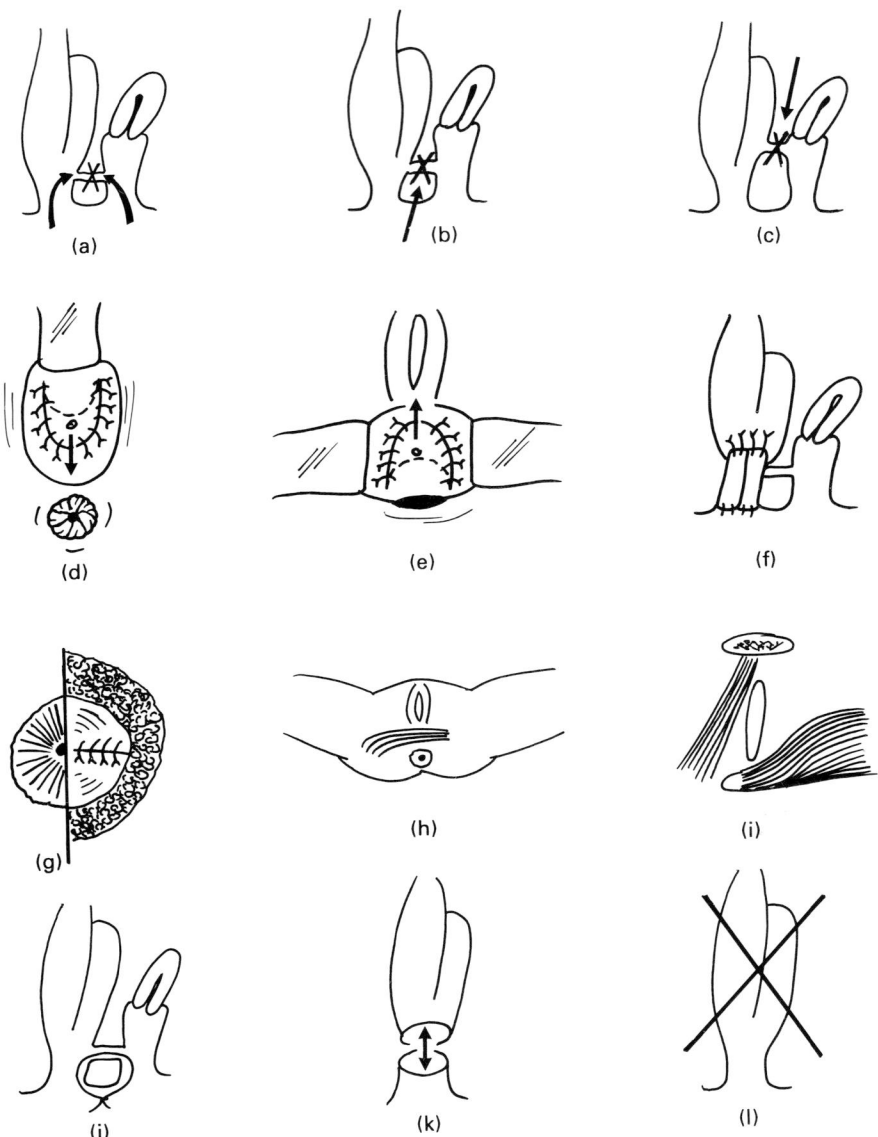

Figure 6.2 Techniques employed in the treatment of pouch–vaginal fistula

instances including the use of a seton (Figure 6.2(j)) (two cases, none successful). Keighley has previously reported the successful use of a Prolene seton in the management of pouch–vaginal fistula (Keighley, Yoshioka and Kmiot, 1988). The gracilis flap (Figure 6.2(h)) was also performed (four cases, two successful), and has been advocated by others (Gorenstein, Boyd and Ross, 1988). In addition use was made of the bulbocavernosus flap (Figure 6.2(i)) (one successful case), and complete pouch reconstruction (Figure 6.2(k)) (one successful case). Others have reported the use of techniques such as anoplasty (Figure 6.2(f)) and transvaginal mucosal flap advancement (Figure 6.2(d)) in the management of this troublesome postoperative complication.

Clearly, such a collection of procedures, each of which was performed in small numbers, precludes statistical analysis. However, this is the largest collection of such fistulas reported in the literature, and its importance lies in its highlighting certain relevant points. First, it appears that pelvic sepsis is an important aetiological factor in the pathogenesis of pouch–vaginal fistulas. This sepsis need not be clinically apparent. Most of these patients have severe proctitis preoperatively, irrespective of whether a preliminary colectomy has been performed. This is a factor known to predispose to postoperative pelvic infection. Secondly, whilst in the male pelvis sepsis may 'point' and drain via the bowel lumen or occasionally into the perineum, in the female the postoperative rectovaginal septum will frequently offer the path of least resistance to such septic collection. In particular, prior weakening of this structure by recent surgery, including midline episiotomy, may further encourage this route to be taken. Technically, the placement of deep sutures during the performance of the anterior section of ileoanal anastomosis must add to the risk of subsequent fistula development.

In any patient presenting with a pouch–vaginal fistula after pouch–anal anastomosis, it is important to exclude Crohn's disease. In those few cases in whom a temporary loop ileostomy had not been performed, intestinal diversion should be provided. Thereafter, if pelvic sepsis can be demonstrated, it should be treated on its own merits. A period of observation of between 4 and 6 months prior to any surgical treatment is to be generally recommended. Thereafter, local treatment should be performed, and it would appear that either sphincteroplasty or endoanal ileal flap advancement are the most efficacious procedures. Should they be unsuccessful, a more aggressive line of management may be required, such as pouch reconstruction or use of the gracilis flap. Ultimately recourse may have to be made to pouch excision in the certain knowledge that this should result in resolution of the fistula.

Pouch–perineal fistula

Fistulas have also been reported between the pouch and perineum, most notably the vulva (Wexner *et al.*, 1989b). The aetiological factors discussed in the above section will obviously be relevant to this complication. Such fistulas-in-ano are treated in a manner analogous to those fistulas not related to previous pouch construction. In the majority of cases simple laying open of the fistula or other local procedures, such as sphincteroplasty, will be successful.

Small intestinal obstruction

Occurring in between 8% and 20% of patients, small intestinal obstruction is the commonest complication in the early postoperative period. Approximately half of these will require a further laparotomy. Some two-thirds of small bowel obstructions requiring surgery will be related to the temporary ileostomy, due to complications such as stenosis, volvulus and parastomal hernia. The remaining third of obstructive problems arise from miscellaneous complications; mostly adhesive obstruction due to a band or volvulus.

Assessing their 17% of patients who developed small bowel obstruction, the Mayo clinic group found that 44% of this group required laparotomy (Francois *et al.*, 1989). Perhaps surprisingly, they found that the presence of a Brooke ileostomy was significantly more likely to be associated with obstruction. Of their patients with such a stoma, 12.5% became obstructed. This compared with 4.6% of their patients with Turnbull loop ileostomies. Numerous other factors, such as age, sex, diagnosis, method of stoma closure, or reservoir type, proved not to be significant. However, a previous subtotal colectomy was associated with an 8.5% incidence of obstruction, compared with only 2.2% in patients who had not undergone previous colectomy.

In the authors' own series, 17% of patients developed small intestinal obstruction. Of these, four underwent laparotomy, three of whom had adhesive obstructions; the other had a volvulus of a loop ileostomy.

Complications related to the loop ileostomy (see Chapter 5)

The commonest complication attributable to the temporary ileostomy is small intestinal obstruction (see above). Other complications such as stomal retraction and stenosis may occur. In the authors' experience these have not usually required formal revision. Frequently, the ileoanal anastomosis will be satisfactory, and the ileostomy can be closed.

Two of our patients have had an excessive ileostomy output in the defunctioned period. We have used various dietary and medical manipulations in these patients, including a somatostatin analogue, but these have met with little success. It is our experience, and that of others, that early closure of the loop ileostomy usually results in a satisfactory outcome in these patients.

Other gastrointestinal complications

Other gastrointestinal complications have ensued after pouch–anal anastomosis, including acute pancreatitis, acute cholecystitis, gastrointestinal haemorrhage, and hepatitis. Gastrointestinal haemorrhage has not been witnessed in the authors' own series, but has been recorded in up to 5% of some other series (Wexner *et al.*, 1990). The majority of these cases involve bleeding from the pouch itself, from the ileoanal anastomosis, or from the site of ileostomy closure. Occasional reports of bleeding duodenal ulcer have been reported.

General complications

After restorative proctocolectomy, nonspecific general complications occur with incidences similar to other major colorectal procedures. As would be expected, complications such as wound infection, urinary retention, chest infection, deep venous thrombosis, pulmonary embolus and myocardial infarction, etc. have all been reported. In addition, we have had a case of transient peroneal nerve palsy. Others have had similar experience (Skarsgard *et al.*, 1989). Wexner has reported brachial palsy. It must be re-emphasized that restorative proctocolectomy is often a prolonged procedure for both surgeon and patient, though the author has performed the whole operation in 90 minutes. Hence, it is important that the patient's pressure points are protected.

Other complications sporadically described include: alopecia (Thompson, 1989), optic atrophy, toxic psychosis (Nicholls and Pezim, 1985), pelviureteric junction obstruction (Taylor, 1987), epididymitis, parotitis (Wexner *et al.*, 1990), and adrenal insufficiency (Fonkalsrud, Stelzner and McDonald, 1988; Thomas and Taylor, 1990; Wexner *et al.*, 1990). Both

our patient, and that of Fonkalsrud, succumbed from this latter complication which occurred some 1 year post operation.

Complications occurring after ileostomy closure

Small intestinal obstruction

After closure of the temporary loop ileostomy, the commonest complication remains small intestinal obstruction. The majority of these are related to adhesions, but it should be remembered that anywhere between the site of closure and the pouch outlet might now be the site of small bowel obstruction. Indeed, stenosis at the site of ileostomy closure, ileal stenosis proximal to the pouch, and stenosis at the ileoanal anastomosis have all been recorded (Francois *et al.*, 1989). Overall, 15% of patients will develop intestinal obstruction after closure of the ileostomy. However, values vary between 6% and 27%. The experience of most surgeons is that approximately half of these patients will require further laparotomy. The importance of exercising meticulous care in the closure of the loop ileostomy cannot be overemphasized. If the stoma is oedematous or fibrosed it should be resected and a two-layer end-to-end anastomosis performed.

Miscellaneous ileostomy closure-associated complications

Other complications which have been reported secondary to the ileoileostomy closure include leakage (2–10%), and on rare occasions bleeding.

Complications related to the pouch

Pouchitis

The subject of clinical pouchitis is discussed fully in Chapter 9. In the reported series, symptomatic pouchitis occurs in between 10% and 30% of patients; overall, the incidence is approximately 15%. The severity and/or frequency of the attacks of pouchitis may necessitate reconstruction of the ileostomy or delay in its closure in some 10% of cases. In less than 5% of the pouchitis group, recourse has had to be made to pouch excision.

Recurrent polyps

The topic of colonic polyposis has been dealt with in Chapter 3. As yet, there are very few reports of recurrent polyps after pelvic pouch construction (Sene *et al.*, 1989). However, further long-term follow-up is very likely to reveal a higher incidence of this phenomenon. Such recurrences have been noted at a straight ileoanal anastomosis (Myrhoj, Bulow and Mogensen, 1989), in a continent ileostomy (Stryker, Carney and Dozois, 1987), and at a permanent Brooke ileostomy after colectomy for familial adenomatous polyposis (Primrose, Quirke and Johnston, 1988). Indeed, in the latter report, an adenocarcinoma was present in one of the polyps. Other benign tubular polyps in this patient had only arisen in areas of colonic metaplasia. As discussed in Chapter 8, colonic metaplasia is extremely common in ileal pelvic reservoirs. It is therefore likely that such recurrent polyps will appear as time progresses, and that they must have a definite, but probably small, malignant potential. This has obvious implications for the follow-up of such patients.

Miscellaneous mechanical complications (Figure 6.1)

Keighley's group have reported the complication of intussusception of the afferent limb into the reservoir itself (Kmiot and Keighley, 1989a). A J-pouch was constructed with a stapled ileoanal anastomosis which was not under tension, and an ileostomy was not utilized. Between the fourth and sixth postoperative days, the patient developed progressively worsening lower abdominal pain. Contrast examination revealed a filling defect within the pouch suggesting an intussusception. An attempt at hydrostatic reduction was unsuccessful. Laparotomy was performed, at which time the pouch was found to be ischaemic and so was excised. Histologically, the afferent limb was ischaemic with venous thrombosis. However, the pouch was otherwise normal, and the point is made that it may have been more appropriate to resect the ischaemic afferent limb and restore continuity by enteroenterostomy.

A clinical syndrome indistinguishable from pouchitis has been reported as a consequence of a solitary ulcer occurring in a J-pouch (Francheschi, Chen and Yuh Jen-Nan, 1986). Lower abdominal pain, diarrhoea and rectal bleeding developed 18 months after stapled construction of the pouch. Endoscopic evaluation revealed an ulcer of the antimesenteric border of the pouch at the junction of the afferent limb with the terminal ileum. There was no evidence of pouchitis. Biopsy of the ulcer showed acute inflammatory changes. The ulcer healed after prolonged antimicrobial treatment, which the authors considered to be probably unnecessary. They suggest that the ulcer was probably due to subnecrotizing ischaemia occurring at the staple line, and so healed spontaneously.

During construction of the duplicated J-pouch, the most terminal closed segment of the terminal ileum is anastomosed to the proximal small intestine. The Mayo clinic group have reported two cases in which, by using a 15-cm linear stapling gun to construct a pouch with limbs slightly longer than 15 cm, this terminal segment is not incorporated into the pouch. It was originally thought that this short isolated distal segment was of little consequence. However, in the cases presented, torsion of these segments occurred, resulting in ischaemia and perforation. Hence, this group now recommends amputation of this appendage (Pezim *et al.*, 1987).

In all patients who present with abdominal trauma, and have undergone pouch construction, it must be remembered that they have within their pelvis a large, somewhat tethered, hollow viscus. The susceptibility or otherwise of this neorectum to blunt external trauma remains unclear, but is probably low. However, traumatic perforation of a J-pouch has been reported (Tzu-Chi Hsu, 1989), in a colitic who presented with severe abdominal pain 24 hours after blunt abdominal trauma. A J-pouch had been constructed 1 year previously. At laparotomy, a perforation was found at the junction of the afferent limb with the pouch. Debridement and primary closure was performed, and a catheter passed per anum to allow for pouch decompression. Recovery was uneventful.

Several important points should be made with regard to ileal pouch injury. First, it is well recognized that distended hollow viscera, such as the urinary bladder, are more prone to blunt external trauma. It could be envisaged that a distended pelvic pouch might be similarly predisposed. In addition, the stretching of the superior mesenteric artery involved in providing adequate length for the ileoanal anastomosis, may make the pouch more susceptible to trauma. Should the pouch wall be breached the bacterial overgrowth associated with reservoir construction may result in a severe peritonitis. There is at present no evidence that an inflamed reservoir is more likely to be damaged by such trauma.

Functional results of the pelvic pouch procedure

Collating the above series, it is obvious that the functional performance of the ileoanal reservoir is generally extremely satisfactory. Of the patients with J- and W-pouches, evacuation is always spontaneous. It is well recognized that the presence of an efferent limb is associated with some necessity to catheterize the pouch (see Chapter 5). Overall, some 80% of S-pouches evacuate spontaneously, so long as short efferent limbs are utilized.

The ability of the patient to defer defaecation varies considerably. No doubt personal confidence and social circumstances have a bearing on this aspect of function. However, most series that comment on this ability report that approximately 50% of patients will be able to defer defaecation for up to 1 hour 1 year after closure of the loop ileostomy. The corresponding figure during the first 6 months or so is less optimistic, with less than a quarter of patients being able to defer. As with the ability to defer, that of fluid/flatus discrimination is also somewhat tempered by other factors. Consequently, there is often a considerable range of ability quoted in the literature. Virtually all reported series document that the ability to discriminate increases significantly during the first year after ileostomy closure. Whether this is due to learning through practice, to growth of afferent nerves across the ileoanal anastomosis, or just due to increasing confidence is at present unclear. Certainly, in the authors' series, in most patients we could elicit a 'neorectoanal' inhibitory reflex. The rectoanal inhibitory reflex, and its possible implications for function, are discussed in Chapter 7. It is our experience

that, even when able, patients frequently do not utilize this ability as a routine, preferring to err on the side of safety. As with our experience, overall about 80% of patients have some discriminatory ability after 1 year.

Approximately 30% of patients have been documented as requiring adjustments in their diets. In the vast majority of cases, this adjustment is of a very minor nature. Our experience is that, rather than altering dietary content, patients more often alter the timing of their meals. In particular, some of our patients have reported the avoidance of meals within a few hours of retiring to bed. Most series document that up to one-third of patients require regular antidiarrhoeal medication. This figure tends to decrease a little as time progresses. Bulk-forming agents appear to be used more frequently over a more prolonged period than do the opiate-derived constipating agents.

Perhaps the major reason for the general decline in the requirement for medications is that most series report that stool consistency improves dramatically during the first year. By this time, up to 80% of patients will be passing a semi-, or even fully formed motion.

During the first few months after ileostomy closure, patients will usually evacuate their pouch between six and twelve times per 24 hours. Of these, between one and five evacuations may occur at night. After the first year, frequency has usually fallen to five or so motions per 24 hours (usual range for any one series is approximately three to eight motions per 24 hours). Of these, up to two nocturnal evacuations may be necessary.

It is heartening that most functional parameters improve during the first postoperative year. In particular, peranal leakage often improves dramatically during this period. It is our experience that, at least initially, most patients suffer some degree of leakage. Within a few weeks this has ceased in a small proportion of patients. This leaves a cohort of some 50–60% of patients who have to wear pads during the day. This is generally in concordance with the reported literature. By 12 months or so approximately half of these patients will no longer require pads as a routine. It should be stressed that the wearing of pads does not in itself imply a functional problem. We have several patients who no longer require pads as a routine, and are frequently without daytime leakage, but who continue to feel safer by using such pads. Approximately 40–50% of patients in reported series do leak initially at some time on most days. Within the first year, this figure will often have reduced to only 10% of patients. Most reports state that up to one-third of patients are likely to continue having some degree of regular nocturnal leakage after 1 year. This is frequently of a minor nature, amounting to little more than spotting. In a small subgroup of patients, perhaps 5%, peranal leakage only occurs during the passage of flatus. In the rest, leakage may occur irrespective of the passage of flatus. Many groups report that up to 75% of their patients are completely continent during the day after 1 year. Nocturnal continence is similarly complete in 50% of patients.

Quality of life after restorative proctocolectomy

As discussed in the opening chapter, the 'gold standard' against which any innovation in the surgery of ulcerative colitis must be compared is the panproctocolectomy and formation of a permanent Brooke everted end-ileostomy. This operation consistently gives good results, with relatively few complications. Patients tolerate the procedure well, and most soon accept their stoma. However, the creation of such a permanent faecal diversion is not ideal, as witnessed by the numerous attempts to avoid such surgery. It is without doubt the ileoanal pouch procedure results in the avoidance of a permanent abdominal stoma in the vast majority of patients so treated. What needs to be answered is whether it gives these patients a better standard of life compared to their fellow colitics with Brooke ileostomies.

Assessments of the effects of these procedures upon the lifestyles of their recipients is of undoubted importance. In particular, procedures such as the permanent ileostomy, potentially seen as mutilating to the patient, must be fully assessed. Where new alternatives to these procedures are devised, it becomes of even greater importance that the effects of each is documented. Where each is shown to be of similar surgical efficacy, variations in their performance with regard to the patient's quality of life might help to determine the procedure of choice for any particular patient.

As discussed in Chapter 1, both the conventional and the continent ileostomies are associated with acceptable lifestyles.

Anecdotally, most workers reporting their experience with pouch–anal anastomosis state that their patients prefer their pouch to their ileostomy. This has certainly been the case in the authors' series. However, this is not altogether a fair comparison. In the vast majority of these patients, a Turnbull asymmetric loop ileostomy has been utilized. Many workers have documented that this technique may be associated with more postoperative problems than the Brooke technique (see Chapter 5). Difficulties with appliance fitting, stomal retraction and skin excoriation are seen more frequently after loop ileostomy construction. Consequently, the direct comparison of the loop ileostomy with pouch construction is not completely valid.

Comparing their patients with permanent Brooke ileostomies with 298 patients after pouch–anal anastomosis, Pemberton *et al.* applied statistical logistic regression analysis to assess differences between these two procedures (Pemberton *et al.*, 1989). In the permanent stoma group, the procedure was performed for colitis or polyposis in 57% of patients, whilst Crohn's disease was the indication in 35%. Miscellaneous indications made up the other 8%. Pouch–anal anastomosis was performed for colitis and polyposis in 99% of patients, of whom 89% were colitics. To exclude elements of bias, only patients in whom permanent ileostomy formation had been performed for colitis or polyposis were included. This provided a population of 406 patients, of whom 95% were colitics. Detailed questionnaires were used in both groups to determine whether any lifestyle changes occurred postoperatively. To exclude bias, postal surveys were performed. Where direct telephone communication had to be performed, a nurse clerk was used. Numerous activity categories were assessed, including social activity, sexual activity, sport, housework, family relationships, general recreation and travel. The patients scored each category on a scale of 1 (severely restricted) to 5 (improvement).

Both operations provided comparably satisfactory lifestyles in their recipients. Ninety-five per cent of pouch patients reported overall satisfaction, compared with 93% of patients with permanent stomas. The extent of dietary restrictions, and numbers of patients returning to work or school were similar in both groups. Attitudes to both of these procedures were also assessed. Approximately 60% of both groups felt that their attitude had improved, whereas in approximately 5% of both sets of patients, the attitude had deteriorated. Thirty-five per cent or so of both groups had an unchanged attitude to their operations. Some 69% of the Brooke ileostomy patients were aware of an alternative to their permanent stoma. Of these, 6% definitely wanted to change their stoma, whereas one-third would change but were otherwise satisfied. Sixty per cent did not favour any alternative to their permanent stoma.

Of the pouch patients, 96% desired no change, whereas 3% desired a change back to their ileostomy but were generally satisfied. One per cent of this group stated that they definitely wanted to revert back to a permanent stoma. In this series, the reoperation rate after permanent ileostomy was approximately double that after pouch construction. Stoma-related complications were the major indications for such further surgery. In addition, persistent perineal wounds accounted for significant morbidity in the former group.

More than 10% of the Brooke ileostomy patients had to empty their bags during the night. This, at least to some degree, negates the criticism of pouch construction that nocturnal evacuation is often necessary. In addition, the number of daily evacuations in the pouch group was very similar to the frequency of bag emptying in the Brooke stoma group. Hence, both procedures result in comparable disruptions to the patients' daily activities.

Cohen *et al.* have used the methods of the Time Trade-off Technique and Direct Questioning of Objectives to assess patients' quality of life after various operations for ulcerative colitis (Cohen, McLeod, Lock *et al.*, 1989). A research assistant questioned patients who were divided into two groups. The first group consisted of patients who were studied preoperatively, and again 12 months postoperatively. In this group of 21 patients, six conventional ileostomies, one continent ileostomy, and 12 ileoanal pouches were constructed. In the 94 patients in group two, patients were assessed at least 1 year postoperatively (mean follow-up 5.2 years). Thirty

conventional ileostomies, 28 continent ileostomies, and 36 pelvic pouches were constructed.

Using both analytical techniques, the quality of life assessment was significantly improved following colectomy, irrespective of the procedure performed. Comparing the three operative procedures, no difference was discernible between any of the three using either analytical technique.

A questionnaire survey has also been used to assess the quality of life status after pouch–anal anastomosis in a series of 75 patients (Skarsgard *et al.*, 1989). A detailed study of occupational, social and sexual function after pouch construction, which was usually of the triplicated form, was carried out. Interestingly, more than 80% of these patients had previously undergone colectomy with rectal stump preservation. All patients had a temporary loop ileostomy.

Written questionnaires were completed during the first 3 months after closure of the ileostomy. At a variable time thereafter (15 ± 11 months), a reassessment was performed by questionnaire. Ninety-four per cent of the patients with a functional pouch felt that their surgery had been worthwhile, and was preferable to their loop ileostomy. In addition, 92% stated that they would be prepared to undergo the procedure again, should it prove to be necessary.

Can we predict the ultimate outcome after restorative proctocolectomy?

Several studies have attempted to find correlations between functional outcomes after restorative proctocolectomy and various clinically definable parameters (Pemberton *et al.*, 1987; Keighley *et al.*, 1989). Whilst several factors have been found to correlate with functional outcome, most of these relate to operative or postoperative factors. Pre-operative predictors of function have been less easy to define.

Pemberton *et al.* (1987) found that older patients evacuated their pouches more frequently during the day than younger patients at more than 2 years postoperatively. However, neither incontinence nor nocturnal frequency were affected by age. Neither sex nor postoperative bowel obstruction correlated with frequency. Postoperative frequency was not found to be correlated with the ultimate development of pouchitis of pouch failure. As would be expected, excessive frequency was associated with postoperative incontinence. In particular, excessive frequency prior to pouch construction was a significant predictor of postoperative incontinence.

In a multivariate analysis of the effects of 14 variables on functional outcome after pouch construction, Keighley found that the patient's age had little adverse effect on function. Similarly, a previous colectomy appeared to be unimportant with regard to ultimate outcome. However, functional outcome was adversely affected by the presence of pelvic sepsis, and by the performance of an endoanal mucosal proctectomy. Failure of the procedure (defined as either the necessity to intubate, reconstruction of an ileostomy, or pouch excision) was also associated with pelvic sepsis and endoanal mucosectomy. In addition, failure was also correlated with a long rectal cuff and the early learning curve of the procedure. Pemberton, however, did not find pelvic sepsis to be a significant predictor of pouch failure.

As discussed in Chapter 12, anorectal physiological assessments prior to ileostomy closure can aid in the prediction of ultimate outcome (Scott *et al.*, 1989). In particular, anal canal resting pressure and pouch compliance significantly affected outcome at 1 year after ileostomy closure.

Can we improve function after restorative proctocolectomy?

Biofeedback is a form of behavioural modification, which is utilized to train a patient to gain control over a specific bodily function. Using some form of instrumentation to demonstrate the success of a particular action, it uses such techniques to reinforce the function in question. It therefore differs from classical Pavlovian conditioning, in which a specific stimulus becomes associated with a function, and hence can be used to stimulate it.

Faecal incontinence is usually secondary to some organic neuromuscular condition. Sensory disturbances of continence are predominantly neurological in aetiology, whereas motor disabilities may be either neurological or muscular in origin. Both forms of incontinence have been successfully treated by biofeedback therapy. Indeed, biofeedback has been described as the treatment of choice for conditions associated with impairment of the neuromuscular apparatus of the external anal sphincter (Engel, Nikoomanesh and Schuster, 1974; Whitehead, Engel and Schuster, 1980).

Utilizing this form of treatment, it has been stated that 70% of patients with such external sphincter impairment regain 90–100% continence. These patients were frequently grossly incontinent prior to biofeedback, and many had previously undergone unsuccessful reconstructive surgery. Importantly, patients with incontinence secondary to direct muscle injury, most often iatrogenic, respond much better than those patients with neurological causes for their incontinence (Cerulli, Nikoomanesh and Schuster, 1979). Such therapy is usually successful if denervation is only incomplete, and when some degree of motor recruitment is demonstrable. It is likely that impulse propagation along alternative nerve pathways is involved in the mechanism for such improvement, since in patients who regain the sensation of rectal distension the new sensation as perceived after biofeedback is described as being different from that as appreciated prior to nerve injury. Hence, this form of treatment lends itself particularly well, at least in theory, in helping to improve continence performance after ileoanal anastomosis. It does of course have the advantage of being free from morbidity and mortality, and does not require any further surgical trauma to the anal sphincter mechanism.

Both anal sphincter function and ileal pouch volume have roles in determining functional outcome after restorative proctocolectomy. In a randomised, prospective controlled study of 40 patients after pouch–anal anastomosis, both balloon dilatation of the pouch and anal sphincter biofeedback were performed during the period of defunctioning (Oresland *et al.*, 1988). Twenty patients underwent the above treatment, whilst 20 did not. Balloon dilatation of the pouch in the early postoperative period resulted in significant improvement in pouch compliance compared to the controls when both were assessed immediately prior to ileostomy closure. However, ileostomy closure resulted in a dramatic increase in pouch volume in the controls, a factor which negated the benefit of preclosure dilatation. Manometrically controlled anal sphincter exercises failed to produce any benefit in the treatment group at any stage. Indeed, throughout the study, stool frequency, peranal soiling and overall functional outcome were unaltered by these treatment modalities. The authors' limited experience with anal sphincter biofeedback is somewhat in dispute with the above. Ten of our patients have undergone sphincter biofeedback exercises after ileostomy closure utilizing a manometry microballoon system. Eight of these patients improved their mean anal canal resting pressure by between 50% and 100%. Two patients did not improve their resting tone. Anal canal squeeze pressure was unaltered by this treatment. This was mirrored in subjective improvements in the incidence of minor degrees of incontinence, in particular nocturnal spotting (P.E. Thomas and T.V. Taylor, unpublished data 1989).

The effects of loperamide and sodium valproate on anal sphincter function and stool frequency after restorative proctocolectomy are discussed in Chapter 7.

Pregnancy and the pouch

A considerable number of patients undergoing pouch procedures are women of child-bearing age. Hence, what are the effects of restorative proctocolectomy on successful implantation and on the subsequent course of the pregnancy? Also, what are the effects of a pregnancy on the function of the ileal reservoir?

For many reasons, it is difficult to quantitate the effects of this procedure on fertility. However, there is evidence from a small series that most women that attempted to conceive were in fact successful (Metcalf, Dozois and Kelly, 1986).

Historically, it is recognized that women with either a conventional ileostomy or a Kock pouch do have more complications during pregnancy and delivery than the norm (Barwin, Harley and Wilson, 1974), such as an increased incidence of perineal tears. What effects restorative proctocolectomy might have are still being defined. It must be realized that childbirth itself can be associated with pelvic floor complications, most notably faecal incontinence (Snooks *et al.*, 1984). Incontinence results from direct sphincter damage, damaged

innervation to the pelvic floor musculature, and pudendal nerve damage. This was particularly noted in multiparous women, and those with prolonged second stages of labour. No such damage was noted in women undergoing caesarean section.

The first report of successful childbirth after restorative proctocolectomy came from St Mark's Hospital (Pezim, 1984). In this detailed case report, it was noted that prior to the pregnancy, this patient with an S-pouch had four or five bowel evacuations in a 24-hour period. All such evacuations required pouch catheterization. She denied faecal urgency or perianal irritation, and had no nocturnal evacuations or leakage. Sigmoidoscopy revealed a 10-cm tortuous efferent limb, and a reservoir of approximately 400 ml. The first trimester of pregnancy was completely normal. However, as the uterus increased in size various changes were recognized in reservoir function.

The first of these changes was an increase in frequency of evacuations, and subsequent evaluations of pouch capacity demonstrated that it had decreased to 250 ml at 25 weeks of pregnancy, and to 180 ml at 32 weeks. During the second trimester, there was also evidence that the pouch was beginning to ride up in the pelvis, as an increased catheter length was required. Further evidence for this was that from 30 weeks occasional spontaneous evacuations occurred for the first time since pouch construction. By 32 weeks, the patient did not need to catheterize her reservoir at all. Sigmoidoscopy at this time revealed that the efferent limb was now straight.

During the last 8 weeks of pregnancy, bowel frequency increased to 12 per 24 hours, with two evacuations occurring at night. The patient also complained of urgency, perianal soiling and irritation. These symptoms were thought to represent that the pouch was now being compressed by the gravid uterus. The patient subsequently underwent full-term delivery by caesarean section, and at 2 months postdelivery pouch function had returned to its prepregnancy state.

The following year, the Mayo clinic group reported their experience with six pregnancies after restorative proctocolectomy with J-pouch construction and closure of ileostomy (Metcalf *et al.*, 1985). Of these initial six pregnancies, three had a transient reduction in anorectal function in the third trimester. In all patients 'normal' function returned after delivery. Four of their patients underwent a normal uncomplicated vaginal delivery. In this group, there were no subsequent problems with continence.

Further experience from this group has recently been provided (Nelson *et al.*, 1989). Since 1981, 354 ileal pouch–anal anastomoses had been performed in women. In this series, 20 women have undergone 22 successful pregnancies and deliveries. However, to maintain statistically independent observations, only the first pregnancies were considered in this report. All 20 patients had J-pouches *in situ*. Nineteen had been constructed for ulcerative colitis, and one for polyposis. Only one of these patients, a colitic, had had a postoperative pelvic infection. Delivery occurred at a median of 27 months after closure of the loop ileostomy (range 12–52 months).

Previous obstetric histories revealed that seven of these women had a successful pregnancy and delivery prior to the pouch procedure. Two patients were delivered by caesarean section. Of the five vaginal deliveries, four had episiotomies. One patient was delivered with forceps. Unfortunately, there was no discussion of anorectal function tests, before or after delivery.

Following pouch formation 14 patients had uncomplicated pregnancies. Complications in the other six were not directly related to the pouch itself, and included deep venous thrombosis (one), pre-eclampsia (one), bladder infection (one), bleeding anal varicosity (one), vaginal bleeding (one) and morning sickness with hypovolaemia (one).

Eleven of the patients delivered by the vaginal route after episiotomy. In eight of these the patients had indicated a preference for this mode of delivery. In two of the other three, the reasons for vaginal delivery were to avoid adhesions or because of rapid delivery. In four patients, the technique of episiotomy was modified to a mediolateral incision, which has been previously reported to be protective of the pouch (Metcalf *et al.*, 1985). Nine underwent caesarean section. In five of these patients the reasons were obstetric, whilst in the other four protection of the pouch was considered to be the indication.

Complications postdelivery in the vaginally delivered group included transient diarrhoea, haemorrhoids and a perineal tear. In the caesarean section group, complications included haemorrhoids and abscess, transient diarrhoea, prolonged ileus and two cases of pouchitis. One of these latter two patients had had pouchitis prior to pregnancy. All babies were reported as normal and healthy at delivery. However, one infant subsequently succumbed to hyaline membrane disease.

Regarding the effect of the pregnancy on the pouch, the mean daytime stool frequency was six (range three to 14). During pregnancy, there was a trend towards increased frequency, though this did not attain significance. The mean nocturnal stool frequency was one (range none to four). The first trimester was not noted to have any effect on nocturnal frequency. During the second trimester, eight patients noted increased nocturnal frequency, whilst nine were worse during the third trimester. Eight patients continued with increased frequency post partum. Only one patient had fewer stools in the third trimester and subsequently. Neither stool consistency, continence performance, perianal irritation nor the need to wear pads were significantly altered during pregnancy or post partum. Similarly, there was no significant difference between any of the above-mentioned factors and the mode of delivery.

It would appear therefore that after an ileal pouch–anal anastomosis, most women will have relatively uncomplicated pregnancies and will proceed to full term. Whilst generally deteriorating pouch function was witnessed during pregnancy, this was neither severe nor protracted. As yet, any precise physiological damage occurring during pregnancy, labour and delivery has to be determined. Such studies may shed light on to which mode of delivery, if any, is to be preferred in these patients.

In a series of 40 female patients from the University of Minnesota, three had become pregnant (Wexner *et al.*, 1989a). All three had been delivered by caesarean section. Two patients had no pouch problems at all, whilst one patient had a transient increase in frequency and incontinence. This resolved after delivery.

Pezim (1984) stressed that caesarean section was to be preferred in patients after restorative proctocolectomy in order to prevent possible sphincter damage. However, the limited data now available would suggest that vaginal delivery can be allowed to progress if there are no obstetric reasons why it should not. Whilst at present such reasons are relative and undergoing continuous reappraisal, it would seem sensible to recommend caesarean section in those women with previous complicated obstetric histories. Multiparous women, particularly with any history suggesting pelvic floor damage, should at least undergo electrophysiological assessment of the pelvic floor prior to any decisions regarding mode of delivery. Even in the face of relatively normal studies of pelvic floor innervation, many would advise elective caesarean section to this group. It would also seem sensible in any woman intending to deliver vaginally, that recourse should be made to caesarean section if the second stage becomes prolonged.

The failing pelvic pouch

The series which have been considered in this chapter have documented a failure rate of approximately 10%. Whilst this figure decreases with increasing experience of the procedure, there is always likely to be a small failure rate following such a complicated procedure. The majority of such failures are due to unsuspected Crohn's disease and pelvic sepsis. Other postoperative complications, such as uncontrollable haemorrhage, and poor functional results account for the few other cases. Depending upon the indication for failure, the pouch may be excised (Figure 6.3(a)), defunctioned or revised. Clearly, the former two options will be associated with loss of a significant length of terminal ileum. This

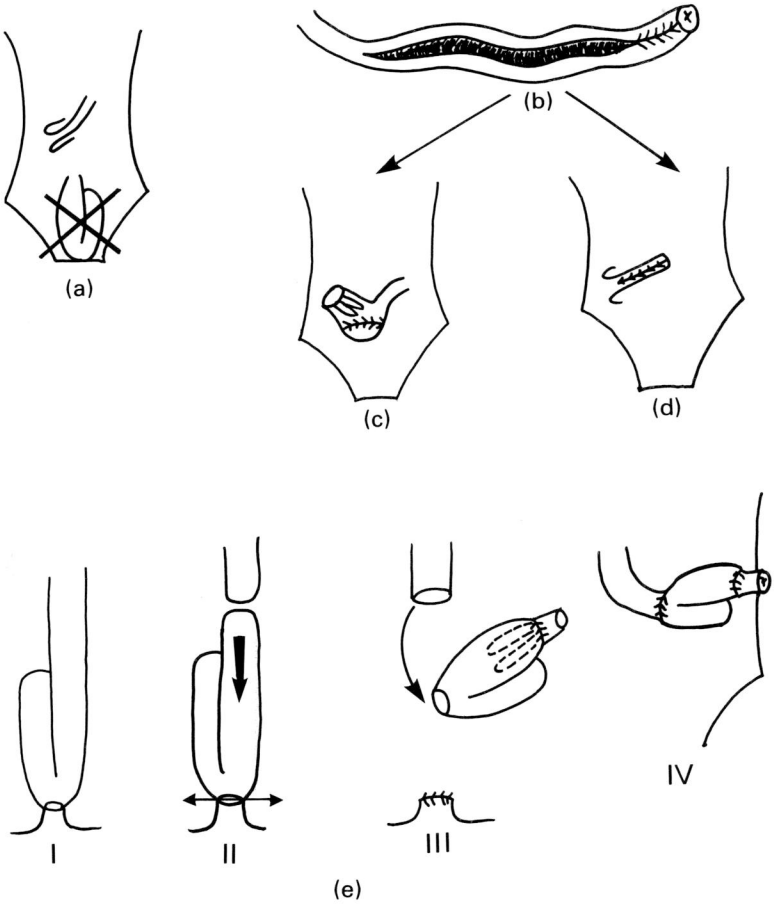

Figure 6.3 The failed pelvic pouch

may be associated with an increased incidence of the recognized complications of terminal ileal disease or excision, such as gall stones and vitamin B_{12} deficiency. In addition, loss of more ileum than necessary, may preclude the patient from procedures such as construction of either a second pelvic pouch or a continent ileostomy. Post-colectomy abdominal complications, such as small bowel obstruction, not infrequently lead to further loss of bowel. It is therefore important to ensure that excessive and unnecessary losses of intestine do not occur.

Complete refashioning of both the malfunctioning pouch and the ileoanal anastomosis have been described, particularly in the presence of a pouch–vaginal fistula (see above). We have no experience with this therapeutic option. More often, such a fistula would be treated by a more conservative procedure, or the pouch would be converted to a permanent ileostomy.

Conversion of a failed J-pouch–anal anastomosis to a continent intra-abdominal ileostomy has also recently been described (Kusunoki *et al.*, 1990a). In this case report, recurring pelvic sepsis necessitated reconstruction of a diverting ileostomy. However, continuing sepsis resulted in a significant reduction in resting anal tone, and it was felt to be unlikely that anal continence could ever be maintained. It was therefore decided to convert the pelvic pouch to an abdominal continent ileostomy. After mobilization of the pouch, the afferent limb was divided, and intussuscepted to form a nipple valve (Figure 6.3(e)). After rotation of the pouch, ileoileostomy restored intestinal continuity. The patient made an excellent recovery, with good pouch function.

Should the pouch–anal anastomosis require formal taking down without reconstruction, Thomson has described his technique for salvaging as much of the terminal ileum as is possible. This has been necessary in 8% of his W-pouches (Thomson and O'Kelly, 1988). His technique is to open the previous anastomoses, therefore forming a long segment of terminal ileum, opened along its antimesenteric border. This is then closed using a single-layer, continuous suture technique (Figure 6.3(b)). This is similar to the technique used for pouch construction, and Thomson states that the bowel used to construct pouches with either two-layer hand-sewn or stapling techniques may be more difficult to salvage. The salvaged small bowel can then be utilized for construction of an ileostomy, be it conventional (Figure 6.3(d)) or continent (Figure 6.3(c)).

Occasionally, in both duplicated J-pouches and in triplicated S-pouches with long efferent limbs, poor reservoir emptying may be due to the presence of a septum within the pouch. Such a septum may be associated with both tenesmus and bleeding per anum. Schoetz and his colleagues have reported that transanal division of the septum using a linear stapling device will frequently lead to the resolution of these symptoms (Schoetz, Coller and Veidenheimer, 1988).

It is now clear that if a high index of suspicion is maintained for postoperative complications, that their presence is meticulously sought, and that they are expeditiously treated, then the majority of failing pelvic pouches can be salvaged (Schoetz, Coller and Veidenheimer, 1988).

7

The anal canal and pelvic floor after restorative proctocolectomy

The anal canal is depicted diagrammatically in Figures 7.1 and 7.2. Varying terminology regarding this structure frequently causes confusion. Interested readers are directed elsewhere for more detailed reviews of this topic (Nivatvongs, Stern and Fryd, 1981; Wood, 1985).

Throughout the rest of this chapter, the anal canal will be considered to run from the upper margin of the anorectal ring (i.e. the puborectalis muscle) to the external anal margin, being some 40 mm long. No precisely definable embryological boundary exists to justify such limits, however the importance of the puborectalis sling as part of the mechanism of continence at least allows for useful conclusions to be drawn from studies based on this definition. Many workers studying patients after restorative proctocolectomy appear to have adopted this basic concept.

The external anal sphincter has been classically divided into three muscular subcomponents (Figure 7.1). The deep part of the sphincter is thought to blend with the puborectalis muscle, and has fibres which decussate and similarly blend anteriorly with the perineal muscles.

The superficial component of the external sphincter is attached posteriorly to the coccyx, whilst anteriorly its fibres merge with those of

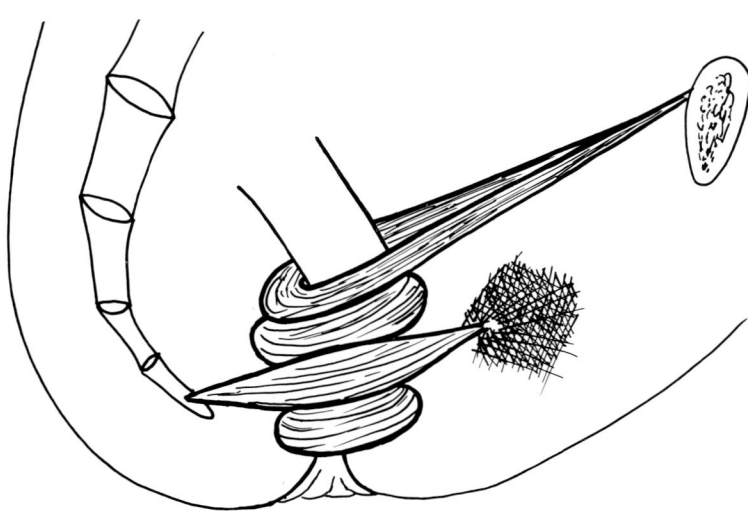

Figure 7.1

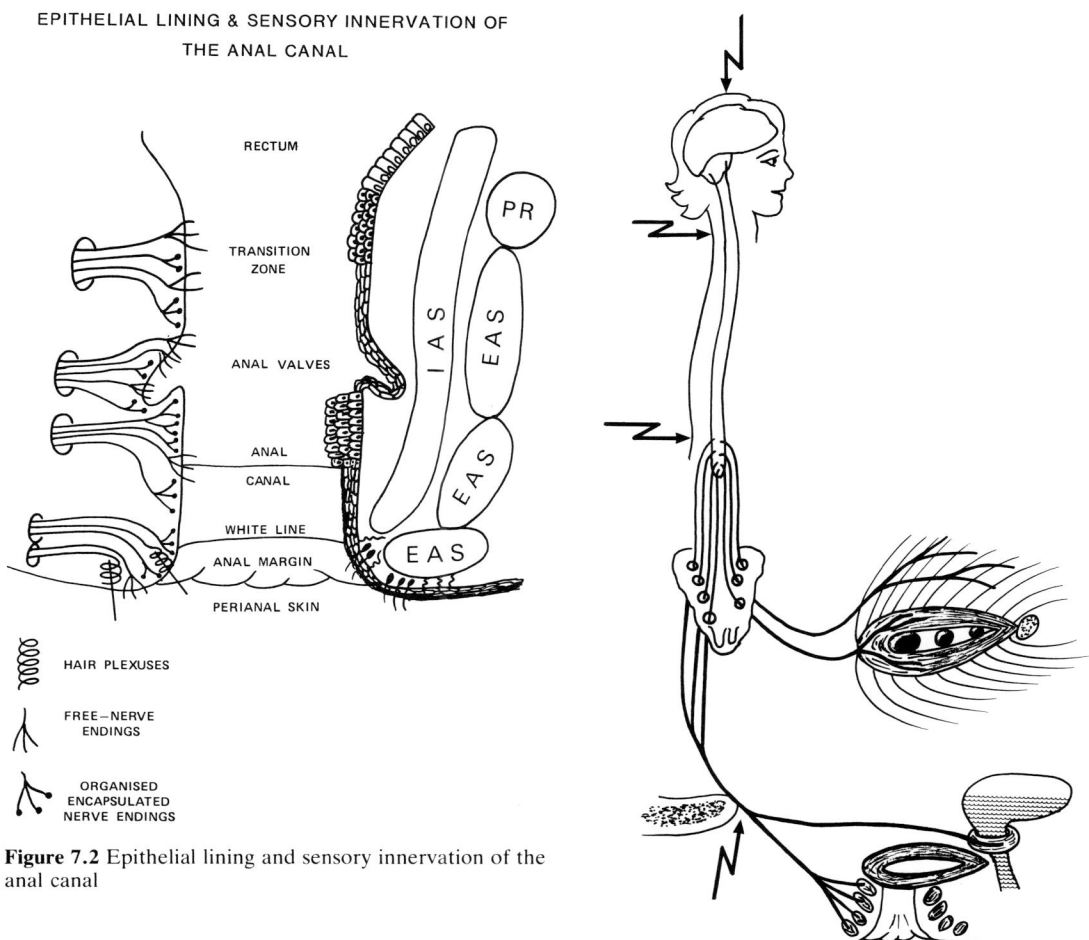

EPITHELIAL LINING & SENSORY INNERVATION OF
THE ANAL CANAL

Figure 7.2 Epithelial lining and sensory innervation of the anal canal

Figure 7.3 Sites of possible stimulation of the nerve supply to the pelvic floor

the perineal body. The subcutaneous external sphincter is an indistinct ring of muscle lying beneath the perianal skin.

The external sphincter has recently been described as consisting of merely two components, namely a superficial (the subcutaneous and superficial parts as described above), and a deep part (the 'deep' external sphincter and the puborectalis) (Oh and Kark, 1972). In addition, the external sphincter demonstrates age and sex differences. Further complexity arises due to the differing form of the external anal sphincter at different sites within the anal canal of any one individual.

The external sphincter is innervated by neurones carried in the pudendal nerve and the perineal branch of S4 (Figure 7.3). The cell bodies of these neurones are in the ventral horn of the spinal cord at the level of S2. In man it is likely that some decussation of these

fibres occurs. Therefore, complete denervation need not result from unilateral transection (Wunderlich and Swash, 1983).

The puborectalis muscle is a sling of muscle, attached anteriorly to the pubis, and passing posteriorly around the rectum (Figure 7.1). There remains a degree of controversy regarding the nervous innervation of this muscle. Historically, but based upon sound research, it was considered that the bulk of the puborectalis was supplied from below by the pudendal nerve via its perineal and inferior rectal branches. In addition, a few specimens demonstrated a varying contribution from the sacral plexus from above (Lawson, 1974a). This would suggest that the puborectalis is not a pelvic floor derivative, but is in fact derived from the embryonic external sphincter.

Recently however, workers from St Mark's Hospital have been consistently able to record electromyographic activity in the ipsilateral puborectalis (but not the external sphincter) by stimulation of the sacral nerves above the levators (Percy *et al.*, 1981). To date, the finer details of the innervation to the puborectalis muscle remain unanswered.

The internal anal sphincter is the accentuated distal 30 mm or so of the inner circular smooth muscle layer of the rectum, as is present along the length of the rest of the intestine. This structure therefore occupies the superior three-quarters of the anal canal as previously defined. The fine structure of the internal sphincter is contentious, and may be divided into separate subdivisions (Lawson, 1974b). However, this topic need not concern us further. It is almost certain that the internal sphincter is innervated by both the sympathetic (via the hypogastric plexus) and the parasympathetic nervous systems (Meunier and Mollard, 1977).

The longitudinal muscle coat of the rectum blends inferiorly with the pubococcygeus muscle at the level of the anorectal ring. The muscle thus formed straddles the external sphincter, aiding in the delineation of the intersphincteric plane between the internal and external sphincters. It is likely that further, somewhat more complicated, arrangements of the longitudinal layer exist, but again these need not concern us. Interested readers may consult the review by Parks (Parks, 1956).

Distal to a line equating to the inferior margin of the internal anal sphincter, often termed Hilton's white line, the canal is lined with hair-bearing skin (Figure 7.2). As would be expected, there is an abundance of sebaceous, sweat and circumanal apocrine glands in this area. Sensory endings are found within this area, and conform to those found in hairy skin elsewhere.

The epithelium covering the inferior 10 mm of the internal sphincter consists of a thick stratified squamous form. Pigmented cells can be found, but this region tends not to bear hair, and is relatively free from the glands found distally. This is the region often termed the 'pecten' in anatomical texts.

In the more proximal canal, the mucosa is thrown into between five and 12 longitudinal folds, termed the anal columns. Their distal limit coincides with a point approximately half-way down the internal sphincter, and is marked by transverse folds of mucosa; the anal valves.

Extending proximally from a point slightly distal to the anal valves, the epithelium becomes more columnar, but is still stratified. However, it is less thick than that in the pecten. It may be that the anal columns consist of stratified squamous epithelium, but that the intervening areas are covered with a more simple columnar epithelium.

This transitional epithelium extends for approximately 10 mm proximal to the anal valves, and ends abruptly at the rectal mucosa. The whole of the region from this level to the anal margin is supplied with an extremely rich sensory nerve supply. Workers vary in their descriptions of the types, concentrations and locations of such endings. However, suffice to say that various sensory modalities (i.e. touch, temperature, pin-prick, etc.) can be discerned within the anal canal to a level probably equivalent to the junction of the transitional epithelium with the rectal mucosa.

The rectal mucosa, with its columnar epithelium rich in goblet cells and tubular glands, lines the most proximal 10 mm or so of the 'long' anal canal. Many non-myelinated nerve fibres can be found in this region. However, receptors within this epithelium are unusual (Duthie and Gairns, 1960). Anatomical doctrine decrees that awareness of rectal distension is transmitted along the S2 and S3 pelvic splanchnic nerves, whereas autonomic pathways (both sympathetic and parasympathetic) convey nociceptive stimuli. As is typical of this region, little totally unequivocal evidence exists for such statements.

Anal canal manometry

Several methods have been used by laboratories studying the physiology of the anorectum. However, the manometric properties of these muscular complexes have attracted most interest. Numerous methods have been used to study such properties, and each has its advocates, and own particular advantages. In addition, each may assess a slightly different aspect of the activity of the anal musculature.

This has obvious relevance to cross-interpretation of data from different centres.

Most systems consist of some form of anal probe connected to a pressure transducer and thence to an amplifier. A little further description of these techniques may aid with the following discussion of those results obtained after pouch–anal anastomosis.

The open-tipped catheter system consists of a piece of low compliance plastic tubing with side ports connected via a closed water-filled system to a pressure transducer. Such systems respond very rapidly to pressure changes, and allow for the precise localization of contractions. They are therefore particularly suited to the assessment of anal sphincter pressure. Conversely, they are of less value for use within the rectum or ileal pouch, since a contraction anywhere within these large, hollow organs will be registered with little, if any, clarity as to the site of contraction (Figure 7.4).

Balloon systems usually consist of large, thin-walled balloons connected via a closed system to pressure transducers. These are of necessity poor localizers of contraction and

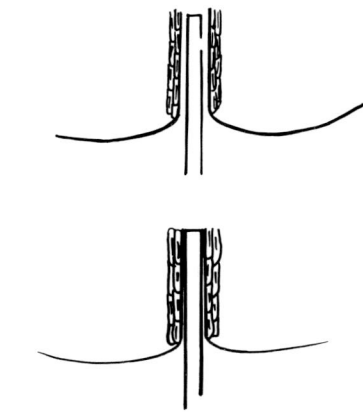

Figure 7.5

hence tend to be used to assess rectal (or ileal reservoir) tone and compliance (Figure 7.8). However, smaller balloons can be used to localize contractions, for example in the rectal ampulla.

Distension of the anal canal may induce sphincteric contraction and subsequent relaxation (Denny-Brown and Robertson, 1935). In particular, heavy water-filled systems may drag on the pelvic floor, stretching the puborectalis muscle. This may result in rectal contraction, and subsequent relaxation of the internal anal sphincter (Scharli and Kiesewetter, 1970).

Scarring of the anal canal is common after ileal pouch–anal anastomosis. Such anal canal fibrosis can be associated with very high anal canal pressures, when assessed with large diameter probes. However, smaller probes may fail to register such pressures (Figure 7.5) (Duthie and Bennett, 1964; Hancock, 1977). Again, this has relevance to data cross-interpretation.

Pressures recorded within the canal vary both radially and longitudinally, which can be explained with a knowledge of the configuration of the anal sphincter musculature. Generally, the pressure in the lower canal is greater than in the upper, presumably due to the bulk of the external anal sphincter. In the upper canal, the pressure is greatest posteriorly, because of anatomy of the puborectalis muscle. In the mid canal, the pressures are equal when measured anteriorly and posteriorly. In the lower anal canal, both the resting and maximal

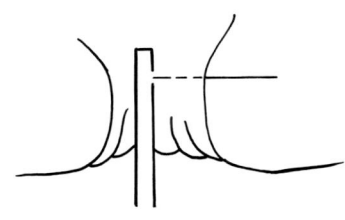

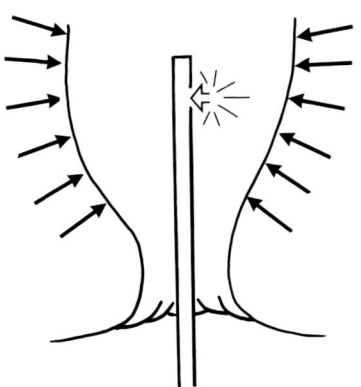

Figure 7.4 Open-tipped catheter

squeeze pressures are greatest anteriorly (Taylor, Beart and Phillips, 1984).

The effects of ileal pouch–anal anastomosis on anal canal manometry have been well described (O'Connell *et al.*, 1987; Johnston *et al.*, 1987; Sharp *et al.*, 1987; Keighley *et al.*, 1988; O'Connell *et al*; 1988; Chaussade *et al.*, 1989c; Emblem, Stein and Morkrid, 1989a,b; Lavery, Tuckson and Easley, 1989; Sagar, Holdsworth and Johnston, 1989; Lindquist, 1990; Miller *et al.*, 1990b). Almost all such studies have utilized water-filled systems, with assessments being performed with the patient in the left lateral position. However, most have involved the use of different types of anal probes.

In a manometric study of 38 pouch–anal anastomosis (31 J- and seven S-pouches), 12 straight ileoanal anastomoses, and 30 controls, O'Connell *et al.* assessed patients at a mean of 22 months postoperation. Mucosal proctectomy had been performed both endoanally and after rectal eversion.

This group utilized a 12-mm diameter rigid polyglass cylindrical probe, through the centre of which was passed a balloon-tipped 4-mm polyvinyl catheter. Four peripheral perfusion channels lying 90 degrees apart were perfused at 0.1 ml/min. Each channel ended in a side port 30 mm from the distal end of the probe. This system therefore allowed for both radial and longitudinal measurements of canal pressure (O'Connell *et al.*, 1987a; O'Connell *et al.*, 1988).

Resting pressure was less in patients than in healthy controls. However, longitudinal analysis revealed that this was purely due to low pressures in the proximal canal. The technique of rectal stripping did not appear to influence the resting pressure. However, resting pressure was significantly reduced at all levels in the anal canal in the incontinent group compared with the continent patients. Importantly, this latter group did not have a significantly lower resting pressure than the control group. Radial assessment of resting pressure could not differentiate either the patients from the controls, or the continent patients from those suffering with poor continence. Squeeze pressure was similar in patients and controls, and again mucosectomy technique did not appear significant in this regard. However, squeeze pressure was lower in the middle and distal anal canal in the incontinent group of patients compared with the continent group. As for resting pressure, radial analysis of squeeze pressure failed to discriminate between the various groups.

Using a 4.8-mm multilumen perfused catheter with a flow rate of 0.6 ml/min, Sharp assessed 28 patients preoperatively, and 12 patients after S-pouch–anal anastomosis. They recorded an approximately 50% reduction in mean preoperative resting pressure from 70.4 mmHg to 43 mmHg postoperatively, whilst the mean preoperative maximal squeeze pressure was less dramatically reduced from 172.3 mmHg to 136 mmHg postoperatively (Sharp *et al.*, 1987).

In an age- and sex-matched control study, simultaneous anal manometry and ileal reservoir pressure recordings were obtained using a four-lumen catheter of 5 mm diameter perfused at a rate of 0.5 ml/min. This probe had side ports at varying lengths from the anal verge (Keighley, Yoshioka and Kmiot, 1988). Median resting pressure was 100 cmH$_2$O in the controls, and 42 cmH$_2$O in the patient group. In seven patients with an imperfect result, the median resting pressure was only 21 cmH$_2$O. This group found that pelvic sepsis was a significant risk factor for poor resting tone, but that reservoir type was not. Similar conclusions were drawn from the median squeeze pressure, being 87 cmH$_2$O postoperatively, compared with 143 cmH$_2$O in the control group. Again, poor functional outcome was associated with a further reduction in squeeze pressure (50 cmH$_2$O).

Comparing 12 patients after an endoanal stapled pouch–anal anastomosis with 24 patients after endoanal mucosal proctectomy and a hand-sewn pouch–anal anastomosis, Johnston found that in the former group, maximal resting pressure decreased from a median of 90 cmH$_2$O to 70 cmH$_2$O. However, after mucosal proctectomy with a hand-sewn anastomosis, the maximal resting pressure decreased from 85 cmH$_2$O to 40 cmH$_2$O. Maximal squeeze pressure in the former group increased from a median of 128 cmH$_2$O to 146 cmH$_2$O, whilst in the mucosectomy group it remained stable (134 cmH$_2$O preoperatively, 137 cmH$_2$O postoperatively). The changes in resting pressure were statistically highly significant, however the differences in squeeze pressure failed to attain statistical significance (Johnston *et al.*, 1987).

Our own observations have provided support for the above findings. In a series of hand-sewn J-pouch–anal anastomoses, resting pressure, as assessed with a closed fluid-filled 6-mm balloon system in the anal canal high pressure zone, was 3.45 ± 1.47 kPa (range 0.9–6.56 kPa). Using a 20-point functional score assessment, patients with more than five adverse factors on clinical grading had a significantly lower resting pressure than those with five or less (2.6 ± 1.0 kPa and 4.73 ± 1.4 kPa respectively, $P < 0.01$). Maximal squeeze pressure was affected to a lesser degree, being 9.40 ± 4.65 kPa (range 2.55–18.13 kPa), and was not found to correlate with clinical score.

Lindquist has also demonstrated that resting pressure is decreased after restorative proctocolectomy (Lindquist, 1990). Using a microtransducer technique in 55 patients, a 1.67-mm catheter was mechanically withdrawn from the anal canal at a constant speed of 2.5 mm/s, allowing for recording of a pressure profile within the anal canal. Thereafter manometry was repeated using the station pull-through technique, allowing assessment of resting and squeeze pressures within different zones. All patients had undergone endoanal mucosal proctectomy, with formation of mostly S-pouches. Postoperatively, there was a marked reduction in resting tone, with no improvement after 12 months. No benefit was noted in patients in whom anal retraction was carefully limited during mucosectomy. In addition, similar results were recorded with regard to length of the high pressure zone. In contrast, maximal squeeze pressure was restored within 12 months, and Lindquist even found that there was a degree of over-compensation of squeeze pressure in male patients.

Twenty-three patients were reassessed after 2 years, and it was found that no improvement occurred in either resting tone or anal canal length. Interestingly, and in contrast to other workers including ourselves, a low resting tone was not correlated with poor continence performance. However, the high pressure zone characteristics did correlate with improved function, especially continence and frequency. It was also found that reduced bowel frequency and the ability to defer defaecation for more than 1 hour were related to higher resting tone. Squeeze pressure, whilst greater in males, did not appear to affect functional outcome.

Hence, to some extent these findings are controversial, and at least part of this discrepancy may be due to differing methodologies. It is unlikely that the system as used by Lindquist was any less 'physiological' than those used by others. Indeed, whilst debate continues as to the ideal method of assessing the anal canal, the method used here should provide for one of the least amounts of canal distension and mucosal irritation. However, assessment was only made in the posterior quadrant of the anal canal, and for the reasons alluded to above it may not be entirely representative. Irrespective of such arguments is the fact that, whilst not correlating with continence, resting tone did correlate with the ability to defer defaecation and with reduced frequency. This, if substantiated, poses more questions than it answers about normal internal sphincter function, particularly its role in relation to rectal sampling and in the maintenance of continence.

Excepting this work, consistently workers have measured significant reductions in resting anal pressures after restorative proctocolectomy. In addition, this fall has been found to strongly correlate with poor functional outcome postoperatively. This is particularly so with regard to continence. However, such reductions have not been completely universal. Both in an experimental study in the dog (Ito *et al.*, 1981) and in a limited clinical study from Italy (Fiorentini *et al.*, 1987), resting and squeeze pressures were found to be preserved after endorectal ileal pull-through.

Less dramatic effects, if any, are generally witnessed on maximal squeeze pressure. Indeed, some patients have shown an increase in squeeze pressure after ileoanal anastomosis, suggesting hypertrophy of the external sphincter (Becker, 1984; Lindquist, 1990). However, Keighley did note that poor continence was associated with lower squeeze pressures. Interestingly, such phenomena were not associated with pelvic sepsis, and were thought likely to be due to damage to the pelvic floor during pouch–anal anastomosis (Keighley, Yoshioka and Kmiot, 1988). Our studies of similar phenomena suggest that neuropathic damage may occur in the external anal sphincter (see below).

What aetiological factors are likely to be important in inducing such changes in internal sphincter function? Excessive retraction during the performance of the endoanal mucosa proctectomy has received much attention (Heald and Allen, 1986). Certainly, Johnston found that mucosal proctectomy was associated with a greater decrease in resting tone than when a stapled anastomosis without mucosal stripping was performed.

Indeed, these same workers using an ambulatory manometric technique have demonstrated that endoanal mucosectomy is associated with significantly fewer spontaneous relaxations of the anal sphincter than after a stapled anastomosis. A 2-mm diameter microtransducer was placed within the anal canal for 3 hours, and the patients encouraged to act as normally as possible. The mucosectomy group demonstrated neither sampling episodes nor spontaneous relaxations of the internal sphincter during the 3 hours of the test. A stapled anastomosis was associated with normal values for both spontaneous relaxations and sampling episodes, as compared to the control group. Hence, the avoidance of mucosectomy was consistent with the maintenance of normal discriminatory function in this group (Sagar, Holdsworth and Johnston, 1989).

Similar conclusions have been drawn by a recent study from the Cleveland Clinic, in which 15 patients underwent manometry with a perfused catheter system of diameter 4.88 mm (Lavery, Tuckson and Easley, 1989). Two groups of patients were specifically assessed to determine the effect of endoanal mucosectomy with a hand-sewn ileal J-pouch–anal anastomosis as compared to the use of a circular stapling device. Both continence and resting tone were significantly better after use of the stapling gun, even though the follow-up in this group was only 3.5 months, as compared to 21.7 months in the mucosectomy group.

Others have found that if care is taken to avoid prolonged endoanal retraction during mucosectomy, often involving an abdominal mucosal proctectomy, the loss of resting tone could be minimized (Keighley, 1987). That anal retraction, particularly if prolonged, is the aetiological force in such poor resting tone and continence performance is still controversial. Conflicting results have been described by Williams' group from the London Hospital (Marzouk, Williams and Hallan, 1989; Williams *et al.*, 1989b). They have found that whilst a stapled anastomosis was both quicker to perform, and associated with a slightly

improved continence performance, it was also associated with the same degree of reduction in resting tone as witnessed after a conventional anastomosis. Clearly, retraction is not the only important mechanism in producing such results, as the Mayo clinic group failed to demonstrate any differences in resting pressure between patients after an everted rectal mucosectomy or after an endoanal mucosectomy with retraction. It has also been postulated that during mucosal proctectomy some of the sphincter musculature itself might be stripped (Sharp *et al.*, 1987). What may be of greater importance is the possibility that mucosectomy and ileoanal pouch-anastomosis might induce long-term sphincteric fibrosis (Emblem *et al.*, 1989). It is well recognized that stenosis at the ileal pouch–anal anastomisis is relatively common, whilst varying in severity. As discussed above, the methods of assessment of anal canal pressure may be important in this regard.

Whilst the stapled ileoanal anastomosis may not solve all the problems associated with this procedure, there is evidence that time might improve resting tone (Kmiot *et al.*, 1989b). This study demonstrated that resting pressure remained lower than its preoperative value for 12 months. It did however improve with time and maintained this improvement for 2 years post pouch construction. Maximum squeeze pressure remained reduced for 6 months after the operation by which time it reached the preoperative level. Thereafter, no further improvement was noted. Even though conflicting results have been described elsewhere (Lindquist, 1990), such findings may at least partly explain the finding that continence performance tends to improve over a protracted period after restorative protocolectomy.

Two recent studies have described the effects of loperamide on the anal sphincter after pouch–anal anastomosis (Becker *et al.*, 1989; Emblem, Stein and Morkrid, 1989b). Loperamide is an opiate, which in *in vivo* experiments has been shown to increase resting anal pressure, presumably secondary to stimulation of the visceral internal sphincter. However, experiments *in vitro* have shown that loperamide reduces resting tone.

Becker has conducted a prospective, randomized, placebo-controlled, blind trial which revealed that patients receiving loperamide had a significantly greater resting anal tone than patients receiving a placebo. No effect could be demonstrated upon maximal squeeze pressure. Emblem *et al.* found that loperamide significantly increased resting tone in those patients who had undergone abdominal mucosectomy sparing the distal 2 cm of mucosa. However, those patients who had undergone a complete endoanal mucosectomy to the dentate line failed to increase their resting tone with loperamide. External sphincter function was similarly unaffected by loperamide in both groups of patients.

In addition to its effects on the anal sphincter, both the above groups showed the faecal weight and daily frequency were reduced by up to 50% by loperamide. By disturbing the coordinated peristaltic patterns of the small intestine, loperamide increases orocaecal transit time, promoting water absorption from the stool. Hence the wet weight of the pouch effluent will be decreased. This effect of loperamide is more pronounced, and probably more relevant in the clinical situation, than that on the internal sphincter. It is therefore perhaps of greater importance that loperamide has been shown not to inhibit the striated external sphincer, an effect which has been demonstrated on the detrusor muscle of the bladder. Should this have been the case, any beneficial effects of its use would have been negated by poor external sphincer function.

Utsunomiya's group have similarly demonstrated that pharmacological manipulations can be used to improve resting tone after mucosal

proctectomy and ileal pouch–anal anastomosis. In 17 patients, sodium valproate or placebo were administered orally up to 4 months after ileostomy closure (Kusunoki *et al.*, 1990b). Whilst placebo was ineffective, those patients who received sodium valproate demonstrated reduced stool frequency, reduced perianal soiling, and alleviation of perianal irritation. These were associated with an elevation in resting anal pressure. Interestingly, this effect appeared to be more significant in patients with polyposis coli, rather than colitics. Whether this effect was statistically significant is unclear. Neither anal canal motility nor maximal squeeze pressure were affected by sodium valproate.

Anal canal length

Manometric techniques, when combined with the endoanal station pull-through technique (Figure 7.6), allow for the definition of the anal canal in terms of the high pressure zone associated with the anal sphincteric muscular complex. As a result, the anal canal has been described as being some 2.5–5.0 cm in length, and is longer in males (Nivatvongs, Stern and Fryd, 1981).

Applying similar methods to patients after ileoanal anastomosis, both with and without a reservoir, the Mayo clinic group described this high pressure zone as being 3.8±0.1 cm in their normal control group, and 3.9±0.1 cm in their patients. Neither the presence of a pelvic reservoir, nor the incidence of postoperative faecal incontinence was correlated with anal canal length in this series (O'Connell *et al.*, 1988).

Johnston found that the site of maximal anal squeeze pressure was in the most distal 1–2 cm of the anal canal in 90% of their control subjects. In addition, the sphincteric high pressure zone began 4 cm from the anal verge. The mean anal sphincter length preoperatively was 4 cm (Johnston *et al.*, 1987). In their patients who underwent a stapled end-to-end ileoanal anastomosis without endoanal mucosal proctectomy, the mean high pressure zone postoperatively was still 4 cm. However, in their patient group who had undergone a conventional stripping of the rectal mucosa and pull-through anastomosis, the mean sphincter length was found to be 3 cm.

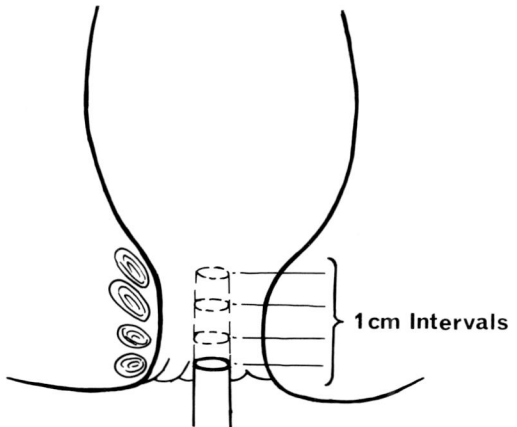

Figure 7.6 Station pull-through technique

1 cm Intervals

Pescatori and Parks (1984a) in their study of 50 patients after mucosal proctectomy and S-pouch–anal anastomosis, found the anal sphincteric length to be 3.2±0.7 cm at a mean of 11±10 months after ileostomy closure, and 3.4±0.6 cm at a mean of 20±16 months postclosure. This compared with a sphincter length of 3.5±0.6 cm preoperatively. The authors' assessments have failed to show any correlation between anal canal length, as measured using the station pull-through technique, and ultimate function outcome after J-pouch–anal anastomosis.

To some degree such conflicting data may be explained by the different methodologies used in such reports. Johnston's group have suggested their results indicate that the entire anal canal should be preserved during ileal pouch–anal anastomosis, and that this is most likely to be achieved by using a stapling technique and avoiding mucosal stripping. Certainly, even though a small decrease in sphincter length was found in Park's patients, this decrease did not correlate with functional outcome, and was still within the range of normality of his laboratory. It would appear that restorative proctocolectomy has limited effect on anal sphincteric length, as assessed from the anal high pressure zone. The precise significance of such effects is presently unanswered. It is our feeling that such effects are of but minor importance to the overall result after pouch–anal anastomosis.

Anal canal motility

Station pull-through of manometry probes may reveal anal canal motility patterns. In the normal canal, such patterns often demonstrate two major types of wave; slow waves of amplitude up to 25 cmH$_2$O and frequency of 10–20 per minute, and ultra-slow waves of amplitude 30–100 cmH$_2$O and a frequency of less than 3 per minute. It is likely that the internal sphincter is responsible for the genesis of both of these waves. Slow wave frequency is greatest in the more distal segments of the anal canal, which may suggest the presence of an inwardly directed contraction gradient from the anal canal back into the rectum. This may facilitate the retrograde passage of small amounts of faecal material into the rectum (Hancock, 1976). Ultra-slow waves tend to be associated with somewhat higher resting pressures, often greater than 150 cmH$_2$O. Consequently, they may be a feature of certain conditions in which a high resting pressure may be an important factor, such as anal fissure (Hancock, 1977).

To date, few reports have documented such anal motility patterns after ileal reservoir formation and ileoanal anastomosis. The Mayo clinic group have recorded that regular slow phasic fluctuations in the resting pressure occurred in 24 of their 30 controls, and in all 50 of their patients. Differences were noticed, however, in the characteristics of these waves between the two groups. First, the slow wave frequency was less in the patient group at 8.6±0.4/min, compared with the controls at 13.8±0.5/min, this being statistically significant. Conversely, the slow wave amplitude was greater in the patient group (28±4 mmHg) compared with the control group (7±1 mmHg), which was similarly significant.

'Giant' slow waves of amplitude greater than 25 mmHg were seen in 23 patients, and interestingly were not seen in any controls. Such giant waves were associated with a slower wave frequency (7.2±0.4/min) than was observed in patients without such waves (9.8±0.5/min). However, giant slow waves were not associated with any differences in sphincter length, maximal resting pressure, maximal squeeze pressure or degree of continence. Ultra-slow waves were also observed in 22% of the patients and in 17% of the controls. In the patient group their frequency was 1.04±0.25/min, compared with 0.74±0.06/min in the healthy controls. Ultra-slow wave activity was not shown to be related to continence after ileoanal anastomosis. The authors' studies of anal canal motility patterns have demonstrated that such large amplitude ultra-slow waves are positively correlated with the presence of faecal leakage, particularly nocturnal leakage.

Such abnormal slow wave patterns may be indicative of an alteration in internal anal sphincter activity after mucosal proctectomy and ileoanal anastomosis. Alternatively, it may be possible that the aberrant slow wave activity as recorded in the anal canal may in fact be produced by the pulled-through ileal segment, and not the internal sphincter itself (Figure

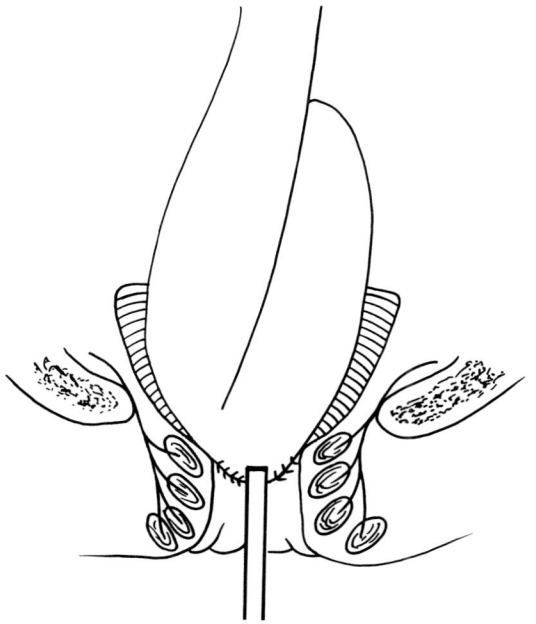

Figure 7.7

7.7). This is supported by the fact that in the Mayo clinic study, the slow wave fluctuation was particularly seen in the proximal and upper anal canal, there being a paucity of such activity in the distal anal canal. Insufficient data exist to answer this question any further at present.

It has been suggested that ultra-slow pressure waves in the anal canal may result from variations in electrical pacemaker potential frequencies of the internal anal sphincter (Ustach, Tobson and Hambrecht, 1970). Such activity is only found in a minority of healthy people, and indeed is seen to be intermittent even in the same subject.

Conversely, there is now evidence that large amplitude ultra-slow waves may occur as a result of spontaneous inhibitory reflex activity (Kestenberg, Becker and Sharp, 1985). Interestingly in the Mayo clinic series, ultra-slow wave activity was seen in some patients without a demonstrable ano- neorectal inhibitory reflex. This group have suggested that either ultra- slow wave activity is not an inhibitory reflex, or that the inhibitory reflex remains postoperatively, but that it is not demonstrable by present techniques.

Anal canal sensation

To date few workers have studied anal canal sensitivity after pouch–anal anastomosis. Those that have have utilized some form of electrical stimulation of the anal mucosa. Holdsworth and Johnston (1988a) studied anal sensation in 14 patients with ulcerative colitis preoperatively, 16 patients after end-to-end ileoanal anastomosis without mucosal proctectomy performed at the level of the puborectalis, and 13 patients after endoanal ileoanal anastomosis performed 1 cm above the dentate line. In these patients, threshold electrosensitivity of mucosa in the upper, middle and lower anal canal (as defined manometrically) was measured using a lubricated bipolar constant current stimulator probe. This group found that in the upper canal, the patients who had undergone mucosectomy had a significantly higher threshold (7.4–17.3 mA, median 9.1 mA), compared with both the end-to-end anastomosis and the control patients (4.5–10.0 mA, median 7.9 mA and 5.4–7.8 mA, median 7.3 mA respectively). In the mid and lower canal there was no significant difference in median electrosensitivity thresholds between the controls (4.5 mA and 5.7 mA respectively), the end-to-end anastomosis patients (5.8 mA and 4.5 mA), and the mucosal proctectomy patients (4.2 mA and 4.0 mA).

With regard to discriminatory function, preoperatively all patients were able to differentiate flatus from faeces. Postoperatively, 100% of patients after end-to-end anastomosis continued with this ability, whereas 77% of those with endoanal anastomosis were able to do so, this was not however statistically significant. Of greater significance was the fact that after end-to-end anastomosis 81% of patients felt confident about releasing flatus safely, compared to only 31% after mucosectomy.

This study demonstrated that end-to-end ileoanal anastomosis at the level of the puborectalis is not associated with any significant impairment of anal canal sensitivity at any level in the anal canal, whereas a significant decrease in sensation is seen in the upper anal canal after mucosal proctectomy. This may be due to the stripping of the rectal mucosa and its replacement with full thickness ileal wall. This factor is strongly associated with the patient's confidence to safely release flatus without fear of faecal leakage. A 'pure' relationship to sensory discrimination of flatus from faeces could not be demonstrated. This group did not report any problems related to the retained mucosa of the transition zone after end-to-end anastomosis or mucosal proctectomy commencing 1 cm above the dentate line, and concluded that preservation of the entire anal canal during restorative proctocolectomy provides definite physiological advantages.

Similar conclusions were drawn by Keighley and his colleagues after comparing anal canal sensation in 30 patients (19 J-, and 11 W-pouches) with a group of age- and sex-matched controls (Keighley *et al.*, 1988). They utilized a monopolar constant-current stimulator to assess the threshold mucosal sensitivity in the proximal, mid and distal canal. In this patient cohort, loss of sensation to electrical stimulation was found in the mid-zone of the anal canal in 25 of the pouch patients. The five patients with normal sensation had an intact anal transition zone, this having been deliberately preserved at operation, the other 25 patients having undergone mucosal proctectomy commencing at the dentate line. This almost certainly explains the disparity between these results and those of Johnston's group as described above. Unfortunately, retention of this region with its concomitant results with regard to sensation, did not result in retention of the rectoanal inhibitory reflex. Keighley's group had however previously shown that discriminatory function is not impaired after excision of the anal transition zone (Keighley *et al.*, 1987b)

The anorectal inhibitory reflex

It is well recognized that rectal distension induces rectal contraction, internal sphincter relaxation and external sphincter contraction. It is possible that this triad of reflexes may facilitate anal epithelial sampling of rectal contents without fear of incontinence. The rectal response is thought to be mediated by a spinal reflex, as it is noted to be decreased or absent in patients with spinal cord lesions (White, Verlot and Ehrentheil, 1940).

Initially, at low rectal distending volumes a transient decrease in anal tone is noted. As the distension volume is increased, the external sphincter contracts resulting in an increase in measured pressure; this being followed by another reduction in pressure as the internal sphincter relaxes. This relaxation is most pronounced in the upper canal, due to the anatomical configuration of the sphincter, and is probably mediated by an intramural reflex, as it is not necessarily abolished by spinal anaesthesia or disease. However, spinal shock does temporarily abolish the reflex, implying that the spinal cord does have a role in modulating the reflex. Haynes and Read (1982) suggested that the internal sphincter response might be mediated by stimulation of in-series tension receptors in the rectal wall.

It is also noteworthy that in the distal 5 mm of the anal canal, the bulk of the external sphincter and its tonic activity may mask any reduction in pressure, having obvious implications with regard to studies of this reflex. Initial distension induces an increase in external sphincter activity, but this is subsequently replaced by relaxation at higher distending volumes (Porter, 1962). Both of these responses are mediated via spinal reflexes, the receptors of which are thought to lie in the pelvic floor, as such reflexes can also be elicited by colonic distension after coloanal anastomosis (Lane and Parks, 1977).

Most methods of registering the normal anorectal inhibitory reflex involve simultaneous anal manometry and rectal distension, for example with a low compliance balloon (Figure 7.8).

Several reports have documented the presence or otherwise of this reflex after restorative proctocolectomy (Pescatori and Parks, 1984a; Sharp *et al.*, 1987; Holdsworth and Johnston, 1988b; Keighley *et al.*, 1988; O'Connell *et al.*, 1988). One such paper documented 100% incidence of the reflex in its control group of healthy volunteers (O'Connell *et al.*, 1988), and in one report where the preoperative patients with ulcerative colitis constituted the control group, the incidence was again 100% (Holdsworth and Johnston, 1988).

Pescatori and Parks (1984) used a soft rubber balloon attached to stiff polyethylene cannula inserted into the lower part of their S-pouches, and a water-filled microballoon system to assess the reflex. The latter was placed 1.5 cm from the anal verge. A decrease in pressure of 20% was required to define the presence of the reflex. They also noted the

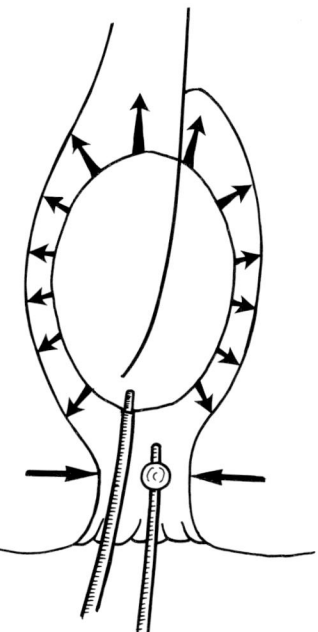

Figure 7.8

minimum volume of distension required to elicit the reflex.

The inhibitory reflex was found in 80% of 15 patients at 7±5 months postoperatively, and 93% at 37±10 months, In a larger group of 49 patients studied at 2 years after operation, the reflex was present in 51%. In these patients where the reflex was present, a positive finding of reflex anal inhibition to ileal pouch distension was associated with a longer duration after pouch construction than in patients without the reflex before the recordings were taken (26 months compared with 15 months), a longer rectal cuff (7±2 cm against 6±1 cm) and a longer efferent limb to the reservoir as delineated at endoscopy (9±1 cm compared with 8±1 cm). However, these differences did not reach statistical significance.

The Mayo clinic group also used a balloon positioned in the ileal pouch, and manometry was performed using a rigid polyglass probe (O'Connell *et al.*, 1988). They found that the 'neorectal anal inhibitory reflex' could be elicited in only 4% of patients. Both of these patients had long rectal cuffs; one had a straight ileoanal anastomosis, the other had undergone J-pouch formation.

Holdsworth and Johnston (1988b) used a low compliance balloon placed at least 10 cm above the anal verge and a water-filled microballoon system, and also defined the reflex as being present if a 20% decrease in pressure was observed. In their patients after end-to-end anastomosis without mucosal proctectomy, the reflex was found in 75%, compared with only 23% after mucosal proctectomy and endoanal anastomosis. The ability to release flatus safely was strongly associated with the presence of the reflex.

Keighley's group, using a balloon and four-lumen perfused catheter system, failed to demonstrate the inhibitory reflex in any of their patients after pouch–anal anastomosis, but again confirmed its presence in 100% of their age- and sex-matched controls (Keighley *et al.*, 1988). In this group of patients 25 had undergone mucosectomy commencing at the dentate line, whilst in five the anal transition zone had been deliberately spared. In the authors' series, the anorectal inhibitory reflex was not elicited in any of our patients, however many retain the ability to discriminate.

It is likely that the inhibitory reflex does indeed represent some form of 'sampling reflex', and as such may be important for retaining normal defaecation. Added weight is given to this arguement in that it can be demonstrated in all control subjects, even when different recording techniques are utilized, and the demonstration that the ability to safely and confidently release flatus is associated with its presence. Others feel that it may provide the individual with an increase in the sensitivity of the discriminatory function.

It is interesting to note that the presence of the reflex appears to increase with time after pouch construction. This, and the fact that it can be demonstrated after this procedure, suggests that there may be growth of intramural nerves across the ileoanal anastomosis (Lane and Parks, 1977). Johnston's results would suggest that if this is indeed the case, then such growth is significantly greater after an end-to-end ileoanal anastomosis, compared with endoanal 'sleeve-type' anastomosis.

This, however, is not the only explanation, and it may be that there is simultaneous distension of the rectal cuff; the pathway for the reflex being via the myenteric plexus. Against this, the St Mark's group did not find any correlation between cuff length and the presence of the reflex, and found that the reflex was sometimes observed when no pressure could have been placed on a short rectal cuff.

The Mayo clinic group have suggested that their consistent failure to demonstrate such an inhibitory reflex, is due to their using a short rectal cuff. Just as likely, is that by using a rigid anal probe within such a short cuff, the reflex may be intact but not detectable.

External sphincter electromyography

Electromyography is a physiological technique permitting the study of the electrical activity generated by muscle fibres, both at rest and during contraction. Upon contraction of a motor unit, the individual action potentials from each muscle fibre summate to form the motor unit action potential.

The pelvic floor musculature consists of a high proportion of small, type I muscle fibres, specialized for tonic contraction, but as with most other skeletal muscle each fibre is innervated by a single motor end-plate.

To proctological practice the major role of electomyography is to provide a functional assessment of the pelvic floor during provocative acts such as coughing and straining, and to study abnormalities of innervation to these muscles, such as in idiopathic faecal incontinence.

Denervation of muscle fibres results in an inability voluntarily to contract that muscle. Hence, electromyographic signs of such a process actually reflect the disordered pattern of reinnervation, and not the denervation per se. Such reinnervation may result from sprouting of unaffected nerves, therefore taking over from the damaged nerves, or possibly axonal regrowth from the damaged nerves themselves. This results in changes in muscle fibre distribution, with loss of the random pattern of motor units, and the formation of small colonies of muscle fibres innervated by the same axon and its branches. This phenomenon can be recognized histologically as fibre-type grouping.

Electromyography requires the use of a recording electrode connected to a pre-amplifier, and hence to an amplifier, an oscilloscope and a loudspeaker. Whilst four forms of recording electrode are available, most proctological studies utilize the two forms of needle electrodes. Such electrodes are inserted into the external sphincter via the perineal skin (Figure 7.9).

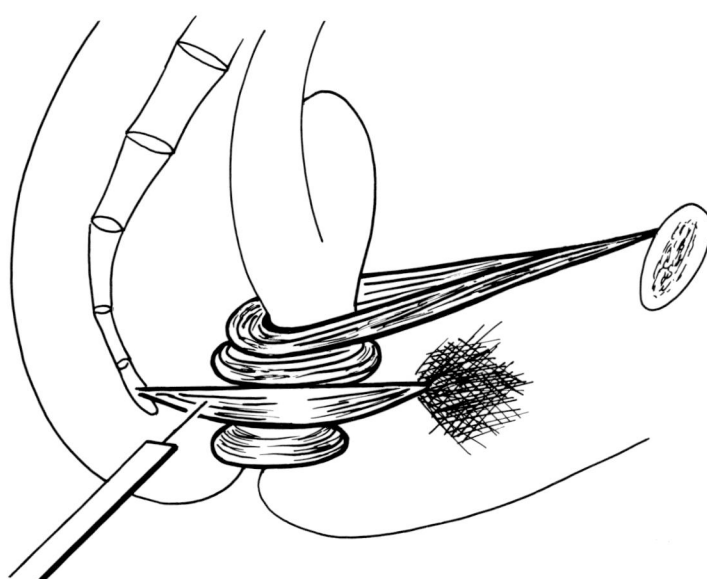

Figure 7.9 External anal sphincter electromyography

The concentric needle electrode consists of a steel wire of diameter 0.1 mm, encased within a thin pointed cannula. Both are separated by an insulating resin. The bare tip of the thin wire is the recording surface of the electrode; the edge of the outer cannula being the reference electrode. This means that the area of uptake of this form of electrode is relatively small, probably involving the territory of several motor units, and provides absolute assurity that any electrical activity monitored is at least from the muscle into which the needle is inserted.

It is therefore evident that should one wish to record the action potentials from a single muscle fibre an electrode with a smaller recording surface is required. Such electrodes have a similar basic design to the concentric needle electrode. Again, a thin needle filled with insulating resin contains a central wire recording electrode. However, in this form of electrode, the latter opens at the mid-shaft of the outer sheath (the reference electrode) presenting a small leading off surface of 25 μm. This device allows the recording of the motor unit potentials of only one or two muscle fibres, and lends itself well to quantitative assessment.

Concentric needle studies of the external sphincter have shown it to have a continuous low frequency activity at rest and during sleep (Floyd and Walls, 1953). Such activity is composed of contractions of individual motor units at low firing rates, and at amplitudes of less than 500 μV. Increases in this basal activity are seen during the rectoanal inhibitory reflex after rectal distension, and on coughing. Defaecation, however, induces electrical silence in the sphincter. Voluntary contraction leads to summation of individual motor unit action potentials, and such potentials may reach amplitudes of 3 mV, with a mean of approximately 500 μV, and a duration of 5–7.5 ms (Bartolo, Jarratt and Read, 1983). Polyphasic action potentials have been found to be present in up to 12% of normal skeletal muscle electromyographs, and have been defined as a potential containing at least four phases (Caruso and Buchthal, 1965). This phenomenon when found in greater numbers in the external sphincter is indicative of reinnervation in a previously partially denervated muscle.

Stryker *et al.* (1985b) studied the electromyographic patterns in 27 patients after ileoanal anastomosis, at a mean of 20 months following closure of the ileostomy. Nine patients had undergone a 3-cm endoanal mucosal proctectomy commencing at the dentate line, rectal eversion being used to facilitate the same extent of mucosectomy in the rest. In 10 patients balloon dilatation of a straight ileoanal anastomosis had been performed, and in 17 patients a pelvic reservoir was constructed (14 J- and three S-pouches). Nine patients were studied who were known to have had poor results with regard to continence (frequent faecal or mucous leakage, the necessity to wear perineal pads, etc.), the remainder having satisfactory continence. At rest, 20 or more motor unit action potentials from all four quadrants of the anal sphincter were characterized as to amplitude, duration, stability, number of turns and number of phases. Recruitment of potentials was also assessed during voluntary contraction and on coughing.

In 18 patients after ileoanal anastomosis, normal patterns of motor unit action potential were observed. Sixteen of these came from the perfect continence group, whilst only two had imperfect continence. In contrast, nine patients had abnormal patterns, such as high-amplitude potentials, prolonged potentials or a high incidence of polyphasic potentials. During voluntary contraction and coughing, three of these nine patients showed decreased motor unit recruitment. Seven of these nine had poor results with regard to continence, whilst only two came from the perfect continence group. There was a significant difference in the duration of potentials between the continent (7.9±2.2 μs) and incontinent groups (6.4±1.3 μs). However, no significant relationship could be demonstrated between both groups in the amplitude/turns ratio, method of mucosal proctectomy, presence of a reservoir or patient sex. Age, however, was significant with all patients over 40 years showing abnormal patterns.

Sharp *et al.* (1987) studied 28 patients preoperatively, and 12 of the same group postoperatively after mucosal proctectomy and ileal pouch–anal anastomosis (26 S- and two J-pouches). Action potential amplitude and duration were assessed in the external sphincter and in the puborectalis muscle using a concentric needle electrode. In the external sphincter the mean resting amplitude was

93 mV preoperatively and 90 mV postoperatively. Values for the contracting amplitude were 260 and 340 mV respectively. The resting puborectalis values were 87 mV before and 71 mV after operation, compared with 323 and 296 mV respectively in the contracting muscle. These figures did not reach statistical significance. It is stated that significance was again not reached with regard to the duration of the action potentials, but the results obtained are not given in this report. Unfortunately, no attempt was made to correlate the results obtained with continence performance or length of follow-up.

The authors' electromyographic assessments of 17 patients at a mean of 26.8±21.1 months after construction of a J-type reservoir (range 6–72 months) have shown a low integrated value for the external sphincter at rest. However, on maximal voluntary squeezing, varying degrees of motor unit recruitment were demonstrated in all patients (75.8±61.4 μVs). On straining, the mean integrated value was 21.9±12.6 μVs.

The Mayo clinic results described above imply that patients with major faecal leakage after this procedure will often demonstrate electromyographic abnormalities consistent with at least partial denervation of the external anal sphincter. It is unlikely that such denervation could occur proximal to the origin of the pudendal nerve, but the precise mechanism involved is as yet uncertain. To date no such abnormalities have been demonstrated in the puborectalis muscle, the exact nerve supply of which is still somewhat contentious.

Pudendal nerve terminal motor latency

The pudendal nerve consists of inferior rectal branches that innervate the external anal sphincter, and perineal branches that innervate the periurethral striated musculature (Figure 7.3). This innervation can be stimulated, and hence quantitatively assessed, at several different levels. This makes this technique a very important research tool.

Pudendal nerve stimulation is performed transrectally, either by utilizing a glove-mounted technique (Kiff, 1983; Kiff and Swash, 1984), or using a bipolar stimulator on the end of a rod (Figure 7.10). Using this technique, square wave stimuli of 0.1 ms

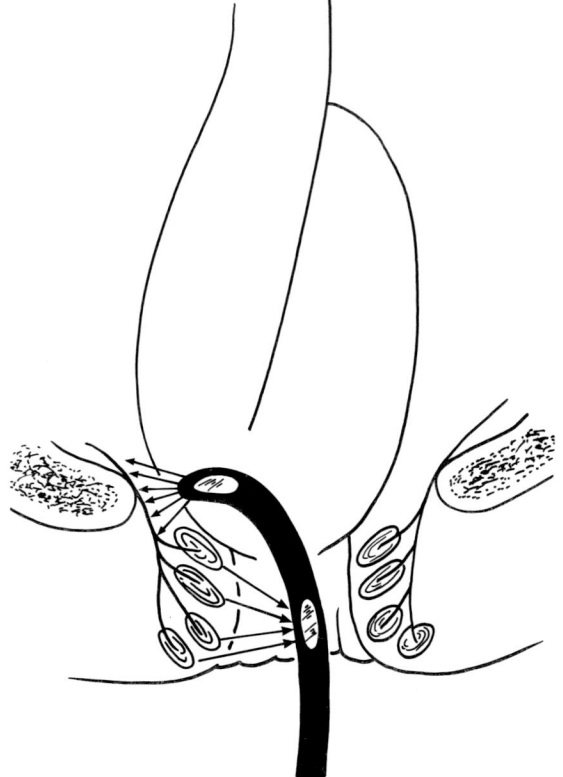

Figure 7.10 Pudendal nerve terminal motor latency

duration and 50 V are given via the stimulating electrodes at 1 s intervals. The optimum site for pudendal nerve stimulation is recognized as that producing the maximum amplitude of the evoked response on the oscilloscope screen, using standard electromyographic amplifier filter settings. Stimulation is performed bilaterally.

After stimulation, the pudendal nerve terminal motor latency of the external anal sphincter response can be calculated from the tracings obtained (Figure 7.11). The normal range as assessed with the glove technique is 2.1±0.2 ms; no correlation being found between pudendal nerve terminal motor latency and increasing age (Snooks and Swash, 1985).

The latency of response off the pelvic floor musculature can be measured from several sites of stimulation (Figure 7.3), for example the cauda equina and the spinal cord. These sites are usually stimulated via transcutaneous

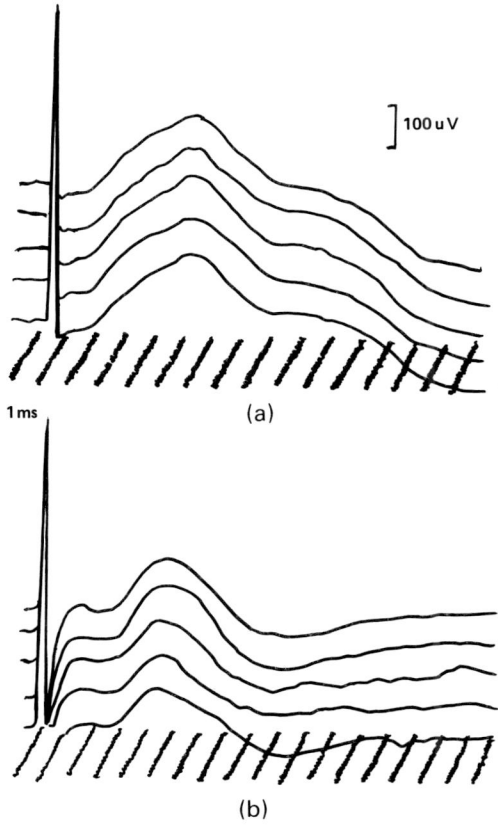

100 µV

1 ms   (a)

(b)

Figure 7.11 Pudendal nerve terminal motor latency tracings

routes in the cervical region and over the first and fourth lumbar vertebrae. Such assessments allow for comparisons of proximal and distal innervation of the sphincter complexes. Research techniques have even been described for electrical transcutaneous stimulation of the pyramidal tract fibres supplying the pelvic floor muscles (Merton and Morton, 1980). Further discussion of these techniques is not relevant to this book, as these research tools are unlikely to be of help in the assessment of patients after restorative proctocolectomy, unless they also have evidence of neurological disease in the spinal cord.

To date the pudendal nerve has received little attention after restorative proctocolectomy. It has been suggested previously that the rectal dissection required for the preparation of the rectal muscular cuff (of whatever length), might result in the loss of the normal pelvic floor support for the abdominal contents (Sharp *et al.*, 1987). This group confirm that in two patients with low resting pressures, pudendal nerve conduction velocity was decreased. However, their method of assessment of pudendal nerve latency, and the values obtained, were not described. Part of their assessment of pudendal nerve function was based upon anorectal sensation to balloon inflation, which they concede is a somewhat imprecise method of assessment.

We have utilized a modified 9-mm endotracheal tube to measure pudendal nerve latency. To this tube are fixed two brass stud receiving electrodes at 4.5 cm from the tip. There are also two stimulating electrodes situated at the tip. Pulsed stimulations of 0.1 ms duration, and between 25 and 150 V were applied to pudendal nerves bilaterally at the level of the ischial spines, thus ensuring supramaximal stimulation of the fastest conducting muscle fibres. Mean pudendal nerve terminal motor latencies to the external anal sphincter were prolonged, and often dramatically so, in patients who had poor functional results. In particular, the inability to defer defaecation correlated with this prolongation. These results suggest that pudendal nerve damage may occur during mucosal proctectomy and pouch–anal anastomosis.

Support for this concept that mucosal proctectomy might be associated with a traction injury to the pudendal nerves has been provided by Emblem *et al.* In an excellent study numerous parameters including external sphincter fibre density, electromyography and histology, anal canal manometry and distal ileal pressure were studied in ten patients who had had to undergo takedown of their ileoanal anastomosis (Emblem *et al.*, 1989). All the patients studied had had straight ileoanal anastomoses, two had undergone abdominal mucosectomy from above with retention of a small segment of mucosa, the other eight had a complete endoanal mucosectomy. The reasons for conversion to a permanent ileostomy were poor continence in seven, excessive frequency in two and mucosal atypia in one. One incontinent patient had normal external sphincter function. In this individual, leakage was associated with high pressure amplitudes in the distal ileum of up to 280 cmH$_2$O. This was more than double the values found in the other nine patients.

This same group had previously demonstrated that incontinence after ileoanal anastomosis was associated with sphincter dysfunction (Emblem, Stein and Morkrid, 1989a). These subsequent studies have demonstrated increased fibre density, excessive external sphincter fibrosis and changes in muscle fibre morphology (see below). All these factors are consistent with reinnervation of the external sphincter after denervation atrophy.

Emblem and his colleagues suggest that traction injury to the pudendal nerves may result from anal dilatation and downward traction. Added weight is given to this argument by the fact that their patients who had undergone abdominal mucosectomy had better clinical and neurophysiological outcomes than in the endoanal mucosectomy group.

Pelvic floor histology

Abnormalities of the pelvic floor musculature have been suggested to be the primary lesion in idiopathic faecal incontinence. The histopathological features associated with idiopathic faecal incontinence have been well described elsewhere (Parks, Swash and Urich, 1977; Neill, Parks and Swash, 1981). Included within these changes are fibre-type grouping (inferring that reinnervation of the external sphincter and puborectalis had occurred), small muscle fibres (suggesting denervation atrophy), hypertrophy of the remaining fibres (especially in the puborectalis) and myopathic changes, such as fibre splitting, fibrosis and fatty degeneration. Abnormalities were not so common, nor so severe in the levator ani muscle in this condition.

Subsequent to the above reports, histometric and histopathological assessments were made of these muscles in patients with rectal prolapse associated with perineal descent. However, features of denervation were less marked, and all abnormalities were less pronounced than in idiopathic incontinence. Rectal prolapse did not appear to be related to abnormalities in pelvic floor muscle morphology (Neill, Parks and Swash, 1981; Henry, Parks and Swash, 1982).

Comparing simple abdominoperineal pull-through with an endorectal pull-through in animals, histological evidence of damage to the pelvic floor was more pronounced after the abdominoperineal approach (Ito *et al.*, 1981). Such features were particularly associated with a more severe reduction in resting anal tone, and loss of the rectoanal reflex, suggesting that the endorectal pull-through was less likely to result in damage to the pelvic floor.

Emblem *et al.* have performed a histological comparison between patients who had to have their ileoanal anastomosis resected, and controls who had undergone a standard extrasphincteric proctectomy for colitis or polyposis (Emblem *et al.*, 1989). Failed ileoanal anastomosis specimens had significantly more fibrosis in the internal sphincter than in the controls. This was particularly prominent adjacent to the submucosa, and was inversely correlated with anal canal resting pressure.

External sphincter dysfunction was also associated with marked, but uniform, external sphincter fibrosis and variations in fibre size, providing further evidence of external sphincter denervation as the aetiological factor (Parks, Swash and Urich, 1977).

Conclusions

Consistently, anal canal resting tone has been shown to be reduced by as much as 50% after mucosal proctectomy and pouch–anal anastomosis. Anal retraction and/or anal canal eversion to facilitate mucosectomy have received much attention as the causal factors. However, recent evidence casts doubt upon this hypothesis. It may also be that denervation of the internal sphincter from above during proctectomy may play a part in reducing resting tone. Inconsistent data pertain to the effects of stapling the ileoanal anastomosis on subsequent internal sphincter function. Clearly more work is required to answer the question of internal sphincter dysfunction after restorative proctocolectomy, but such dysfunction is consistently demonstrated to effect adversely the ultimate functional outcome after this procedure.

Anal canal maximal squeeze pressure as an indicator of external sphincter function is less severely affected after pouch–anal anastomosis. However, many groups have recorded some degree of reduction. Whilst this reduction is not shown reliably to result in a deterioration in function postoperatively, studies have suggested that injury to the nerve supply of the external sphincter may occur, presumably during endoanal retraction and mucosectomy.

8

Pathophysiology of the ileal pelvic reservoir

In Chapter 5, technical aspects regarding the construction of pelvic reservoirs were discussed. In the present chapter, the pathophysiological characteristics of these pouches will be presented.

Pouch capacity and sensation

Using similar basic techniques as those employed in the investigation of anal canal manometry (see Chapter 7), studies can be undertaken to assess numerous parameters of the ileal pouch itself. To aid subsequent comparison, pouch volume has been measured often at the time of construction. The precise relevance of the latter, and how it might change with time, is at present somewhat uncertain, and may vary with pouch design and efferent limb configuration.

In order to attempt to assess the temporal relationship of pouch volume in isoperistaltic side-to-side reservoirs, 20-cm length pouches were created in dogs. Subsequently, pouch volume was measured over several months (Kawarasaki, Fujiwara and Fonkalsrud, 1985). The volume of an isolated 20-cm segment of ileum at a pressure of $10 \, cmH_2O$ was 69 ml. Four weeks after pouch construction, the reservoir had a volume of 203 ml. This had increased again to 458 ml at 8 weeks. During this period, bowel frequency in these animals had decreased from 18 bowel actions per 24 hours to five.

In a series of 25 dogs, both isoperistaltic side-to-side reservoirs and triplicated S-pouches were evaluated to determine which physiological parameters might be of greatest importance to ultimate functional outcome after restorative proctocolectomy (Rosemurgy, Schraut and Block, 1983). Both pouch configurations had either long (6 cm) or short (2 cm) efferent limbs. Comparing the pouches with straight ileoanal anastomoses, a laparotomy was performed at 2-monthly intervals to assess pouch volume, which was defined as the volume required to raise the luminal pressure to $25 \, cmH_2O$. Initially, both the straight anastomosis group and the reservoir groups had similar capacities (82–110 ml). However, by 6 months, both types of reservoir were of significantly greater volume than the straight anastomosis group. In addition, the S-pouch was of significantly greater volume than the double-barrelled pouch. Similarly, those pouches with long efferent conduits attained greater volumes than those with 2-cm efferent limbs, presumably secondary to reservoir outflow obstruction.

Using the technique of saline infusion (Figure 8.1), Keighley has assessed intraoperative volume in 18 stapled J-pouches with 20-cm limbs, and compared these with 15 hand-sewn W-pouches constructed from four 10-cm lengths of ileum (Keighley, Yoshioka and Kmiot, 1988). Mean intraoperative volume was 190 ml (J-pouches) and 230 ml (W-pouches). Functional results in both groups were similar. In particular, no difference was

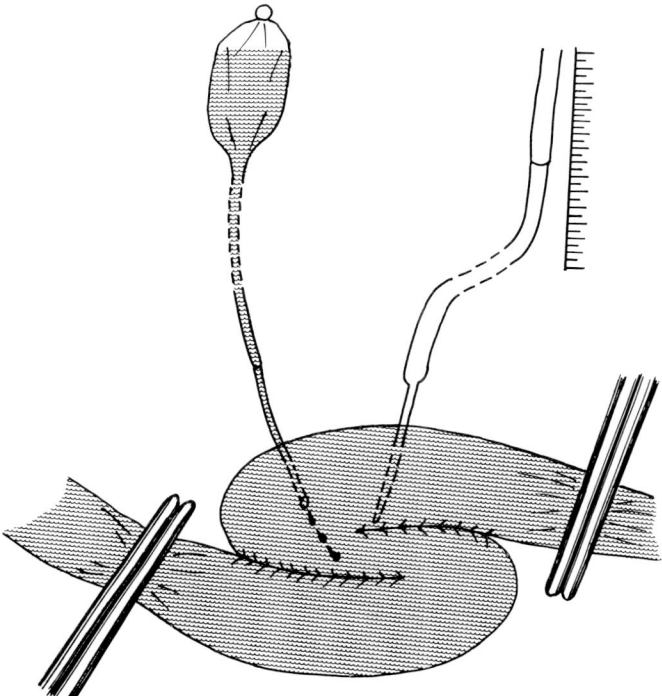

Figure 8.1 Saline-infusion technique

noted with regard to daytime frequency and nocturnal evacuation. This contrasts with the experience from St Mark's Hospital, where W-pouches were associated with a significantly lower evacuation frequency as compared with the S- and J-pouches in the same series (Nicholls and Pezim, 1985). Whilst intraoperative volumes in the S- and J-pouches were similar (177 ml and 172 ml respectively), that in the W reservoir was 325 ml. Further evaluation of reservoir volume was undertaken post ileostomy closure, when respective volumes were 416, 197 and 322 ml. In this series, all pouches were handsewn in two layers, whereas Keighley in his series had used a single layer extramucosal suture technique.

Further assessment of intraoperative volume in W-pouches has come from Everett, who described his clinical results in 60 patients (Everett, 1989). Fifty-three patients had handsewn W-pouches of the staggered configuration, with limb lengths of 12, 15, 12 and 12 cm. Intraoperative volumes were 150–300 ml, figures which were similar to those described elsewhere for a staggered W-pouch of limb lengths 12, 9, 9 and 9 cm (Harms, Pellett and Starling, 1987). In Everett's report, functional results were uniformly satisfactory, tending to negate any possible correlation between volume and function.

Harms and his colleagues from Wisconsin have compared their duplicated and four-loop reservoirs to determine the physiological differences between them (Harms, Pahl and Starling, 1990). In this group of 50 patients, 38 had undergone W-pouch formation. The technique of saline inflation was used to determine intraoperative volume, which for the W-pouches was 199±4 ml. In the S-pouches, the corresponding value was 185±6 ml. A loop ileostomy was used in all patients for an average of 2 months. Interestingly, their operative procedure lasted 7.3±1.1 hours (range 6–10 hours). A double-lumen catheter was used to assess reservoir volume and pressure, allowing for calculation of pouch compliance. Various sensations were recorded, such as initial sensation, normal urge to defaecate, and maximum tolerated volume. Assessments were performed 2 and 12 months after ileostomy closure. The normal volume which produced an urge to defaecation in

J-reservoirs increased from 218 ml at 2 months to 310 ml at 12 months. A similar trend was seen in duplicated reservoirs (201–291 ml). The pressure within the pouches at this volume did not differ between the two designs throughout this period.

The normal evacuation volume was found to correlate inversely with 24-hour stool frequency, which decreased by an average of three in both groups throughout the first year after ileostomy closure. In addition, the reduction in frequency appeared to be correlated with an increase in pouch compliance, as the increase in normal evacuation volume was achieved without any significant increase in intrapouch pressure. Both these pouch designs appeared, in these surgeon's hands, to produce very similar functional outcomes, which were associated with similar compliance profiles.

Thomson has developed a mathematical equation for the assessment of ileal pouch capacity (Thomson, Simpson and Wheeler, 1987). Starting from the premise that both J- and W-pouches can be considered as closed cylinders (one long and narrow, the other short and wide), then it should be theoretically possible to calculate volumes for any given length and radius of pouch. The following equations were developed, where $b=$ ileal circumferences:

for a J-pouch with 20-cm limbs:

$$\text{volume} = \frac{2b^2(30-b)}{3\pi^2}$$

for a W-pouch with 10-cm limbs:

$$\text{volume} = \frac{8b^2(30-2b)}{3\pi^2}$$

If the ileal circumference is taken to be 5–7 cm, then the J-pouch volume calculates to 150–290 cm^3, whilst the W-pouch is 250–440 cm^3. This would therefore suggest that for any given length of ileum utilized, the more nearly spheroid W configuration of pouch will result in the greatest subsequent volume. These calculations assumed that a one-layer anastomosis, or using stapling devices, will result in a small but quantifiable loss in available ileal cicumference. Assuming a loss of 2 mm of ileum at each inverted suture line, Thomson calculates that J- and W-pouch volumes will be reduced by 15% and 13.6% respectively.

O'Connell and colleagues have correlated pouch volume with functional outcome in 23 patients (19 J- and four S-pouches) at a mean of 2 years after pouch construction (O'Connell *et al.*, 1987a). These particular patients were chosen as they represented a suitable cross-section of clinical outcome. Ten patients (seven J- and three S-pouches) had a good result, i.e. six or fewer stools per day and perfect continence, whilst 13 (12 J- and one S-pouch) had a fair result. This was defined as more than six stools per day and only episodic minor incontinence. Eight controls were also studied. Capacity was assessed using a 600-ml non-compliant, thin-walled flaccid bag. Without formal bowel preparation, other than a phosphate enema in the controls, the bag was inserted into the rectum or ileal pouch and inflated with 10–20 ml increments of air up to the maximum tolerated capacity. This was perceived by the patient as a continuous discomfort associated with the desire to defaecate. The maximum pouch capacity was 320±36 ml, whereas in the controls the rectal capacity was 330±29 m. These figures did not reach statistical significance. However, the maximum capacity was statistically greater in those patients who had a good functional result compared to those with imperfect continence and excessive frequency (409±33 ml and 290±27 ml respectively). This compares with a capacity of 248 ml, which this same group had recorded 4 months after straight ileoanal anastomosis (Heppell *et al.*, 1982).

It would appear from this report, that in order to obtain a satisfactory result after restorative proctocolectomy the maximum tolerated pouch volume should be significantly greater than that of the normal rectum. Whilst overall the patient group had similar results to the controls, those patients with maximum volumes similar to the controls tended to have had a poor functional result.

Using a soft rubber balloon attached to a stiff polyethylene cannula, Pescatori and Parks (1984a) measured pouch capacity in 50 S-pouches at 20±16 months after closure of the loop ileostomy. Functional capacity was defined as that volume at which a desire to defaecate was reported, whilst maximal capacity was recorded when urgency or pain occurred. The effect of time on volume was quantitated in 17 patients who were assessed at 7±5 and 37±10 months. Pouch functional capacity was 267 ± 121 ml, whilst maximal capacity was 450 ± 204 ml of air at 20 months, and had increased to 487 ± 190 ml at 37 months. Few patients in this group were able to evacuate spontaneously their pouch, and required the use of routine catheterization. Comparing temporal changes between W- and S-pouches, pouch evacuation volumes 2 months after ileostomy closure were 218 ± 9 ml and 201 ± 14 ml respectively (Harms, Pahl and Starling, 1990). Corresponding volumes after 12 months were 310 ± 12 ml and 291 ± 22 ml. This group found that this measured volume was the strongest predictor of stool frequency.

Pouch compliance

As mentioned in the previous section, synchronous measurement of reservoir volume and intraluminal pressure allows for calculation of the vessel compliance, by the equation V/P. Rectal distension induces an initial pressure rise within the normal rectum. Thereafter, reflex rectal contraction may result in a further pressure rise (Duthie and Bennett, 1963). This is one part of the anorectal inhibitory reflex discussed in the previous chapter.

After this secondary, reflex-induced pressure rise, the rectal intraluminal pressure slowly falls back to a new baseline. Further increments of volume increases induce similar changes. A stage is eventually reached where further rectal accommodation to volume increases cannot occur. Any subsequent volume increases are followed by proportional increases in intraluminal pressure. It is at this stage that lower abdominal discomfort and the intense desire to defaecate may be felt.

If the volume/pressure relationship is plotted, the gradient of the curve achieved equates to rectal compliance. As with all such techniques, methodological variations may affect the results obtained. For example, the material from which the intrarectal balloon is made, and its elastic properties, may be important. Consequently, we feel that the value of these techniques is not at its greatest when comparing results between the differing reservoirs used by various surgeons. Their value is more in allowing the determination of the importance of compliance with regard to poor and satisfactory functional results in individual

series, particularly if different reservoirs have been utilized or other correlations made. In addition, reservoir compliance is dependent upon the surrounding structures. Such compliance measurements taken after pouch excision demonstrate that the ileal pouches are more compliant *ex vivo* (Thayer *et al.*, 1990).

Assessing these characteristics after ileoanal anastomosis with balloon dilatation, Stryker *et al.* studied 12 controls against 12 young patients (Stryker, Telander and Perrault, 1985). Six of the patients had good functional outcomes, whereas six had imperfect results. A four-channel probe was used to assess distensibility at an intraluminal pressure of 25 mmHg. In the controls, normal rectum had a compliance of 330 ml at 25 mmHg, whereas the patients with satisfactory results had a neorectal compliance of 200 ml. This compared with the value of 150 ml for those patients with a less than satisfactory result. This early study showed that after straight ileal anastomosis, ultimate neorectal compliance is important with regard to ultimate functional outcome.

Specifically assessing important factors in determining functional outcome, 23 patients (19 J- and 14 S-pouches) were studied at a mean of 2 years postoperatively (O'Connell *et al.*, 1987a). These patients were selected to represent a reasonable spectrum of functional results, and were compared with eight healthy controls. A 600-ml non-compliant, thin-walled floppy balloon was inserted into the pouch or rectum with the patient in the left lateral position. Within this balloon was a non-perfused catheter connected to a water-filled strain gauge transducer. This allowed for measurement of the intraluminal pressure, and hence compliance could be calculated. In the ileal pouch group, compliance was 14.7 ± 1.4 ml/mmHg compared with 18.6 ± 2.8 ml/mmHg in the controls. There was no significant difference between these results. Similarly, no significant difference was determined between the good result group of 10 patients and the poor result group of 13 patients (16.2 ± 2.5 and 13.4 ± 1.6 ml/mmHg respectively). This therefore confirmed reports that ileal reservoir compliance is like that of the healthy rectum. Also that in this group compliance did not appear to relate to outcome.

In a controlled study, 30 patients (19 J- and 11 W-pouches) were assessed at a mean of 28 months postoperatively (Keighley *et al.*, 1988).

A specially designed clinical scoring system allowed subdivision of these patients into those with good and those with imperfect results. Pouch manometry was performed using a four-lumen catheter. Rectal compliance was found to be significantly better than the ileal pouches (12 ml/cmH$_2$O and 6 ml/cmH$_2$O respectively). When considering the pouch subgroups, the corresponding values were 10 ml/cmH$_2$O for the W-reservoirs, whilst the duplicated pouches had a mean value of 4 ml/cmH$_2$O. It was concluded that the four-limb W-pouch has a pressure/volume advantage over the duplicated J-pouch.

Pouch motility patterns

Under normal resting conditions the rectum exerts a low basal pressure of some 5 cmH$_2$O. In addition, the maintenance of an intraluminal rectal pressure catheter reveals that there is little basal rectal motility. Rectal distension results in three patterns of contractility: simple non-propagated contractions (frequency 10/min), slower non-propagated contractions (3/min), and propagated slow contractions (3/min). Amplitudes ranged up to 100 cmH$_2$O. Whilst non-propagated contractions were universal, propagated contractions were absent in 85% of individuals (Scharli and Kiesewetter, 1970).

The St Mark's group have assessed 11 patients with S-shaped ileal reservoirs and compared them to seven patients with ileostomies (two Brooke and five loop). They recorded pressures at three sites within the reservoir system as described in Chapter 17 (Rabau, Percy and Parks, 1982). A balloon attached to a double-lumen water-filled polyethylene tube was introduced into the pouch. This facilitated filling of the pouch and synchronous pressure recording. Single phasic waves were witnessed in both groups, and the characteristics of these waves did not significantly differ between them. Their duration ranged from 3 to 9 seconds, with an amplitude of 5–30 cmH$_2$O. In the efferent limb the amplitude was 10–60 cmH$_2$O, with a similar duration. In addition, tonic waves were observed, which tended to last longer than the phasic waves (15–120 seconds with an amplitude of 10±5 cmH$_2$O). This was less than that

recorded in either the terminal ileum or the efferent limb of the pouch (20–50 cmH$_2$O, and 35±20 cmH$_2$O respectively). These tonic waves tended to occur in a sequential manner between the pouch and the efferent limb. The instilled volume required to induce tonic contractions was 322 ml for the reservoir and 30 ml for the terminal ileostomy. Hence, the ileal reservoir demonstrated features of a capacitance organ, whilst retaining its ileal characteristics.

The relative proportions of tonic wave forms varied throughout the study. In the fasting state, phasic waves were the predominant form, occupying 31.3% of the time in the reservoir and 51% in the efferent limb. Very little time was occupied by tonic wave forms. Eating increased the total time occupied by activity to 57.1%, with a modest increase in tonic activity. A similar result occurred in the efferent limb. Reservoir distension during fasting resulted in a marked increase in both total activity and, to a greater degree, tonic wave contraction duration. This was witnessed in the pouch and efferent limb. Even more pronounced effects were seen in the pouch upon postprandial reservoir distension, with total activity increasing to 78.1% of the time and tonic activity occupying 49.9%.

Tonic waves resulted in the passage of effluent from the ileostomy, and in the desire to defaecate in the pouch patients. That such waves are propulsive was shown by the observation that if external sphincter contraction was voluntarily resisted, their presence resulted in faecal leakage.

Experimental evidence of reservoir motility came in the following year (Rosemurgy, Schraut and Block, 1983). Twenty-five dogs, six with straight ileoanal anastomoses and 19 after ileal reservoir construction, were studied. Nine animals had S-pouches (six with long and three with short efferent legs), and ten had antiperistaltic double-barrelled reservoirs (seven with long and three with short efferent legs). Reservoir motility patterns were studied by using a compliant latex balloon introduced into the pouch or distal ileum under light anaesthesia. Water was instilled into the balloon to a pressure of 20–25 cmH$_2$O. The balloon was connected to a strain gauge transducer allowing continuous pressure recording. Records were obtained synchronously with electromyographic recordings, allowing for the corrrelation between such electrical activity and any resultant pressure changes within the reservoir lumen. Strong and frequent pressure waves were seen in all animals studied, and appeared to be the initiating stimulus for defaecation. In those animals with a straight anastomosis, propulsive pressure waves with an amplitude of 20–50 cmH$_2$O and frequency of 6–10 per hour were witnessed. Such waves followed bursts of electrical spike activity. In the reservoir group, only synchronous limb contraction generated propulsive pressure waves. Not surprisingly perhaps, these were more commonly seen in the isoperistaltic double-barrelled reservoir as compared to the triplicated pouch with its antiperistaltic segment. Dysynchronous spike activity within the reservoirs was associated with only minimal increases in intraluminal pressure. This tended to result in a churning type of movement within the pouch.

In empty or only partially filled pouches, very little motility or electrical activity was seen. Contractions were at one or less per hour and with an amplitude of 10 cmH$_2$O. Filling of the reservoirs to a pressure of 25 cmH$_2$O, resulted in repetitive bursts of synchronous spike activity, with an associated increase in both amplitude and frequency of the recorded pressure waves. At the time of construction, the double-barrelled reservoir generated more frequent, stronger waves (amplitude 20–40 cmH$_2$O at a frequency of 6–8 per hour) than did the S-pouch. The presence of a long efferent limb resulted in a decrease in such activity, which in the case of the triplicated reservoir caused it to become an atonic bag by 4 months. The double-barrelled reservoir tended to retain both its contractile and electrical properties, particularly when it was placed proximal to a 2-cm efferent spout (2–8 waves per hour, amplitude 15–45 cmH$_2$O).

Using a double-lumen catheter to which a large floppy balloon was fixed, pouch motility was found to show a steady increase in low amplitude waves (5–19 mmHg). As the volume of the balloon was increased over 150 ml, higher amplitude tonic contractions were recorded (25–50 mmHg). As the volume reached 350 ml or so propulsive contractions increased (Harms, Pahl and Starling, 1990). This group found that low frequency contractions of less than 10 mmHg in general were not associated with any clinical desire to evacuate the pouch.

Amplitudes greater than 25 mmHg, especially if associated with waves of higher frequency, were important in inducing the desire to defaecate. This sensation was related to the contraction wave itself, rather than to the increase in intraluminal pressure per se. Interestingly, 60% of patients with S-pouches felt the desire to defaecate synchronous with these waves, whereas only 40% of patients with W-pouches did so.

Using an isobaric manovolumetric method in order to assess J-pouch motility, Oresland and colleagues reported pronounced motility within the reservoirs as compared to normal rectum. Even at higher distension volumes, such activity was easily recorded. Importantly, such high pressure patterns were associated with a poor functional outcome (Oresland *et al.*, 1990a).

Pouch absorption

Decreased water absorption has previously been described in the continent ileostomy (Philipson, Kock, Robinson *et al* 1975). Regarding the ileal pelvic pouch, in a study of 18 dogs (six after S-pouch formation, six after lateral reservoir formation, and six controls), water absorption was assessed using polyethylene glycol (Kojima, Sanada and Fonkalsrud, 1982b). Water absorption was found to be significantly greater in both reservoir groups as compared to the controls. That in the lateral reservoir group was slightly greater than that in the S-pouch group. In a further study, Fonkalsrud studied 12 dogs (Kawarasaki, Fujiwara and Fonkalsrud, 1985). A colectomy and ileorectal anastomosis was performed, or a 20-cm double-barrelled isoperistaltic reservoir constructed. Saline absorption was quantitated by injecting a known volume into either the normal ileal segment or into the reservoir. After 1 hour, the residual volume was measured. For a normal 20-cm ileal segment, the saline absorption was 29 ml/hour/20 cm. At 4 weeks post construction, the reservoir value was 74 ml/hour/20 cm, and at 2 months this had increased further to 106 ml/hour/20 cm. Over the same period, pouch volume had increased to 458 ml, compared to 69 ml for the control ileal segment.

Studying the long-term effects of both S-pouches and antiperistaltic double-barrelled reservoirs in 19 dogs, six animals were compared after straight ileoanal anastomosis (Rosemurgy, Schraut and Block, 1983). Water absorption was assessed using 14C-labelled polyethylene glycol as a non-absorbable marker. At 6 months, dogs with a straight ileoanal anastomosis had an absorption of 55 ± 10 ml/hour. This compared with 35 ± 5 ml/hour in those animals with S-pouches. These figures were significantly different. The double-barrelled pouches were not significantly different from either of the other groups (44 ± 12 ml/hour). Interestingly, animals with clinical features of pouch outlet obstruction had the lowest values of water absorption within their pouches. Unfortunately, this group did not correlate these results with histological features and long efferent conduits which were also assessed in this report. It is likely that their histological findings, such as villous atrophy, are responsible for the finding of reduced water absorption.

Pouch electrical patterns

In a study of myoelectrical activity of lateral and J-pouches, these reservoirs were constructed in rabbits (Stone *et al.*, 1986). In ten animals J-pouches with 10-cm limbs were fashioned, whilst 10-cm-limbed lateral isoperistaltic reservoirs were created in a further ten animals. These were compared with three controls. Electrodes and strain gauges were connected to the afferent limb of the pouch, to both limbs of the pouch itself, and to the efferent limb. Two forms of electrical activity were noted, short spike burst complexes (SSBC) characterized as lasting for longer than 25 seconds but less than 3 minutes, and long spike burst complexes (LSBC) which lasted for longer than 3 minutes. SSBC appeared to be synchronous with intestinal contractions, and LSBC were associated with prolonged propulsion. LSBC were only infrequently observed in all three groups. In the controls, they were synchronous with propulsion, however in the reservoir groups they appeared to occur in random fashion until at least 12 weeks after pouch construction. After this period they began to be associated with propulsive activity. Such electrical patterns were more frequently seen, and were of longer

duration, in the lateral reservoirs as compared to the J-pouches. SSBC were propagated through the lateral reservoir as early as 2 weeks after pouch construction, whereas in the J-pouch at least 8 weeks passed before such electrical activity was witnessed.

This study therefore demonstrated that there is a period of healing during which reservoir electrical activity is abnormal. The lateral type of reservoir construction appears to return to normal quicker than the J-pouch. However, both groups were effective in allowing propagation of such activity within 3 months of pouch formation. It is likely that this may be due to the antiperistaltic segment of the J-pouch. In addition, this reservoir configuration requires a distal end-to-side anastomosis to restore continuity. This may infer that a longer healing time might be required for J-pouches as compared to the lateral isoperistaltic reservoir.

Similar results were provided by the same group from UCLA working with dogs (Kawarasaki, Fujiwara and Fonkalsrud, 1983, 1985). In these studies, animals underwent either colectomy with a two-layer ileorectal anastomosis to a 5-cm rectal cuff, or formation of a 20-cm-limbed lateral isoperistaltic reservoir. Standard electrocardiograph electrodes were placed on the bowel to assess electrical activity. In the ileorectal anastomosis group, slow electrical waves were seen at a frequency of 15/min. Immediately after pouch construction, such patterns were observed at 10.2/min, increasing to 13.5/min at 8 weeks post reservoir construction. Throughout this period, slow wave amplitude was also reduced as compared to normal. Both amplitude and wave frequency attained virtual normality after 8 weeks. It was noted that pouch distension resulted in a reduction in the rhythmicity of these wave forms.

Further experimental evaluation of reservoir myoelectrical properties has been combined with motility recording in order to assess the physiological significance of such electrical activity (Rosemurgy, Schraut and Block, 1983). In this series, 25 dogs underwent either straight ileoanal anastomosis (six), S-pouch construction (nine) or isoperistaltic double-barrelled reservoir construction (ten). In both pouch designs, both long and short efferent limbs were assessed. After 8 weeks, a laparotomy was performed and bipolar electrodes were implanted on the serosal surface of the terminal ileum of the straight anastomosis, or onto all limbs of the reservoirs. This allowed for frequent recordings of both slow waves and spike discharges. Neorectal motility was monitored by a compliant water-filled balloon. Interestingly, strong and frequent pressure waves were seen to initiate defaecation. In those animals with a straight anastomosis, propulsive pressure waves with an amplitude of 20–50 cmH$_2$O and frequency of 6–10 per hour, followed bursts of electrical spike activity.

In the reservoir group, only synchronous limb contractions generated propulsive pressure waves. Not surprisingly perhaps, these were more commonly seen in the isoperistaltic double-barrelled reservoir as compared to the triplicated pouch with its antiperistaltic segment. Dysynchronous spike activity within the reservoirs was associated with only minimal increases in intraluminal pressure, this produced a churning action within the pouch. Filling of the reservoirs resulted in repetitive bursts of synchronous spike activity, with an associated increase in both amplitude and frequency of the recorded pressure waves. At the time of construction, the double-barrelled reservoir generated more frequent, stronger waves than did the S-pouch. The presence of a long efferent limb resulted in a decrease in such activity, which in the case of the triplicated reservoir caused it to become an atonic bag by 4 months. The double-barrelled reservoir tended to retain its contractile and electrical properties, particularly when proximal to a 2-cm efferent spout (2–8 waves per hour, amplitude 15–45 cmH$_2$O).

Reservoir electrical pacing

All gastrointestinal reservoirs tend to function at less than optimal predicted levels. In Chapter 10, studies using radiolabelled media document the efficiency of ileal pelvic reservoir emptying. Whilst results vary, even within the same series, it is not uncommon for patients to evacuate less than 60% or so of the pouch contents. It is well documented that the normal rectum empties virtually completely upon defaecation (Heppell *et al.*, 1987).

Electrical stimulation of various intestinal segments has been described (Gillespie, 1962; Fox *et al.*, 1984). Such stimulation has tended to be used in order to control the slow wave frequency (i.e. intestinal pacing), and may induce the secretion of motilin from the gut wall (see Chapter 10). Several workers have attempted to control small bowel motility *in vivo*, and have been successful in improving such parameters as transit time and absorption (Sawchuk, Nogami and Goto, 1986). However, such stimulation has not been shown to induce genuine peristalsis.

We are aware of only one report in which an attempt has been made to control an ileal pouch by electrical stimulation (Grundfest-Broniatowski *et al.*, 1988; Moritz *et al.*, 1989). After initial experiments to determine the optimal features of the stimulating electrodes and their placement, J-configuration ileal pouches with 7-cm limbs were constructed in four dogs. The distal outlet of the pouch was situated some 15 cm proximal to the caecum. Four pairs of flat stimulating electrodes were sewn to the pouch serosa, one each at the entry and exit of the pouch, and one each at 5-cm intervals along the pouch. Three pairs of nonpolar disk electromyography electrodes were fixed to the bowel, one at the apex of the pouch, one 1 cm proximal to the afferent opening, and one 1 cm distal to the exit of the pouch. Intestinal intraluminal pressure was monitored by three perfused catheters. Electrical stimulation was applied in pulse trains of 30 seconds duration. By varying the frequency, amplitude and pulse width the optimal values were assessed. This group did not attempt to coordinate their simulation with the slow wave, and have therefore termed their technique 'coordinated electrical stimulation', rather than intestinal pacing. Coordinated electrical stimulation resulted in reliable pouch contraction. Contrast studies demonstrated that the pouches were static and failed to empty in the unstimulated state. Stimulation, however, resulted in complete reservoir emptying in approximately 12 seconds. The mechanism was though to be related to activation of intrinsic neurones within the bowel wall, with subsequent motilin release.

With the use of biocompatible materials, using appropriate electrical parameters for stimulation, and insulating the system from other muscles, the authors of this report feel that there may be a clinical role for this technique. The results obtained showed that ileal pouches can be emptied completely upon voluntary contraction induced by coordinated electrical stimulation. It appeared to be important that optimal characteristics are used (30-s trains of 6 Hz, 50-ms pulses of amplitude 15–20 mA). However, it was not necessary formally to 'pace' the small intestinal slow wave.

Pouch mucosal blood flow

It has been well documented that the blood supply to the ileal pelvic reservoir is critical with regard to such factors as pouch healing and avoidance of ileoanal anastomosis dehiscence. As a consequence of this, the anatomy of the superior mesenteric artery, and the surgical techniques which may result in mesenteric lengthening have received much attention (see Chapter 5). To date, however, pouch mucosal blood flow has received little such attention.

Fluorescein flowmetry has been utilized to study mucosal blood flow at the time of pouch construction (Perbeck, Lindquist and Liljeqvist, 1985). This group from the Karolinska Institute constructed a mathematical model to distinguish between mucosal and seromuscular blood flow. Fluorescein flowmetry allows measurement of relative capillary blood flow in the intestine. However, it is only accurate to a depth of 0.6 mm. This implies that the mucosal layer must be exposed if its blood flow is to be determined. By producing a reliable mathematical model which allows prediction of the mucosal blood flow from that in the seromuscular layer, intraoperative assessment of pouch mucosal blood flow can be obtained after ileoanal anastomosis. They termed this predictive model 'indirect mucosal fluorescein flowmetry'. Having validated this model, these investigators went on to study pouch mucosal blood flow in 14 patients, and fluorescein flowmetry in the ileoanal anastomosis in eight patients. Compared with the normal controls, the pouch mucosal blood flow was reduced to 88% if the ileocolic artery or the distal mesenteric branch of the superior mesenteric artery were left intact. However, if any of these vessels was sacrificed, mucosal blood flow was reduced to 58% of normal. This reached statistical significance ($P<0.05$). Compared with the normal intestine, the blood flow to the ileoanal anastomosis at the time of construction was only 23%. The mucosa at the anastomosis had a blood flow of 30% of that of the normal mucosa. No difference was noted in the blood flow to J- or S-type pouches (five and three cases respectively).

These results re-emphasized the importance of the vascular supply of the ileal pouch, particularly in relation to the ileoanal anastomosis. Unfortunately, no attempt has been made to correlate intraoperative mucosal blood flow with subsequent clinical performance. At the admission of the authors, this technique, whilst obviously reproducible, is very time consuming. It is therefore unlikely to be widely adopted in the clinical situation. What might be of importance is whether pouch mucosal blood flow can be correlated to any specific postoperative problem, or to a poor functional result in general.

Keighley's group has attempted to shed more light on this subject (Sakaguchi et al., 1989; Keighley et al., 1990). Using a laser Doppler probe passed via the biopsy channel of a flexible sigmoidoscope, multiple readings of flux were taken from the four quadrants of the pouch itself; from the afferent limb of ileum, and from patients with permanent ileostomies. Pouch flux was found to be lower than in permanent ileostomies. In those patients with clinical pouchitis, the flux was lower than in normal pouches. There was no difference between the fluxes in J- and W-pouches. These findings suggest that reservoir ischaemia may be an aetiological factor in the pathogenesis of pouchitis.

In order to assess whether relative tissue ischaemia may occur during ileal pull-through, the technique of intraoperative tissue oxymetry has been utilized. This is an easily performed technique allowing for the evaluation of tissue oxygen levels at several sites within the pouch. It has been demonstrated previously that a low tissue oxygen level predisposes to anastomotic dehiscence (Sackier and Wood, 1988). Recent evidence suggests that tissue oxygen is reduced after pouch construction, especially at the apex of the reservoir. Interestingly, stapled pouches may be associated with a localized reperfusion injury. It is suggested that this may potentiate subsequent ischaemia (Fozard, Lowndes and Young, 1990).

Reservoir histology

Early in the relatively short history of restorative proctocolectomy, came recognition that histopathological abnormalities were relatively common (Kojima, Sanada and Fonkalsrud, 1982b). In this experimental study, 18 dogs underwent colectomy. Six animals did not undergo reservoir formation, whilst six animals each had either an S- or a lateral pouch constructed. Both conventional light and electron microscopy were used to assess pouch morphology. Inflammatory changes were frequently seen, particularly within the S-pouches. Precise morphometric analysis was not provided in this report. Shortening of villi, mucosal ulcerations, and submucosal inflammation were common features in a further experimental study (Rosemurgy, Schraut and Block, 1983). Such features were particularly common in reservoirs with long efferent conduits, especially if associated with faecal stasis. Additional confirmation of the presence of such abnormalities came from a study of eight patients from Italy (Fiorentini *et al.*, 1987). This group noted that seven patients had evidence of mild inflammation within their reservoirs, whilst one patient demonstrated subtotal villous atrophy. Hence, abnormalities were universal within this small series. However, further investigation of these findings was not provided.

Studying a cohort of 92 patients from St Mark's Hospital, mucosal biopsy specimens were assessed for the appearance and severity of both acute and chronic inflammation, villous atrophy and histochemical staining for mucins (Shepherd *et al.*, 1987). This group included 78 patients who had undergone ileal reservoir construction for ulcerative colitis, 12 patients with familial polyposis, and two patients for whom a pouch had been fashioned for 'functional' bowel disease (one patient with Hirschsprung's disease, and one young adult with an ileostomy after having necrotizing enterocolitis as a child). Sigmoidoscopic biopsies were taken of the pouches at 6-monthly intervals for the first year after ileostomy closure. Standard methods for fixing and processing the specimens were employed, prior to staining with haematoxylin and eosin.

Apart from 13% of the initial biopsies taken at 6 months, all specimens demonstrated histological and architectural abnormalities. The former mentioned samples showed a relatively normal small intestinal mucosa. In the rest, the majority demonstrated chronic inflammatory changes and abnormal villous architecture.

Assessing the chronic changes in more detail, all cell types associated with chronic inflammation (lymphocytes, eosinophils, histiocytes and plasma cells) were witnessed. Such changes were usually associated with varying degrees of villous atrophy. The more severe forms of villous atrophy were predominantly related to acute inflammatory changes, and were always accompanied by pronounced crypt hyperplasia. As a consequence, an appearance resembling colonic mucosa was produced. This, when compounded by extensive chronic inflammation, produced a picture not unlike that associated with chronic ulcerative colitis in remission.

Even in the face of acute and severe inflammation, the intraepithelial lymphocyte count rarely exceeded 5% of the total epithelial cell count. This was a significant difference between the appearances of the pouch mucosa from that in untreated coeliac disease. Otherwise subtotal villous atrophy and crypt hyperplasia led to similar histological features. Chronic inflammatory bowel disease in either the small or large intestine, may result in pyloric metaplasia. Again the St Mark's group demonstrated such findings, if only rarely, in the ileal reservoirs. In these patients it was associated with previous episodes of acute inflammation. Histological features consistent with the diagnosis of mucosal prolapse of the rectum, and solitary ulcer syndrome (villous atrophy, fibromuscular obliteration of the lamina propria and crypt cell hyperplasia) were found in two of the biopsies. Both of these patients had clinical evidence of mucosal prolapse within the pouch.

Acute inflammatory changes were less common. A mild, superficial inflammation occurred in 64% of the colitics and 50% of the polyposis patients. Extensive acute changes, including crypt abscesses and ulceration, were seen in 7% of the patients, all of whom were colitics. Such histological findings were always associated with clinical pouchitis. Reactive hyperplasia was associated with severe acute inflammation, however no evidence could be found of dysplasia within the reservoir. Two mildly dysplastic adenomatous polyps were found within the pouches of two patients with polyposis.

Apart from the above described inflammatory features, this group also studied intestinal mucin in 32 patients within the same series. For

25 of these patients, specimens of terminal ileum obtained at the original colectomy were available for comparison. Assessment was performed using high diamine–alcian blue (HID-AB) and periodate borohydride–potassium hydroxide–periodic acid Schiff (PB-KOH-PAS) stains. The PB-KOH-PAS stain was not found to be particularly useful, as the normal small intestinal mucosa also tended to stain well.

Using HID-AB, each specimen was graded for blue predominance (small intestinal goblet cell type), a mixed pattern, or brown predominance (colorectal goblet cell type). The blue staining implies that there is a high content of sialic acid within the mucin. A change to brown staining indicates an increased sulphate content.

The small intestine at the time of colectomy was normal in 96% of cases. In one patient, a significant terminal ileal inflammation was associated with a predominantly brown reaction using HID-AB. After 6 months, the first biopsy usually showed a predominantly blue reaction. In many patients, subsequent specimens demonstrated a change to a predominantly brown staining. Utilizing HID-AB, 50% of specimens (80% of which were from patients with ulcerative colitis) demonstrated extensive brown predominance. This change was associated with chronic inflammation. Half of the colitics with acute pouchitis developed a similar pattern.

This then was the first major description of the epithelial changes which accompany the pelvic pouch procedure, and emphasized that the pouch lining was not normal. Further surveillance was therefore required, and has come from other groups performing such procedures.

The Leeds group recently reported their results of a detailed study of, amongst other things, pouch mucosal morphology and its possible relationship to parameters such as functional result and reservoir ecology (Nasmyth *et al.*, 1989a). Twenty-nine patients with ulcerative colitis were studied. Fifteen of these had undergone ileoanal pouch construction, and were at a median of 6.4 months post ileostomy closure (range 3–31 months). The other 14 had undergone conventional procto-colectomy with Brooke ileostomy formation at a median of 59 months previously (range 4–204 months). Control ileal mucosa was obtained from patients undergoing right hemicolectomy for neoplasm. Sigmoidoscopic biopsies were taken from the pouch patients, whilst a Watson capsule was utilized to procure samples from the ileostomy patients. Standard histopathological techniques were used to process the samples which were stained with haematoxylin and eosin. Each specimen was assessed by a pathologist without prior knowledge of the clinical details of the patient. A scale of 0 (absent) to 3 (severe) was used to assess four criteria for mucosal inflammation (chronic inflammatory cell infiltrate, acute inflammatory cell infiltrate, crypt cell hyperplasia and fibrosis of the lamina propria). In addition, a quantitative analysis of villous atrophy was performed using an image analyser. This allowed appraisal of features such as the length of the mucosal surface, area of the lamina propria, mucosal thickness, crypt depth and villous height. Villous atrophy was defined in terms of the ratios of mucosal surface length to area of the lamina propria, and of the villous height to mucosal thickness.

The ileal pouches showed several abnormalities, including inflammation of the lamina propria, villous flattening, and elongation of the crypts. There was no significant difference between the duplicated and triplicated reservoirs in the series. Other parameters such as faecal bacterial counts, faecal volatile fatty acids, clinically defined function or scintigraphic assessment of pouch emptying did not correlate with these histological findings. With regard to morphometric analysis, the controls did not differ from the ileostomy patients. However, villous atrophy was a feature of patients with pouches, and was directly related to the number of *Bacteroides* sp. isolated from the pouch effluent. Villous atrophy was inversely related to the concentration of faecal butyrate. Crypt depth was greater in the reservoir group than in either of the other groups. Such morphometric indices were not related to the time period since the original colectomy, nor did they differ between the two pouch designs.

In an ultrastructural study of 12 patients after J-pouch–anal anastomosis, Lerch confirmed transformation from an ileal to a more colonic form of epithelium (Lerch *et al.*, 1989). In a patient cohort which did not exhibit clinical pouchitis, various stains were used for light microscopy, including PNA lectin and

ULEX lectin. As previously described by others, the villi were flattened, and intestinal crypts were lengthened and increased in number. Goblet cell numbers were dramatically increased, with a much accentuated production of mucus. In addition, Paneth cell numbers were increased with some alteration in their fine structure. This group found no alteration in endocrine cell numbers.

There is now considerable evidence that the mucosa of surgically created ileal reservoirs is commonly, if not almost universally, abnormal (Figures 8.2, 8.3). However, to date it is difficult to define precise causative roles to

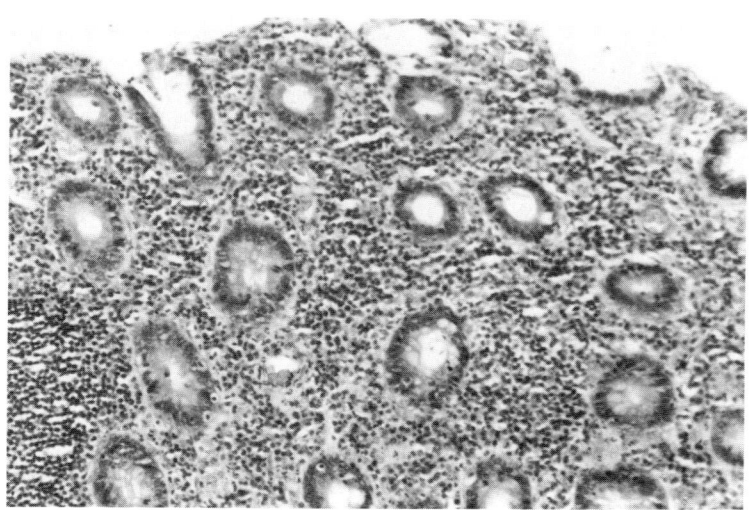

Figure 8.2 Biopsy of ileal pouch showing superficial ulceration, colonic metaplasia and marked active chronic inflammatory cell infiltration of the lamina propria (H & E; ×260, reduced to 55% on reproduction). (Courtesy of Dr R.F.T. MacMahon, University of Manchester)

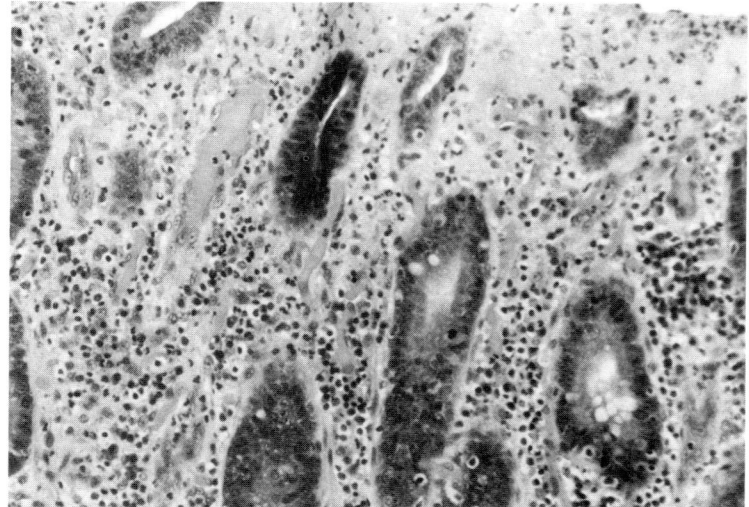

Figure 8.3 Ileal pouch biopsy in which there is fibrosis of the lamina propria and a mixed acute and chronic inflammatory infiltrate; there is hyperplasia of the crypt epithelium with depletion of goblet cells (H & E; ×360, reduced to 55% on reproduction). (Courtesy of Dr R.F.T. MacMahon, University of Manchester)

factors which might be important in the genesis of these abnormalities. Equally difficult at the present is determination of what deleterious effects such changes might have for the patients with ileal reservoirs.

Inflammatory changes of varying degrees appear to be extremely common. Chronic inflammatory cell infiltrates become more common 6 months after ileostomy closure, and are witnessed in both colitics and in patients with polyposis. When these changes become increasingly severe, such infiltrates are associated with extensive villous atrophy and crypt cell hyperplasia. This results in an appearance like that seen in colonic mucosa, particularly that in ulcerative colitis in remission, and is found almost exclusively in patients with ulcerative colitis.

Acute inflammatory changes are observed in all groups of patients. However, when these infiltrates are associated with crypt abscesses and ulceration, it is only those patients with previous ulcerative colitis who are so affected. Clinically symptomatic pouchitis is again mostly, if not only, found in colitic patients.

Assessments of intestinal mucin histochemistry infer that there is a conversion in all patient groups to a colonic type of pattern (Corfield, Warren and Bartolo, 1990). Whilst epithelial hyperplasia has been witnessed in these patients, frank dysplasia has not been previously reported.

Unfortunately, little study has been made of the defunctioned pouch, either prior to closure of the ileostomy or after re-defunctioning for whatever reason. Keighley's group have recently provided evidence of the role of the faecal stream in promoting such changes in the neorectal mucosa (Kmiot *et al.*, 1989c). In this study, 15 patients were studied both prior to pouch formation, and again 6 months thereafter. Seven of these patients subsequently had their pouch defunctioned, and their investigations were repeated at that time. The crypt cell production rate (an assessment of cell kinetics within the reservoir) was assessed *in vitro* using a tissue culture technique. The results were correlated with standard morphometric analysis of villous height and crypt depth. The crypt cell production rate was found to be significantly elevated in the pouch mucosa compared with normal ileum. Upon defunctioning, the value for this parameter decreased, only to rise if continuity was again restored. Perhaps not surprisingly, a direct relationship was found between crypt cell production rate and crypt depth, whilst an inverse relationship was found with villous height. This important study therefore demonstrates that there is an increase in the production of crypt cells after ileal reservoir construction, and that the faecal stream has a positively trophic effect upon such ileal adaptation.

Reservoir microbiology

The normal terminal ileum is a relatively sterile environment. Conventional permanent ileostomies are associated with a change in bacterial flora to one which is both quantitatively and qualitatively intermediate between normal ileal content and normal stools (Gorbach, Nakas and Weinstein, 1976).

The construction of an ileal pouch, irrespective of its anatomical site, is associated with an even greater tendency to mimic the flora of the normal colon and rectum (Brandberg, Kock and Philipson, 1972; Philipson *et al.*, 1975; Schjonsby *et al*, 1977; Kelly *et al.*, 1983). In particular total bacterial counts are elevated after ileostomy formation, and proportionately the number of anaerobes are increased more than aerobes.

Studying the effects of a pelvic pouch, three separate groups of 15 patients were assessed. The ecologies of conventional ileostomy, Kock pouches and ileoanal anastomosis with J-pouches were described (Luukkonen *et al.*, 1988). Two of the Kock cohort and four of the pelvic pouch group had a syndrome definable as clinical pouchitis.

Fresh faecal samples were quantitatively assessed with results expressed as logarithm (base 10) of the numbers of colony-forming units of aerobic and anaerobic organisms per gram of ileal effluent.

The flora in the ileostomy and pouch groups was predominantly colonic in nature. Whilst the commonest aerobes were coliforms (especially *Escherichia coli*), enterococci and *Streptococcus viridans*, *Haemophilus parainfluenzae* was noted to be the predominant aerobe in one of the Kock pouch and two of the ileostomy patients. Proteus was dominant in one pelvic pouch, whilst one Kock pouch had klebsiella as the predominant aerobe. Five of the ileoanal pouches had small amounts of *Clostridium difficile*. Whilst total anaerobe counts were similar in both pouch groups, they were significantly greater than those in the ileostomy group. Five of the Kock pouch and four of the ileoanal pouch groups had what might be termed 'normal' anaerobe counts, i.e. less than 10^7. All other patients had evidence of bacterial overgrowth, with counts above 10^7. *Bacteroides* sp., especially *B. fragilis*, were the most common anaerobes in every patient group. However, there was no significant difference between the concentrations in the three patient groups. There were no significant differences between 'normal' patients and those with pouch ileitis.

Nasmyth has studied 11 patients after creation of an ileal pelvic reservoir at a median of 6.4 months (range 3–31 months) after closure of an ileostomy. This group was compared to 12 patients after conventional ileostomy. As above, quantitative analysis was performed quoting results as logarithm (base 10) of the numbers of colony-forming units of aerobic and anaerobic organisms per gram of ileal effluent. The ratio of anaerobes to aerobes in pouch effluent was significantly greater than in faeces from ileostomies. The median number of bifidobacteria and especially bacteroides was greater in the pouch group. There was no significant difference between the flora from either the J- or S-pouches, and no recognized pathogens were observed in any of the samples from either group (Nasmyth *et al.*, 1989a).

Faecal volatile fatty acids

Faecal volatile (or short chain) fatty acids are, along with hydrogen and methane, the metabolites of anaerobic fermentation of carbohydrate by intestinal bacteria. The precise role of these products is debatable, however certain of their properties have been documented. In most assessments of these compounds, particular emphasis has been placed upon the study of those acids with between two and five carbon atoms, namely acetic, propionic, butyric and valeric acids respectively. Such compounds are the major anions of faecal water, and only very low concentrations are normally found in human ileal effluent.

As a group they are known to stimulate the motility of the human ileum, and this has obvious potential implications for the ileoanal

pouch procedure. Whilst acetic acid is the most potent of these short chain acids, butyrate has also been demonstrated to have a trophic effect upon the colonic mucosal cells, and to have an important positive effect on sodium absorption (Roediger, 1988; Roediger and Rae, 1982). However, to date, their pathophysiology in relation to the ileoanal reservoir has yet to be determined.

In the normal anatomical state, the colon is the site of both synthesis and absorption of volatile fatty acids. Hence, their concentration in normal stools is a poor guide to their rate of production. However, by comparing those patients with Brooke ileostomies, with those patients with an ileoanal reservoir, it might be possible to discern any possible role of these compounds in the latter group of patients. It has previously been demonstrated that overgrowth of anaerobic bacteria occurs to a greater degree in patients with a pelvic pouch (see above). On theoretical grounds it might be expected that this phenomenon should be mirrored in an increased production of volatile fatty acids. If this is indeed the case, then it may be possible to correlate such an increase in one or all of these compounds with clinical or pathophysiological parameters of pouch function.

Johnston's group have described such experiments in 12 patients after restorative proctocolectomy and 11 patients after construction of a Brooke ileostomy (Nasmyth *et al.*, 1989a). Much of this report has been alluded to above. Faecal volatile fatty acid concentrations were measured using gas–liquid chromatography, and compared with the results from faecal specimens from 17 healthy control subjects. Compared to the Brooke ileostomy, median concentrations of both propionate and butyrate were significantly greater in the pouch patients. Also, the normal controls had greater amounts of propionate, butyrate and isobutyrate than the ileostomy group. Interestingly, little difference was noted between the controls and the pouch patients, other than that a higher concentration of acetate was found in pouch effluent.

Utilizing a scintigraphic method to assess pouch emptying, correlation was found between poor pouch evacuation and an increased concentration of propionate. Otherwise, these compounds did not appear to affect pouch function. There was no significant relationship between the concentration of volatile fatty acids and the bacterial counts in the effluent from either the ileostomies or the pouches. Unfortunately, none of the patients examined in this study had clinical pouchitis, so that further conclusions are difficult to draw.

Ambrose and colleagues have studied random stool specimens from six controls and six patients at a mean of 55 ± 9 months after ileoanal pouch anastomosis. Again, estimation of these compounds was performed using gas–liquid chromatography. Compared with the normal group, total volatile fatty acids were 61% in the pouch patients. Acetic acid was found in similar concentrations in both groups, and was the major faecal volatile fatty acid in these groups. However propionic, butyric and isobutyric acids were significantly reduced in the pouch group. No valeric or isovaleric acid was detected in any of the samples from the pouch patients. Again, no mention was made as to the pattern of these compounds in acute pouchitis (Ambrose *et al.*, 1989, 1990b).

Effluent characteristics after pouch–anal anastomosis

In Chapter 6, the subject of pouch absorption, particularly of water and simple electrolytes, was discussed. It is not intended to repeat such a discussion here. Suffice to say that it is possible that stool consistency may be at least partially related to the absorptive capacity of the reservoir. To date, there are conflicting results of such a capacity, in that the group from UCLA have consistently found that reservoir absorption increases with time (Kojima, Sanada and Fonkalsrud, 1982b; Kawarasaki, Fujiwara and Fonkalsrud, 1985). Others have recorded a decrease in pouch absorption, both in the Kock pouch (Philipson, Kock, Robinson *et al* 1975) and in the ileal pelvic pouch (Rosemurgy, Schraut and Block, 1983).

One study has quantitated the nitrogen and fat content of the effluent from 20 ileal reservoirs (O'Connell *et al.*, 1986). These patients were at a mean of 2 years after pouch construction, and had a range of functional outcomes, including six patients with recurrent pouchitis, as previously described. After an overnight fast, a standard diet of protein

(20%), carbohydrate (40%) and fat (40%) was taken. During the last 24 hours of the study, stool volume was recorded. Specimens of effluent were collected for nitrogen and fat analysis.

Stool volumes were greater in patients with a poor result than in those with either pouchitis or a satisfactory result (1136 ± 278, 627 ± 75 and 594 ± 24 ml/24 hours respectively). The nitrogen content of the effluent held a similar relationship (2.9 ± 0.3, 2.2 ± 0.3 and 2.0 ± 0.3 g/24 hours respectively). Stool volume directly correlated with jejunal anaerobic growth. The fat content of the effluent was similar in all three groups.

The same group also documented various parameters pertaining to pouch effluent in 23 patients at a mean of 2 years after pouch construction (O'Connell *et al.*, 1987). After 48 hours on a standardized diet, 24-hour stool collections were performed. Records were kept of the number of stools passed, the volume of each stool, and the total volume of effluent passed in the 24-hour period. The mean stool frequency in this series of J-pouches was 9 ± 1 per 24 hours (range 4–20). The 24-hour stool output was 776 ± 90 ml (371–2380 ml), with a mean stool volume of 99 ± 8 ml (30–222 ml).

Attempts were made to correlate such findings with other determinants of pouch function. It was found that stool frequency was directly proportional to the 24-hour stool volume, and indirectly proportional to pouch threshold volume and maximum capacity. However, pouch compliance did not affect frequency. The efficiency of pouch emptying was weakly correlated with stool frequency. The mean stool volume was not related to the efficiency of pouch evacuation, 24-hour stool volume or to reservoir compliance. However, it was correlated with pouch maximum capacity and threshold volume.

Empirically, clinicians have attempted to alter stool consistency in the hope that this might help to improve function after ileoanal pouch anastomosis. However, there is little evidence regarding the efficacy of such methods, or the effects of stool consistency on efficiency of pouch emptying.

A recent abstract has described the effects of altering stool consistency in six patients and 12 healthy volunteers (Ambrose *et al.*, 1989a). Patients were at a mean of 55 ± 9 months post pouch construction. Artificial stools of three consistencies were made from aluminium magnesium silicate gel labelled with ^{99m}Tc. Thin, medium and thick consistencies were used incorporating 5%, 7.5% and 11.25% w/w of the gel respectively. The anorectal angle was assessed scintigraphically during the investigation, and the maximum tolerable volume measured by air insufflation of an intrarectal or intra-pouch balloon.

There were no significant differences between either ano(neo)rectal angles or in maximal tolerable volumes between the groups. Overall the mean evacuation percentage was greater in the control group. In the control group, patients were able to evacuate the medium consistency stool more efficiently than either of the other stools. In the pouch group, there was no significant difference in the efficiency of evacuation of any of the stools. Therefore the conclusion made by this group was that ileal reservoir patients evacuate less efficiently than controls. Whilst stool consistency affects evacuation efficiency in health, there appears to be little evidence that it does so after ileoanal pouch construction.

9

Inflammation in ileal reservoirs

Introduction

Inflammatory changes of varying degrees have been recognized historically within capacitance vessels constructed from terminal ileum, whether they be placed within the pelvis or within the abdomen. Indeed, prior to the development of Brooke's modification of the then standard end-ileostomy, stomal ileitis was a common finding. Initially, it was assumed that this represented the technical failure to site the stoma away from an area of 'backwash ileitis'. However, it soon became apparent that this condition could be successfully managed by stomal dilatation, usually combined with lavage (Warren and McKittrick, 1951). It became obvious that stomal ileitis was for the most part secondary to subacute obstruction of the stoma. This obstruction was part of the process termed 'maturation', as discussed in Chapter 1. The development of the Brooke everted ileostomy has meant that such obstruction is now a rarity, however, when it does occur, further ileal resection and ileostomy refashioning are usually required (Weakley and Farmer, 1964; Knill-Jones, Morson and Williams, 1970).

Inflammation within intestinal reservoirs, and specifically the ileal pelvic reservoir, remains a somewhat contentious issue. To date, most reports documenting clinical pouchitis have tended to focus upon faecal microbiology. Whilst this is understandable in that antimicrobial therapy against anaerobes often results in great benefit, there is as yet little specific evidence that bacterial overgrowth per se is the fundamental abnormality in this syndrome. Separate consideration will therefore be given to a number of factors such as pouch ecology, bacterial metabolites and bile salt metabolism. Attempts will be made to define any possible role which these and other factors might have on the incidence of reservoir inflammation.

Incidence

Even in early experimental studies of the ileal pelvic reservoir, pouchitis of some degree was frequently witnessed, and appeared to be related to faecal stasis within the pouch (Kojima, Sanada and Fonkalsrud, 1982b; Luukonen et al., 1988a). In the former series, pouchitis was more frequently seen in S-pouches than in Fonkalsrud's lateral side-to-side reservoirs. In contrast to the early experience of Fonkalsrud, pouchitis has not generally been found to relate to faecal stasis, which is usually quantified as residual pouch volume. This same author has also described an early transient pouchitis in 50% of his patients who had undergone isoperistaltic lateral reservoir formation (Fonkalsrud, 1984a). In all cases, remission was readily induced by metronidazole. Interestingly, it was found that this form of pouchitis became a rarity 6 months after pouch construction.

Subsequent clinical reports continued to document a regular occurrence of acute pouchitis, with an incidence of between 8% and 33% (Dozois *et al.*, 1986). This, however, pertains to the clinical syndrome of acute pouchitis. It has also become apparent in recent years that subclinical reservoir inflammation may occur after restorative proctocolectomy, and that its subclinical nature does not preclude it from being severe.

In addition to these acute changes, chronic inflammatory changes are frequently witnessed, at least histologically, in pelvic pouches. Our own experience, and that of others, reveals an incidence of such changes in up to 90% of individuals (Nicholls, Moskowitz and Shepherd, 1985). It is therefore important that studies shoud define diagnostic criteria for pouchitis, and that separate emphasis is placed upon these varying presentations. Thus, pouchitis was one of the first clinical sequelae to be described after restorative proctocolectomy. It remains an enigmatic condition, occasionally presenting difficult management problems to the surgeon.

Aetiology

Early studies consistently reported that acute pouchitis is found almost exclusively in patients who suffered with ulcerative colitis prior to their colectomy. Indeed, it is extremely unusual to find pouchitis in patients with adenomatous polyposis coli. In particular, those patients who had a pancolitis are more likely subsequently to develop pouchitis than are those patients whose colitis was predominantly distal (Madden, Farthing and Nicholls, 1990). It was therefore tempting to ascribe pouchitis to the presence of 'backwash ileitis' seen in ulcerative colitis.

However, in a study of 131 patients after restorative proctocolectomy, only 15 patients had the non-specific inflammatory changes in the terminal ileum diagnostic of backwash ileitis (Gustavsson, Weiland and Kelly, 1987). In this series 20 patients developed acute pouchitis, but only two of the latter had backwash ileitis. Hence, 90% of the patients with pouchitis did not have backwash ileitis. In addition, of those 15 patients with backwash ileitis, only 13% subsequently developed clinical acute pouchitis. This compared with an incidence of 16% in those patients without backwash ileitis. No relationship could be

found between the presence of backwash ileitis and acute pouchitis, and the Mayo clinic group have not considered backwash ileitis to be a contraindication to ileal reservoir formation.

In agreement with the experience from UCLA discussed above (Fonkalsrud, 1984a), many surgeons have found that pouchitis usually responds well to antimicrobial treatment, most notably metronidazole. Emphasis has therefore been placed upon bacterial overgrowth within the pouch as being a prime factor in the genesis of pouchitis. Several studies have attempted to document the presence or otherwise of bacterial abnormalities within ileal reservoirs, and their relationship to pouchitis. These studies are detailed in Chapter 8.

Comparing patients with either conventional ileostomies, continent ileostomies or ileal pelvic pouches, Luukkonen found the flora in all three groups to be predominantly colonic in nature. Aerobes (especially coliforms) were not uncommon. Anaerobe counts were greater in the pouch groups, with most patients having counts suggestive of bacterial overgrowth. However, neither total counts nor particular pathogen concentrations were associated with the presence of clinically definable pouchitis (Luukkonen *et al.*, 1988b). Keighley has measured cell production rate within the pouch crypts in patients with and without pouchitis (Kmiot, Youngs and Keighley, 1989; Keighley, Kmiot and Youngs, 1990). This correlated with the degree of villus atrophy but not with pouch bacteriology. In addition, anaerobe counts were unaffected by the presence of pouchitis. Treatment with metronidazole improved the indices of both crypt cell production and villus atrophy. This same group has suggested that pouch ischaemia may be a factor in the development of pouchitis (Sakaguchi *et al.*, 1989). Using a laser Doppler probe, flux within inflamed pouches was significantly lower than in normal pouches (see Chapter 8).

Whilst bacterial pathogens themselves might not be incriminated in pouchitis, it is possible that some product of their metabolism may be. Both volatile fatty acids (see Chapter 8) and products of bile acid metabolism (see Chapter 13) are undergoing scrutiny. Some bacteria are known to produce volatile fatty acids from their metabolism of carbohydrate. These acids are thought to be trophic for enterocytes, and their absence may be responsible for so-called diversion proctitis (Harig *et al.*, 1989). Chronic inflammation appears to correlate histologically with depressed volatile fatty acid levels, but more detailed investigation is required before their role in either the pathogenesis or management of pouchitis can be defined.

Conjugated bile acids are secreted in the bile, where they undergo bacterial hydrolysis within the gut, back to the deconjugated primary form. Alternatively, secondary bile acids can be formed from bacterial dehydroxylation. Some of these products are potentially damaging to the enterocytes, hence forming a putative mechanism for the development of pouchitis. Again, further work is required to unravel this problem.

In a controlled study, Stelzner has assessed rates of nutrient uptake *in vitro* using an everted sleeve technique on small mucosal segments, which were exposed to radiolabelled nutrient solutions (Stelzner *et al.*, 1989; Stelzner and Fonkalsrud, 1990). Absorption rates for bile acids and short chain fatty acids were similar in controls and pouches (both normal and inflamed). Carbohydrate uptake was decreased in pouch patients compared with controls, but amino acid uptake was significantly greater in inflamed pouches. It was concluded that increased bacterial degradation of carbohydrates and proteins, rather than bile acids, contributes to the diarrhoea and inflammation in pouchitis.

Recent evidence suggests that alterations in stool chemistry may be important in the genesis of some of the symptoms and signs of acute pouchitis. Assaying stool PAF (an endogenous phospholipid produced by inflammatory cells as a reaction to bacterial endotoxin, and known to be spasmogenic to ileal myocytes), it was found that the presence of this compound was related to previous colectomy. In particular, patients with pouchitis had significantly higher concentrations of this compound than either those patients with normal pouches or those with conventional ileostomies (Chaussade *et al.*, 1990).

It has been felt that acute pouchitis may represent 'ulcerative colitis' arising within the ileal pouch, presumably in areas of colonic metaplasia. As pouchitis occurs virtually exclusively in colitics, this is a powerful argument. Lohmuller and colleagues have recently reported that 31% of their colitic patients developed pouchitis, whilst this complication was found in only 6% of polyposis patients. This group found that those colitics who had suffered extraintestinal manifestations of their colitis (either before or after pouch construction) were significantly more likely to develop pouchitis. Further, the exacerbations of such extraintestinal manifestations were frequently related temporally to the episodes of pouchitis (Lohmuller *et al.*, 1990).

Why metronidazole is so efficacious in pouchitis, but has little role, if any, in ulcerative colitis remains unclear. It has also yet to be shown that, in cases where pouchitis is patchy, such a distribution is related to areas of colonic metaplasia. In addition to its antimicrobial activity, metronidazole has immunosuppressive properties; a possible role for this mechanism of action in acute pouchitis has not yet been established.

Interesting recent work has utilized monoclonal antibodies to assess possible microphage subpopulations with the lamina propria of pouches (Gionchetti *et al.*, 1989). Pouchitis was associated with an increase in RFD9 positive cells; a pattern which has previously been recorded in active ulcerative colitis and Crohn's disease (Mahida, Gionchetti, Vaux *et al* 1986). Similar results have been reported by others in patients with clinical pouchitis (de Silva *et al.*, 1990).

To complicate matters further, there is emerging evidence that the terminal ileal pouch may have effects upon other parts of the gastrointestinal tract, particularly the normal stomach. Such interrelationships may have implications for the development of pouchitis. Dube has reported that those patients developing pouchitis may have a high gastric pH, even in the presence of a normal gastric biopsy (Dube and Heyen, 1989). One patient in this study required pouch excision for toxic dilatation, and intragastric pH returned to normal in this individual. In addition, two patients requiring H2-receptor antagonists for duodenal ulcer developed pouchitis. It would appear that there may be an interrelationship between relative gastric hypochlorhydria and clinical pouchitis. Whilst the endocrine studies outlined in Chapter 10 might ultimately shed some light on this relationship, clearly more work is required.

It now appears to be increasingly likely, however, that the aetiology of reservoir ileitis is more related to the aetiology of chronic ulcerative colitis than to a mechanical effect within the pouch per se. It may be that both represent abnormal host responses to a specific stimulus, such as a change in the bacterial flora, or a hypersensitivity reaction to a bacterial cell wall protein.

Clinical features

Generally, patients present with changes in bowel habit, especially diarrhoea and urgency. In our experience, the passage of blood per anum is uncommon. Otherwise, symptoms are often negligible, but may include abdominal pain, malaise, anorexia and fever (Figure 9.1). Occasionally more severe systemic manifestations, such as arthralgia and skin lesions, may occur (Klein, Stenzel and Katon, 1983). In such circumstances, the severity of these symptoms often mirrors that of the inflammatory process within the pouch (Lohmuller *et*

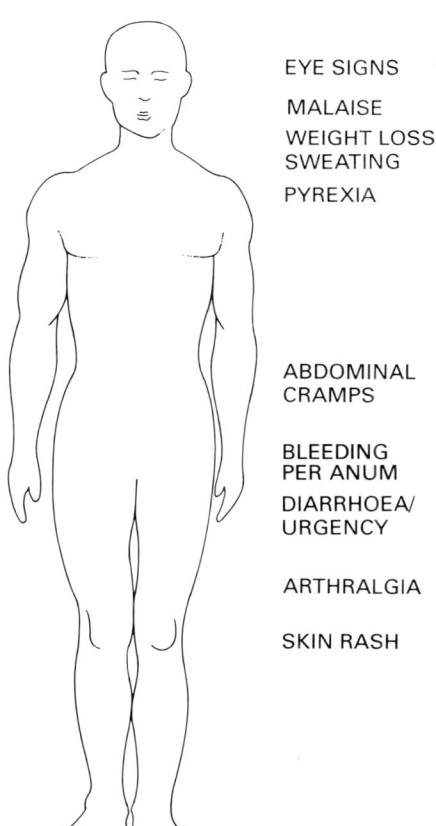

EYE SIGNS

MALAISE
WEIGHT LOSS
SWEATING
PYREXIA

ABDOMINAL
CRAMPS

BLEEDING
PER ANUM
DIARRHOEA/
URGENCY

ARTHRALGIA

SKIN RASH

Figure 9.1 Clinical features of acute pouchitis

al., 1990). It is well recognized that asymptomatic subclinical pouch inflammation can occur; indeed, the most severe inflammatory changes which we have witnessed in a pelvic pouch were found in a patient who was completely asymptomatic. It is important to realize that, in patients with these symptoms, efferent limb obstruction, reservoir ischaemia or Crohn's disease may also enter the differential diagnosis, particularly if the inflammatory process is resistant to treatment. However, in such cases, there would appear to be little evidence that pouch inflammation reflects an original misdiagnosis of colitis, rather than Crohn's disease (Subramani *et al.*, 1990).

Investigation

It is our practice to adopt a policy of routine endoscopic assessment of these patients, along with biopsy of several sites within the pouch, particular attention being placed upon any suspicious areas. The endoscopic appearance of pouchitis can be highly variable. Numerous features have been described, including areas of congestion, mucosal petechiae, excessive mucous secretion and frank ulceration. In approximately 15% of cases of pouchitis, a pseudomembranous-type picture of inflammation may be seen. Interestingly, it has been shown that in up to 80% of asymptomatic individuals, various microscopic features may be found on routine biopsy. Further, some 20% of such individuals may also have focal macroscopic lesions. In patients with pouchitis, such lesions are seen in all cases, with the afferent limb above the pouch also affected in up to 50% of cases (Di Febo *et al.*, 1990). In experimental animals, such jejunoileitis may be associated with abnormalities of mucosal function, in particular ion transport (Perdue, Marshall and Masson, 1990).

Whilst frequently performed, we have not found either microscopy or culture of pouch effluent to aid in diagnosis or management. However, as a cautionary note it should be remembered that stool culture should be performed if there is any doubt as to the diagnosis, or if there is little response to treatment. Lontoft (1986) has described an extremely severe *Salmonella typhimurium* pouchitis, which resulted in pouch perforation and generalized peritonitis. In the vast majority of patients little further investigation is necessary. Even unusual causes of 'pouchitis-like' symptoms should be excluded (Franceschi, Chen and Yuh Jen-Nan, 1986). Recently, the use of [111]indium-labelled granulocyte scanning and faecal granulocyte excretion has been described (Kmiot *et al.*, 1989a; Keighley *et al.*, 1990b). It was found that these methods were of particular value if inflammation was patchy. The findings correlated with those patients who improved following treatment with metronidazole.

Treatment

In the majority of patients, treatment of pouchitis is symptomatic. Antidiarrhoeals are used to reduce stool frequency, which may be excessive. In addition to metronidazole, other broad spectrum agents have been shown to be effective, especially tetracycline. Some surgeons advocate the use of antibiotics in order to test the diagnosis (Tytgat and van Deventer, 1988). However, a therapeutic response is not universal.

What of the asymptomatic individual? In our limited experience, antimicrobial therapy does not confer much, if any, benefit, and endoscopic improvement appears to be obstinate. Others have suggested that treatment is unnecessary in such circumstances (Madden, Farthing and Nicholls, 1990).

If pouchitis is refractory to antibiotics, corticosteroid enemas are given, with or without salicylates or their modern derivatives (Miglioli *et al.*, 1989). Oral corticosteroids may be required for a limited period. We have limited experience with the successful use of azathioprine in the management of a particularly severe case of acute pouchitis. Others have described the use of the irrigation of short-chain fatty acids into the pouch (de Silva *et al.*, 1989). We have had marked success with such a treatment modality in one particularly obstinate case of pouchitis. This patient instilled medium-chain triglyceride oil into his pouch twice daily, resulting in a complete cessation of his pouchitis symptoms, including marked urgency and severe perianal excoriation, within 2 weeks. Whether other cytoprotective agents, such as misoprostol, will prove to have any role in the management of pouch inflammation is yet to be evaluated (Fedorak *et al.*, 1990).

Fonkalsrud has described the long-term prophylactic use of metronidazole in his patients (Fonkalsrud, 1987). We have followed this advice in patients with less severe, but none the less refractory pouchitis, with very satisfactory results over periods of up to 1 year.

Conclusions

Clinical pouchitis is one of the most troublesome complications after ileal pouch–anal anastomosis. Whilst its aetiology remains obscure, treatment with metronidazole is often efficacious. In refractory cases, corticosteroids or other immunosuppressive therapy may be indicated.

10

The small intestine after restorative proctocolectomy

Jejunoileal motility

Restorative proctocolectomy has been found to modify the motility patterns of the small intestine (Stryker, Borody, Phillips *et al* 1984, Chaussade *et al.*, 1989a). It can be envisaged that there may be at least two potential mechanisms for such modifications. First, the anal canal muscular complexes are in a state of tonic contraction, relaxation being a transitory event. In this respect it differs markedly from the normal ileocaecal valve, implying that the small bowel might be chronically, subacutely obstructed. Further evidence for this comes from the fact that pelvic ileal pouches can increase their volume by some 250% in the first 6 postoperative months (Chaussade *et al.*, 1989a). Secondly, it is well recognized that bacterial overgrowth in the pouch is, to some degree, a virtually universal phenomenon (O'Connell *et al.*, 1985). Such overgrowth may be associated with jejunal bacterial overgrowth, and subsequent modification of jejunal motility. It is becoming increasingly apparent that such obstructed intestine can act as a focus for more severe systemic infections (Deitch *et al.*, 1990).

More recently, attention has been turned to the possible role of endocrine mediators in such phenomena (Greenberg *et al.*, 1989; Soper *et al.*, 1990). Whilst such work is still in its infancy, the utilization of the pelvic pouch procedure provides an interesting clinical model with which to study developing aspects of gastrointestinal physiology.

Intestinal motility probes have been used to assess motility after pouch construction (Figure 10.1). Workers from the Mayo clinic compared eight colitics (who were studied up to 2 years post pouch construction) with six healthy controls (Stryker, Borody, Phillips *et al* 1985).

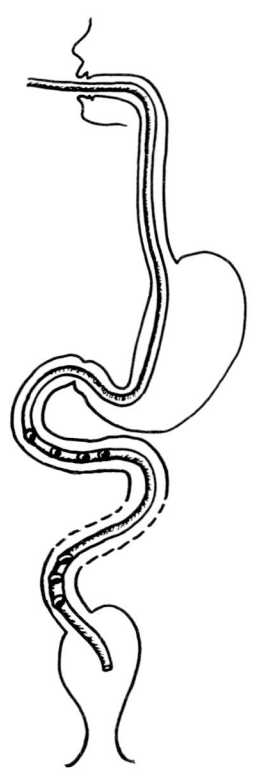

Figure 10.1

Patients were selected to represent a wide range of clinical outcomes after pouch construction, with stool frequency ranging from 2 to 17 per 24 hours. The motility probe which they used consisted of an assembly of nine polyvinyl tubes, with an additional radiopaque channel and a latex balloon at its end. The overall diameter of the probe was 3.6 mm. In each tube a side port was cut at 10, 20, 30, 40, 50, 75, 100 and 125 cm from the tip. A low compliance pneumohydraulic system was utilized for catheter perfusion. In the patient group, the tip of the probe was placed, via the nasal or orointestinal routes, just cephalad to the pouch; in the controls, it was allowed to enter the caecum. In the patients, a separate three-lumen assembly was placed transanally into the pouch in order to monitor complex migration into the pouch.

Fasting recordings were made over a period of approximately 20 hours. Subsequently, recordings were made over a 6-hour period after the subject had eaten a test meal. No differences were noted in the frequency, duration or velocity of migratory motor complexes in either the patient or control groups. Interestingly, 3% of jejunal complexes reached the terminal ileum in controls, whereas none passed into the pouch in the patient group. Propagated contractions were readily identified in both groups. In the fasting state, they were infrequent in both groups, being slightly more common in the pouch group. Whilst durations and velocities were similar, the distribution was different in the two groups. In the controls, such patterns were only witnessed in the distal ileum, that is the region of bowel used to construct the pouch in the patient group. However, in the pouch group, they were observed in three patients at the most proximal recording site, i.e. 125 cm cephalad to the pouch. Discrete clustered contractions were witnessed in all of the controls, and in just over half of the patients. In both groups, the frequency, duration and velocity were similar. In this study, no correlation was found between motility patterns and frequency of pouch evacuation, nor did the presence of any of these motility patterns coincide temporally with individual bowel movements.

In a recent study from France, an attempt was made to document jejunal motility patterns, and to identify any specific patterns which might be suggestive of partial intestinal obstruction. An attempt was also made to define a correlation between such patterns and bacterial overgrowth in the proximal jejunum (Chaussade *et al.*, 1989a). Eleven patients (four S- and seven J-pouches) and six controls were studied. In all patients a total excision of the rectal muscular cuff was performed (Chaussade *et al.*, 1989c). Studies were performed at either 6 or 12 months after closure of the ileostomy, and patients were selected to represent a reasonable cross-section of clinical outcomes.

Jejunal motility patterns were recorded using a four-lumen probe, with channels of internal diameter 1 mm. A further radiopaque channel allowed fluoroscopic visualization, and the inflation of a terminal latex balloon which aided the propagation of the tube through the bowel. The four side ports were located at 0, 30, 60 and 90 cm from the tip, the study commencing when the proximal port was at the level of the ligament of Treitz. A low compliance pneumohydraulic system was utilized for catheter perfusion. Recordings were taken over a 4-hour period after an overnight fast, and after a standardized test meal.

Using standard criteria for defining the motility patterns, no difference was noted between the patients and the controls with regard to the frequency, duration or velocity of the migrating motor complexes.

Propagated contractions were infrequent in the control group, never being seen postprandially. However, four patients demonstrated numerous such contractions, two of whom had evidence of jejunal bacterial overgrowth. Of possible importance is the fact that three of these patients had S-shaped reservoirs, two of whom required intubation to promote evacuation.

In the fasting state, discrete clustered contractions were witnessed equally between the patients and controls. However, postprandially such contractions were never witnessed in the control group, whilst they were to be seen in all seven patients studied. One of these patients had evidence of jejunal overgrowth, but saline infusion tests with evacuation studies failed to demonstrate incomplete pouch emptying in any patient.

From these and other similar studies, it appears that fasting jejunal motility patterns remain normal after ileal pouch formation. However, if one excludes the migrating motor complexes, variations from the norm are witnessed postprandially.

Excessive propagated contractions, and their electromyographic equivalent (the migrating action potential complex), were not uncommon after eating. Such patterns, originating in the proximal small intestine, are known to propel intestinal contents over long distances; they have previously been witnessed in patients with secretory diarrhoea (Coremans *et al.*, 1987), and during bacterial overgrowth (Burns *et al.*, 1978). Hence, they may be responsible for the efficacy of antibiotics in treating the high stool output witnessed in such patients. The Mayo clinic group did not correlate such motility patterns with bacterial overgrowth (Stryker, Borody, Phillips *et al* 1984). It has been postulated that propagated contractions may be either the consequence of bacterial overgrowth or a response to the storage of chyme in the ileal pouch. It is also possible that small intestinal distension has a role in the genesis of these patterns (Sjogren, Wardlow and Charles, 1984; Camilleri, 1989).

There is some disparity between the two reports discussed above regarding discrete clustered contractions (Chaussade *et al.*, 1989a; Stryker, Borody, Phillips *et al* 1984). In the former paper, such contractions in the fasting state were infrequent in both patients and controls. In the postprandial period, discrete clustered contractions were not witnessed in controls, but were common in the patient groups. This contrasts with the results from the Mayo clinic, and, differing methodologies are likely to be important in such discrepancies. The former groups studied motility patterns in the upper jejunum, whilst Stryker and his colleagues studied the distal jejunum and ileum. Also, meal types varied between studies; a solid test meal being used by the Mayo clinic, and a liquid test meal being utilized by the French group. Gastric emptying after the liquid meal would be faster, a factor which has been shown to facilitate the appearance of discrete clustered contractions. This is not to negate these results, as studies have also documented such patterns as being common in patients with partial small intestinal obstruction (Summers, Anuras and Green, 1983). This then supports the hypothesis that the ileoanal anastomosis might be responsible for producing a chronic partial small intestinal obstruction.

What then are the likely mechanisms for such an obstruction? It is unlikely that incomplete pouch emptying is responsible as no correlation between these factors has been noted. The same holds true for the case of bacterial overgrowth in the pouch as being a possible aetiological factor.

Under normal conditions, the ileocaecal valve merely represents a zone of tonic activity. After ileoanal anastomosis, the 'outlet' of the small intestine is the anal sphincter. This muscular complex is closed at most times, and may be the causative agent in producing the high incidence of discrete clustered contractions after pouch construction. It would certainly seem likely that the improving sphincter function postoperatively does result in partial obstruction, as the capacity of pelvic pouches increases more than two-fold in the first 6 months or so after ileostomy closure.

Therefore, restorative proctocolectomy results in little alteration in jejunoileal motility, particularly in the fasting state. However, it is likely that propagated contractions may subsequently originate from a more proximal site in the bowel than in the normal state. This presumably reflects a physiological response to ileal distension, secondary to its new storage function. Whilst it remains possible that increased small bowel transit has a role in the frequency and pattern of defaecation after restorative proctocolectomy, no relationship has been described between motility patterns and such parameters.

Small bowel transit after restorative proctocolectomy

Small intestinal transit continues to demand much attention from gastroenterologists, as it is highly likely that aberrations of gut motility are of paramount importance in the genesis of gastrointestinal symptomatology. Small intestinal transit, or orocaecal transit time, has been variously assessed using hydrogen breath testing and radioisotope assessment using gamma scintigraphy (Gilmore, 1990). Such methods are necessary when the colon remains *in situ*, but after colectomy with ileoanal anastomosis, assessments using the direct counting of ingested particles can be utilized.

Rosemurgy and colleagues assessed small

bowel transit using such a non-absorbable marker in 25 dogs after either S- or lateral isoperistaltic pouch construction (Rosemurgy, Schraut and Block, 1983). At 3-monthly intervals, intestinal transit was assessed after an overnight fast. Both reservoir types significantly prolonged the intestinal transit time when compared to the straight ileoanal anastomosis group (235 and 135 minutes respectively). The lateral side-to-side reservoir prolonged transit time compared with the S-pouch (254 and 215 minutes respectively), however, the animals with S-pouches retained the marker for much longer than did the former group, who rapidly cleared it. No effect was noted as being related to the efferent limb length.

Using the hydrogen breath test, Lerch has measured intestinal transit in 20 controls and 12 patients after J-pouch–anal anastomosis (Lerch *et al.*, 1989). Lactulose and mannitol were used as non-absorbable carbohydrates, and it was found that intestinal transit was significantly accelerated in the pouch group. Therefore, both intestinal transit and motility patterns show changes after pouch–anal anastomosis. Greenberg has recently reported elevated plasma motilin levels after restorative proctocolectomy (Greenberg *et al.*, 1989). Whilst the other gut hormones assessed were equivalent in both patients and normal controls, both basal and postprandial motilin concentrations have also been recorded in cases of ulcerative colitis prior to any surgical intervention (Besterman *et al.*, 1983). It is possible that motilin initiates certain intestinal motility patterns, such as migrating motor complexes. In addition, its elevation in ulcerative colitis may be responsible for rapid intestinal transit. However, it appears to be unlikely that colectomy results in either potentiation or suppression of this action. Based upon these studies, accelerated intestinal transit after pouch–anal anastomosis may possibly be a consequence of the underlying colitis.

Further evidence of an endocrine influence on intestinal motility and transit had been provided by studies of the 'ileal brake' mechanism (Holgate and Read, 1985; Miglioli *et al.*, 1989). It has been reported that small bowel transit and gastric emptying can be slowed by direct intraluminal infusion of certain nutrients into the ileum. The mechanism by which the 'ileal brake' functions is not understood, although various peptides, including several putative neuroendocrine mediators, are most favoured at present.

The intestinal infusion of nutrients induces release of one identifiable peptide from the ileum, termed peptide YY. This has been demonstrated to reduce intestinal transit and to slow gastric emptying. Using ileal pouch–anal anastomosis as a model, several groups have quantified peptide YY levels (Armstrong *et al.*, 1989; Mariani *et al.*, 1989; Soper *et al.*, 1990). Soper *et al.* have infused the pouch with a fatty acid and demonstrated both slowed gastric emptying and reduced small bowel transit. In addition, it appeared that the pouches became more capacious after such infusion, although the mechanism for this is far from clear. The occurrence of these phenomena was associated with prolonged deferral of defaecation without impaired efficiency of evacuation. Others have reported similar findings in patients with intact colons (Fone *et al.*, 1990).

Whilst the hormonal profiles measured during infusion were inconclusive for a mediator role for either peptide YY, enteroglucagon or neurotensin, Holgate's study has confirmed that the 'ileal brake' mechanism is still present after colectomy and pouch–anal anastomosis. Armstrong found that pouch construction in experimental animals was associated with significant elevations of both enteroglucagon and peptide YY levels (Armstrong *et al.*, 1989). Basal levels of these hormones were elevated, however the effect was most pronounced postprandially. Whilst somewhat conflicting results have also been reported (Marianai *et al.*, 1989), these results provide a potential mechanism for small bowel adaptation after colectomy and pouch–anal anastomosis, in that enteroglucagon is trophic for enterocytes, and peptide YY slows intestinal transit. As a consequence ileal chyme might be in contact not only with a greater surface area, but also for a longer period. Hence, stool volume, consistency and frequency might be improved. There is evidence of impaired intestinal absorption of carbohydrate after pouch construction (Lerch *et al.*, 1989). Both lactulose and D-xylose absorption were found to be abnormal on breath hydrogen testing. One-third of the patients assessed developed abdominal pain and diarrhoea after administration of the carbohydrate load. However, maintenance of a balanced diet enabled patients to avoid biochemically discernible malabsorption. Therapeutic manipulation of the 'ileal brake' may be possible in the future, as may dietary manipulations (Higham and Read, 1990). Such advances may benefit patients with rapid transit, associated with excessive stool output and frequency.

Small bowel bacterial overgrowth after restorative proctocolectomy

Bacterial overgrowth within the small intestine results in a syndrome associated with malabsorption. However, its diagnosis can be problematical. To date, there is little agreement as to which assessment is to be preferred. Perhaps the 'hardest' evidence for such a diagnosis may be provided by aspiration and culture of intestinal juice. However, the complexity and invasiveness of this method limit its practical application. Consequently, many workers have advocated the use of more indirect assessments, most notably breath hydrogen testing. However, the efficacy of this latter method remains in doubt (Corazza *et al.*, 1990).

Jejunal bacterial counts have been studied in 20 pouch patients at a mean of 2 years after closure of ileostomy (O'Connell *et al.*, 1986). Seventeen had 12–15-cm-limbed J-pouches, three had 10-cm-limbed S-pouches with 5-cm efferent limbs. The patients were specifically chosen to represent a spectrum of results; eight good, six poor and six had recurrent pouchitis. A good result was defined as six or fewer stools per 24 hours with perfect continence. Patients were deliberately chosen such that pelvic sepsis could not be the cause of their varying clinical outcomes. After an overnight fast, an orojejunal aspiration tube was passed, 5 ml of jejunal fluid aspirated and immediately placed in a special anaerobic transport tube. A 5-g sample of fresh ileal effluent was placed in a similar container. The samples were quickly transported to the microbiology laboratory where processing occurred within 2 hours. Both aerobic and anaerobic cultures were performed using several different culture media. A Gram stain was performed on each morphological type cultured, allowing placement into one of four categories: Gram-positive cocci or bacilli, or Gram-negative cocci or bacilli. Further subculturing allowed

detection of true anaerobes. The effluent specimens were processed in a similar manner after prior serial dilutions to 10^{-8}.

Patients with good clinical results did not differ in their jejunal counts from those with recurrent pouchitis, in either total aerobe or total anaerobe counts. Both were within the values expected for healthy controls. Those patients with a poor clinical result demonstrated overgrowth of both aerobes and anaerobes. Specifically, jejunal anaerobic Gram-negative bacilli, and aerobic Gram-negative cocci were responsible for the overgrowth. Conversely, effluent culture revealed both aerobic and anaerobic overgrowth as compared to healthy ileal chyme. However, there was no difference between the values for any of the clinical groups. Gram staining failed to demonstrate any particular causative organisms. The jejunal bacterial overgrowth was found to correlate significantly with large stool volumes, increased frequency and an elevated stool nitrogen concentration. There was no such correlation with stool fat concentration or with efficiency of pouch emptying.

Recently, further evidence of proximal small intestinal overgrowth after ileal reservoir formation has been provided (Kmiot, O'Brien and Keighley, 1989). This group found that the absolute number of bacteria in ileal reservoir chyme and the anaerobe to aerobe ratio increased after pouch construction. They utilized hydrogen breath testing to assess anaerobic overgrowth in 30 age- and sex-matched controls. Tests were carried out at 5-minute intervals for 1 hour, following a 20-hour fast. Ileal reservoir patients had a higher mean fasting breath hydrogen value than controls (16.4 and 5.7 p.p.m. respectively). Six pouch patients did not exhibit such a rise either on repeated testing or on direct intrapouch instillation of glucose. These six patients had significantly lower faecal bacterial counts than the rest by at least 20 p.p.m. All patients with counts greater than 10 p.p.m. had evidence of bacterial overgrowth in the pouch. There was no relationship between pouch overgrowth and frequency of defaecation.

Conclusions

The construction of an ileal reservoir at the end of the small intestine clearly has implications for the normal functioning of the more proximal small intestine. As such, this operation provides for a very exciting model of small intestinal physiology, and one which can be studied with relative ease. Such studies are likely to reveal much in ensuing years. To date, changes in motility patterns and evidence of small bowel overgrowth have both been reported, possibly resulting from chronic subacute intestinal obstruction.

11

Radiology of the ileal pelvic reservoir

Roentgenographic assessments

Several studies have investigated the use of a static form of contrast study of the ileoanal reservoir both before and after emptying (Pescatori, Manhire and Bartram, 1983; Lindquist, Liljequist and Sellburg, 1984; Hillard *et al.*, 1985; Kremers, Scholz and Schoetz, 1985; Bank, White and Coran, 1986; Hennild, Kjaergard and Hansen, 1986; Brown *et al.*, 1990; Thoeni *et al.*, 1990). Of undoubted importance is the role of such techniques in the investigation of postoperative complications, such as fistulas, abscesses, pouchitis and strictures. In addition, radiological investigations have also been used as research tools to assess the anatomy and function of the ileoanal reservoir.

It is some 9 years since the first report of contrast radiology after ileoanal pouch anastomosis, when such studies were used to assess postoperative healing and the presence of complications in five patients after S-pouch construction (Fonkalsrud, 1980).

The St Mark's group studied 34 patients after S-pouch–anal anastomosis at a mean of 21 months (range 1–72 months) after closure of the ileostomy (Pescatori, Manhire and Bartram, 1983). They divided the patients into two groups, those who could spontaneously evacuate, and those who practised self-catheterization. There was little difference in age or bowel frequency between the two groups. The pouch was catheterized with the patient in the left lateral position. Barium was instilled until reflux in the afferent loop was seen. The patient then sat upright on a commode such that lateral views of the pelvis could be taken. A lateral film was obtained at rest with the pouch full, and the patient encouraged to empty the pouch. A second film was taken to record the empty reservoir. Pelvic floor and pouch descent on straining; filling of the distal segment (which they defined as the region between the pouch and the anal margin, thus including the efferent limb and the anal canal); the length and configuration of the distal segment; and the angle between the pouch and the distal segment, were measured. In S-pouches, filling of the distal segment both at rest and on straining was associated with the ability to evacuate the pouch spontaneously. Spontaneous evacuation was also associated with a shorter distal segment (mean 8 ± 3 cm) than in the self-catheterization group (11 ± 4 cm). Pouch configuration within the pelvic cavity, i.e. horizontal, oblique or vertical, did not relate to the ability to evacuate spontaneously. Similarly, perineal descent on straining and the angle between the distal segment and the pouch appeared to be unimportant in this regard. Nocturnal leakage was associated with the need for self-catheterization, a distal segment of 10 cm or longer, and perineal descent of less than 1 cm. Hence, this group recommended that a short distal segment be constructed to increase the likelihood of spontaneous defaecation.

A study from the University of Copenhagen described further aspects of the radiological appearances of S-type reservoirs (Hennild, Kjaergard and Hansen, 1986). They constructed 26 S-pouches, the first 13 having 12-cm efferent limbs, the subsequent 13 having efferent limbs of 3–5 cm. Several radiological investigations were performed, including a small bowel contrast study, and a pouch enema via the efferent limb. Cold barium sulphate suspension was used for the small bowel study, and serial radiographs taken to assess the rate of progress to the reservoir. The range of such transit was up to 7 hours (mean 2 hours), two patients having a paralytic ileus. Jejunal diameter was noted to be within normal limits. In almost all patients, the ileum was somewhat dilated (range 3–8 cm, mean 4 cm), however throughout the small bowel the mucosal pattern was normal.

Either a barium sulphate suspension or Urografin 30% were used for the pouch enema. Long efferent limbs were measured at 10–20 cm (mean 15 cm), whilst the short limbs were 5–11 cm long (mean 9 cm). Stenoses between the efferent limb and the pouch were noted in 50% of patients (70% long and 30% short efferent limbs). Long limbs were associated with a tortuous course to the reservoir. This group therefore concluded that whilst potentially useful if inflammation is suspected, the diagnostic yield of the small bowel study was so low as to preclude its routine use in such patients. Interestingly, the efferent limb almost universally appeared to be longer than when measured at operation, presumably as a result of ileal relaxation and lengthening.

Radiological evaluation of J-pouches was provided by Hillard *et al*, who examined 42 patients mostly at about 4 weeks after ileoanal pouch anastomosis (Hillard *et al.*, 1985). Their assessment was carried out to provide information regarding continence, integrity of the anastomosis, pouch anatomy, and distal ileal motility. After catheterizing the efferent limb of the loop ileostomy, contrast was injected under fluoroscopic control. The ileum was assessed for motility, and the reservoir measured for maximum length, width and fold thickness. The presacral space was also measured and any external impressions on the pouch noted.

The ileum forming the afferent limb of the pouch demonstrated normal motility and folds. Pouch length varied between 7.7 and 17 cm (mean 13.8±0.8 cm), and the maximum width was 2.7–6 cm (mean 4.3±1 cm). In 78% of patients, spiral folds were seen running from the middle third of the pouch down to the ileoanal anastomosis. These were thought to represent tension on the ileum. Ninety-one per cent of examinations revealed a lucent band running through the centre of the pouch, probably representing the pouch suture line.

Other radiological observations included an extrinsic 'mass effect' caused by the ileal mesentery, and pseudopolyps which were seen in 40% of the patients at the point where the ileoanal anastomosis was crossed by the previously mentioned spiral fold. As none of the patients studied were incontinent, conclusions are difficult to draw from this report. However, it clearly demonstrates what might be considered the 'normal' appearances of a J-pouch in the early postoperative period.

We have routinely performed videofluoroscopic assessment in our patients, and we and others have found this technique useful in several respects (Bank, White and Coran, 1986; Kmiot *et al.*, 1990). The patient has the opportunity to evacuate his/her pouch for studies performed after ileostomy closure. In patients assessed during the period of defunctioning, no bowel preparation is used. With the patient in the left lateral position, the anastomosis is assessed digitally, then a lubricated urinary catheter is inserted into the reservoir. The patient then sits on a specially constructed radiolucent commode sited in front of the X-ray machine. A pad is placed over the loop ileostomy, to provide a seal, then a dilute barium solution is run into the pouch. Fluoroscopic screening takes place during filling of the pouch, and the patient notes any sensations felt at particular volumes. When the pouch is distended, several features are noted, including pouch size, orientation, mucosal pattern, motility pattern and the presence or otherwise of leaks. The ileoanal anastomosis is similarly assessed for leaks, and for any other mucosal patterns present at this site. Both standard films and cinematic copies of the study are taken.

The patient has explained to him or her the manoeuvres used to aid pouch emptying. Initially, the Valsalva manoeuvre is explained, as often this proves to be both easily understood and sufficiently efficient to provide satisfactory pouch evacuation. After this brief instruction, the patient attempts to evacuate the pouch, whilst being shown the fluoroscopic monitor. In spite of having a defunctioning stoma for several months, these patients frequently evacuate their pouches very success-

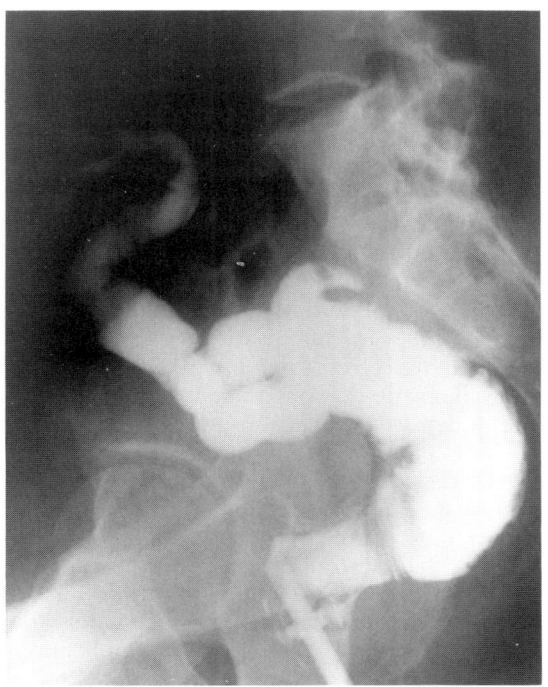

Figure 11.1

fully at their first attempts. Should this not be the case, we have found that a timed forward and backward rocking movement during the Valsalva manoeuvre is frequently beneficial. During the act of defaecation 'hard' copies are taken, for assessment of perineal descent and pouch emptying. At the end of defaecation further films are taken.

Using the technique of videopouchography prior to ileostomy closure, in our experience ileal pelvic pouches usually lie in a vertical plane. On instilling barium, the afferent limb of the pouch always fills spontaneously (Figure 11.1). There is usually little of note regarding the mucosal pattern in the pouch. We have not perfomed formal double-contrast studies. In approximately 10% of our reservoirs, the diffuse motility pattern shown in Figure 11.2 is seen. Such motility of the pouch is non-propulsive.

These preclosure examinations allow the assessment of the ileoanal anastomosis itself, in two of our patients a constant mucosal fold was seen at the site of the anastomosis (Figure

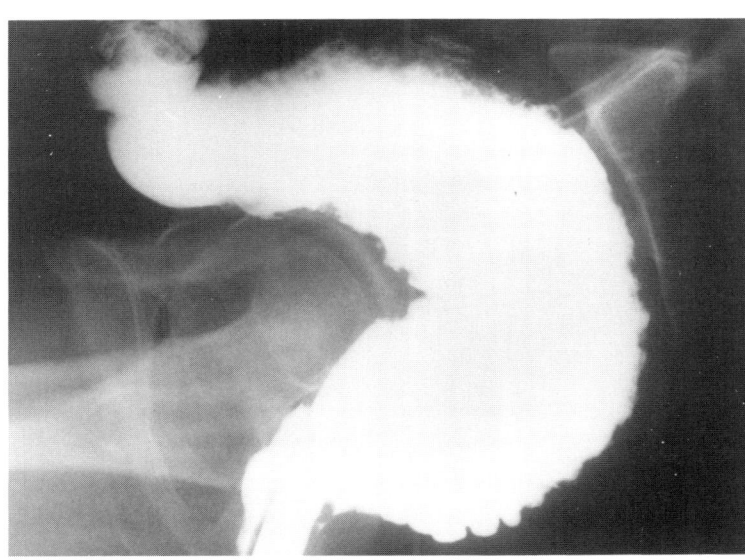

Figure 11.2

11.3). In neither of these patients, have these folds proved to be symptomatic. In addition, postoperative complications such as pouch–vaginal fistula (Figure 11.4), pouch–perineal fistula, anastomotic strictures (Figure 11.5) and pouch leaks can be demonstrated. With long anastomotic strictures, the barium may have to be instilled via the distal limb of the loop ileostomy.

Ileal pelvic pouches are well recognized to increase in volume after ileostomy closure. The change in pouch dimensions occurring in the first 6 months after ileostomy closure in one of our patients can be seen in Figures 11.3 and 11.6.

Upon defaecation, it is our experience that the afferent limb and the pouch act as one functional unit, emptying simultaneously (Figure 11.7). In our patients, the Valsalva manoeuvre is required for pouch emptying, there being no demonstrable inherent ability of the pouch to aid evacuation.

Thoeni and his colleagues have attempted to assess the relative merits of contrast pouchography, as discussed above, with both computerized scanning of the pelvis and [111]indium-labelled leucocyte scanning, in the evaluation of postoperative complications after restorative proctocolectomy. Overall, pouchography was least sensitive (60%) for all complications, such as abscess, fistula and pouchitis. This compared with values of 78% for CT and 79% for scintigraphy. Abscesses were consistently diagnosed by CT scanning (100% sensitivity), whereas pouchitis was best diagnosed by scintigraphy (80% sensitivity). Fistulae were frequently missed irrespective of the technique used. When tests were combined, the combination of CT with scintigraphy proved most efficacious, increasing the overall sensitivity to

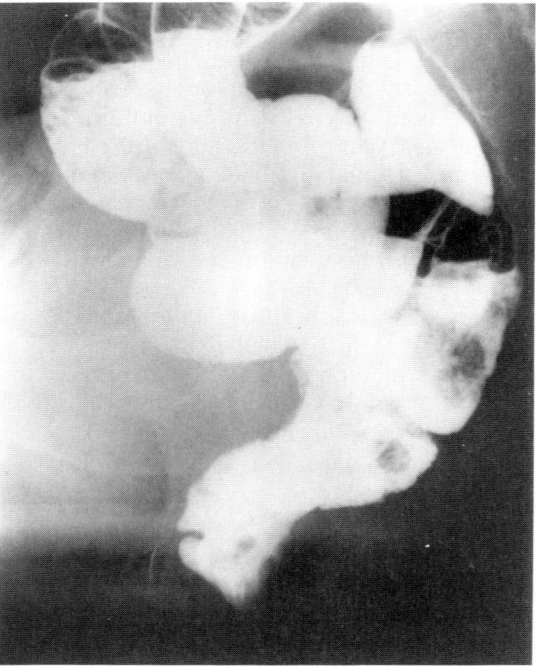

Figure 11.3

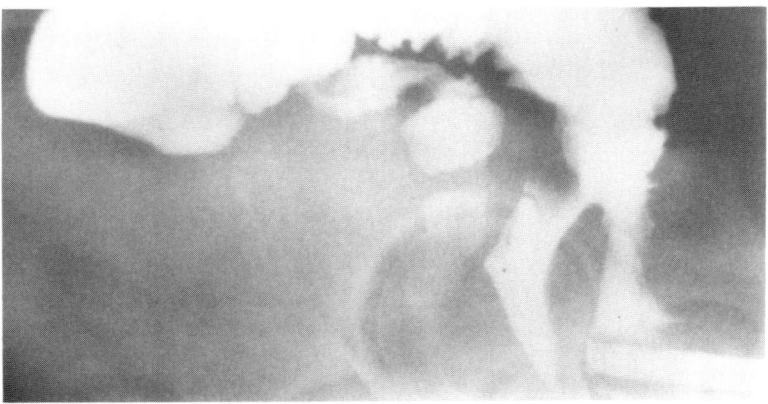

Figure 11.4

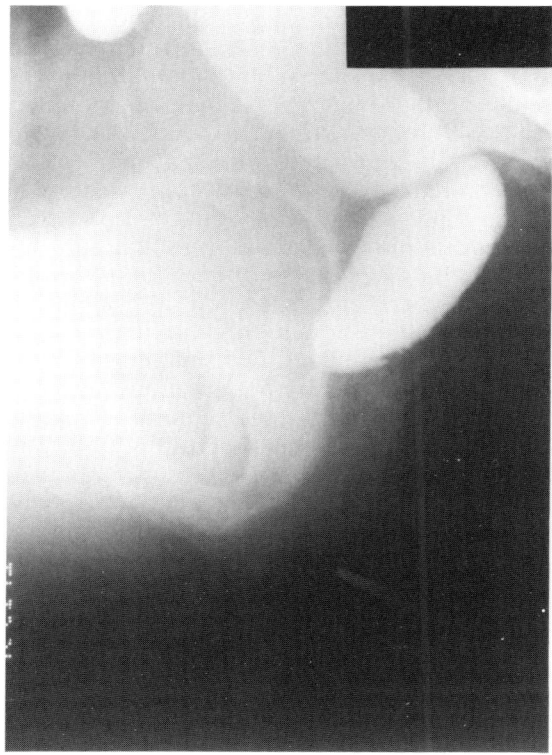

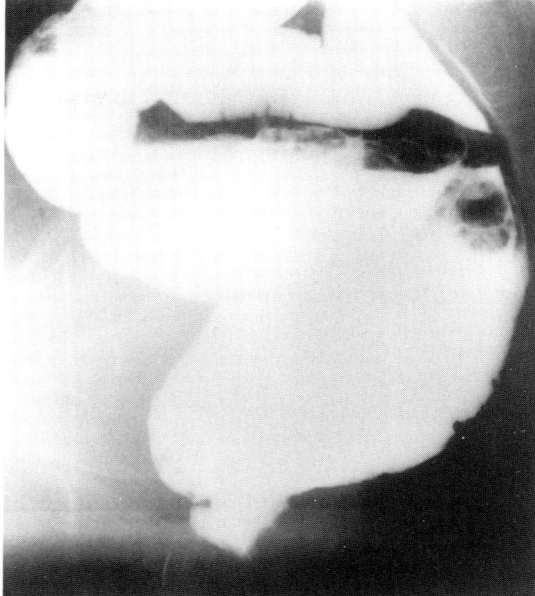

Figure 11.6

Figure 11.5

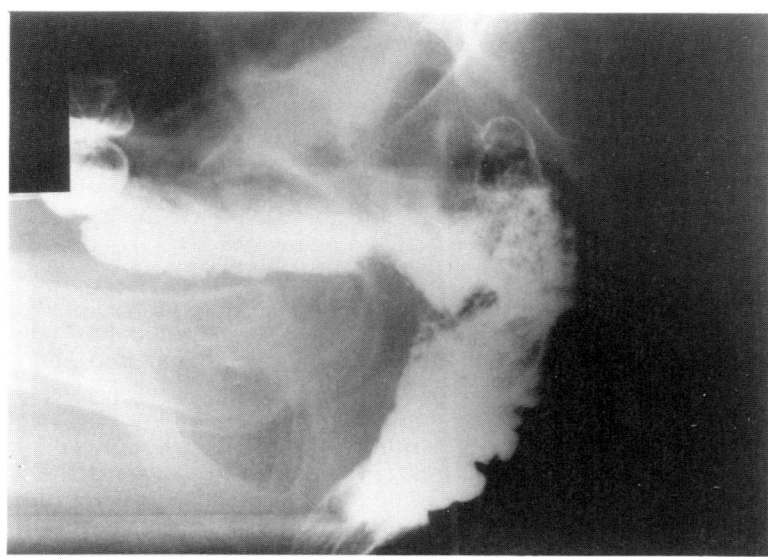

Figure 11.7

93%. This group therefore concluded that for patients presenting with complications of ileal pouch formation, computerized scanning should be the initial investigation. Others have reported similar findings (Brown *et al.*, 1990). This will reliably exclude abscess formation. If this is negative, scintigraphy should be performed (Thoeni *et al.*, 1990).

Radioisotopic assessments

Radionuclide imaging has to date been used infrequently in proctological practice, but would appear to be particularly well suited to the functional assessment of pelvic reservoirs. Initial studies involved its use in attempting to quantitate emptying efficiency after straight ileoanal anastomosis (Stryker, Telander and Perrault, 1985). This group used a labelled viscous load, comprising PSP-labelled Veegum to assess emptying efficiency in 12 controls and 12 patients after endorectal ileoanal anastomosis and balloon dilatation. Six patients had what would be considered an acceptable result, whilst the other six had a poor functional result. There was little difference between any of the groups with regard to efficiency of emptying (controls emptied 65%, good result patients 54%, and poor result patients 58%).

O'Connell and his colleagues were the first group to develop a reproducible labelled artificial stool which could be used to assess reservoir function after restorative proctocolectomy (O'Connell, Kelly and Brown, 1986). They utilized aluminium magnesium silicate, which was known to be inert, and to form a colloidal suspension in water. At a temperature of 37°C, it forms a paste resembling ileostomy effluent. The gel was made up to 7.5% concentration, which is the closest consistency to semisolid. A preliminary *in vitro* study assessed several isotopes, including [$^{99}T^m$]pertechnetate and [$^{99}Tc^m$]albumin, however it was found that [$^{99}Tc^m$]sulphur colloid had the greatest binding affinity for the silicate gel, and was therefore utilized at a dose of nCi. Seven controls and 23 patients were died. The patient group was at a mean of 2 months post pouch formation, with a age of 38±2 years. Nineteen patients had uch *in situ*, whilst four had an S-pouch. ntrols had a mean age of 37±6 years. the test, the activity per gram of the

labelled stool was measured. Rectal or neorectal capacity was first assessed using balloon manometry. No special bowel preparation was utilized, other than a phosphate enema in the controls. Using a syringe, a volume of labelled silicate gel, equivalent to the maximally tolerated volume as previously assessed, was injected per anum. A 5-minute anterior scan was taken pre-evacuation, with the subjects standing in front of the gamma camera. The patient was then seated on a radiolucent commode. A 5-minute pre-evacuation right lateral scan was taken. Dynamic images were then obtained during defaecation, every 2 seconds over 4 minutes. Finally 5-minute lateral and anterior scans were repeated. The total radioactivity of the excreted material, and its activity per gram were calculated. This allowed assessment of whether faecal material had diluted the silicate gel. The volume of material injected was similar in both groups (controls 330±29 ml, patients 320±36 ml). In all patients the gel was seen to reflux into the ileum at a mean of 46±6% of injected isotope. The pouch retained 54±6%. In the controls, 71±5% remained in the rectum, whilst 29±5% passed into the colon.

Little difference was found between the evacuation figures as assessed in the anterior and lateral scans. However, the lateral scan provided a clearer anatomical picture of the ileum and pouch. Pre- and post-evacuation counts per gram were similar, indicating that faecal contamination did not occur and allowing valid assessment of efficiency of emptying from the weight of gel recovered. This correlated well with efficiency assessment as determined by pouch scintigraphy. Defaecation lasted a median of 20 seconds in the patient group (lasting less than 90 seconds in 20 out of 23), and 40 seconds in the controls. These patients emptied 61±3% of colloid-labelled gel. The other three patients took more than 90 seconds to evacuate, and emptied 37±5% of the gel. This was associated with the passage of small stools and impaired continence.

In the controls, whilst evacuation efficiency was not dissimilar from the pouches (60±6%), the pattern of defaecation differed. The sigmoid colon first emptied into the rectum which became distended, and then evacuated. In the ileal pouch patients, the ileum and reservoir emptied as one functional unit.

Heppell *et al.* studied 33 patients (17 S- and 16 J-pouches) at a mean of 17 and 13 months respectively after closure of the ileostomy (Heppell *et al.*, 1987). There were 16 males and 17 females. Interestingly, in this series of patients, 12 males received S-pouches, whilst 12 females received J-pouches. The mean age was 30.4 ± 1.9 years. Fifteen of the S-pouches had short efferent limbs, being less than 3 cm long. Ten controls (seven males and three females) of mean age 28 ± 2 years were also assessed.

Without prior bowel preparation, patients were injected with a radionuclide marker consisting of 1 mCi of $[^{99}Tc^m]$sulphur colloid added to 350 ml of beaten eggs. This mixture had been precooked to a consistency resembling ileostomy effluent. A 2-minute posterior view pre-evacuation film was taken with the patient in the upright position. The patient then evacuated in a washroom, and a 2-minute post-evacuation image was taken. This allowed calculation of the emptying fraction. Functional results were analysed using a detailed questionnaire.

The mean emptying fractions of J-pouches was $72\pm4\%$, compared with $67\pm5\%$ for the S-pouches. These figures were not significantly different, however the controls emptied significantly better at $90\pm3\%$. There was no correlation between efficiency of emptying and sex, age, postileostomy interval and stool frequency. Also, in a group of seven patients with documented clinical pouchitis, there was no evidence of inefficient emptying of their reservoirs. However, the two patients with S-pouches and long efferent limbs had emptying fractions of less than 30% and poor functional results, which have been improved by the instigation of catheter intubation of the pouch. This also resulted in an improved emptying fraction.

The Mayo clinic group have used similar techniques to study the ano-pouch angle after restorative proctocolectomy (Barkel *et al.*, 1988). In six patients (all men at a mean age of 38 ± 5 years) and 13 controls (seven men and six women, aged 35 ± 3 years), a balloon device was utilized. This consisted of a low compliance latex balloon of length 16 cm and diameter 2.24 cm. Inside this balloon was a semirigid rubber catheter with an external diameter of 5.33 mm. Connected to the balloon was a large bore tube leading to a fluid-filled reservoir, containing 500 ml of water labelled with 40 mCi of $[^{99}Tc^m]O_4$. The height of the reservoir could be varied, thus dictating the pressure within the balloon. Radiolabelled markers were placed over the tip of the coccyx and the symphysis pubis, allowing localization of the pubococcygeal line. The balloon was inserted per anum, such that the distal portion projected from the anal verge. The proximal portion was situated within the rectum or pouch. With the patient in the left lateral position the balloon was filled by elevating the reservoir. Images were collected for 30 seconds, then subjects were requested to squeeze against the balloon and to perform a Valsalva manoeuvre. Both such actions were monitored in the sitting and standing positions.

In the left lateral position, the anorectal angle was $102\pm18°$, compared to an ano-pouch angle of $108\pm19°$. In both groups moving to a sitting position resulted in straightening of this resting angle. However, studying the patient standing upright did not result in such a straightening. In controls, voluntary squeezing and the Valsalva manoeuvre resulted in a sharpening of the anorectal angle in all positions. In the pouch group, a Valsalva manoeuvre resulted in sharpening of the angle in the sitting position only, whilst voluntary squeezing resulted in sharpening both in the standing and sitting positions. In both groups, the ano-pouch or anorectal junction remained below the pubococcygeal line in all positions. Sitting resulted in descent of the anorectal junction in controls, but not in patients. Standing resulted in an elevation of the ano-pouch junction, whilst having no effect in the controls. In all positions, voluntary contraction of the external sphincter caused elevation of the anorectal junction in controls; whereas Valsalva's manoeuvre resulted in elevation in this group in the sitting position only. Neither manoeuvre had any effect in the pouch group of patients, regardless of position.

Filling pouches above the threshold volume (i.e. the volume first discernible to the patient), resulted in afferent limb reflux (O'Connell *et al.*, 1987a). This volume corresponds to that at which large pressure waves can be recorded. Afferent limb reflux is associated with similar large pressure waves within the more proximal ileum itself. The clinical corollary of these events is that in pouch patients, the postponing of defaecation results in generalized abdominal discomfort and marked urgency. This same group found that the pouch and distal ileum empty as one functional unit. If intrinsic pouch motility were to be responsible for pouch evacuation, then one would expect that proximal reflux would occur during defaecation. However, both ileum and pouch act as a common capacitance vessel. It is therefore likely that ileoanal pouches empty by Valsalva's manoeuvre.

Many studies have now demonstrated that reservoir emptying efficiency is related to stool frequency (Cranley and McKelvey, 1982; Stryker *et al.*, 1986). However, O'Connell's multivariate analysis has suggested that the threshold volume and 24-hour stool volume are more important factors in stool frequency.

12

The defunctioned state

As discussed in Chapter 3, most surgeons continue to utlize the temporary, defunctioning ileostomy in order to protect the healing pouch–anal anastomosis, and to limit any consequences of anastomosis dehiscence. The topic of staging of this procedure has similarly been considered elsewhere. However, what of the effects of adding a proximal diverting enterostomy above the pouch–anal anastomosis? Whilst being protective, a loop ileostomy may add considerably to the surgical trauma placed upon these already often compromised patients.

Metabolic

Few studies have attempted to detail such consequences of the defunctioned state after restorative proctocolectomy. Max *et al.* have formally assessed patients during their period of defunctioning (Max *et al.*, 1987). Numerous parameters, mainly of a biochemical nature, were assessed in the immediate postoperative period, and after 6 weeks of defunctioning, just prior to closure of the ileostomy. The group studied consisted of 21 patients (17 with ulcerative colitis and four with familial polyposis), all of whom had undergone restorative proctocolectomy with J-pouch formation. There were 11 males and 10 females, with a mean age of 34 years (range 26–57 years). This group found that the haemoglobin concentration remained unchanged throughout the period concerned. The platelet count, however, increased from a mean of 304 000 in the immediate postoperative period to 447 000 just prior to ileostomy closure. The aetiology of this rise is unclear.

The authors' studies have shown that during pouch–anal anastomosis, the intraoperative transfusion requirement was 3.08±1.1 units. Two of our patients remained anaemic in the defunctioned period, however a consistently normal haemoglobin was recorded in both within the first year thereafter. Of seven of our patients who were thrombocythaemic preoperatively, two remained so, but to a lesser extent, prior to ileostomy closure. Otherwise, routine full blood counts were normal throughout the defunctioned state. Serum iron, ferritin, total iron binding capacity, vitamin B12, folate and red cell folate were normal in all patients throughout this period.

Interestingly, Max *et al.* also found that in 19 of the 21 patients, body weight was reduced by a mean of 7.2 kg during the study. In only one patient did the weight remain unchanged, and in the last patient the weight was noted to have increased slightly. Others have similarly noted a reduction in body mass index, arm muscle circumference and triceps skin fold thickness during this period (Pironi *et al.*, 1989).

Max determined the serum cholesterol to fall from a mean of 183 iu/l to 120 iu/l, whilst serum triglyceride levels rose from a mean of 95 iu/l to 190 iu/l. Our own patients have retained a normal cholesterol level throughout their period of defunctioning, and similarly thereafter (Thomas and Taylor, 1989a).

Indices of hepatic function may become elevated. Max found that liver enzymes (SGOT, SGPT and LDH) were all increased during the 6 weeks of defunctioning, as was the serum alkaline phosphatase. As the preoperative values for these parameters were not given, their precise meaning is difficult to evaluate, particularly with reference to colitis-associated cholestasis. In our patients only three patients biochemically demonstrated cholestasis preoperatively, and in all these patients complete improvement was seen during the period of defunctioning. Blood urea nitrogen was found to have risen from 11 mg/100 ml to a mean of 22 mg/100 ml, whilst serum creatinine increased from 0.97 mg/ml to 1.5 mg/ml. Serum uric acid rose from 5.6 mg/100 ml to 7.5 mg/100 ml. Our own assessments demonstrate remarkable normality in serum electrolytes throughout the whole pelvic pouch procedure. Serum sodium, potassium, calcium phosphate, urea and creatinine were normal in all patients.

Recent studies have demonstrated that the period of defunctioning may be associated with an increased susceptibility to the formation of uric acid and calcium oxalate renal stones (Caudarella *et al.*, 1989). This group found that the urinary excretion of sodium, potassium, magnesium, calcium and citrate was significantly reduced, when compared to both the preoperative and postileostomy closure states. The urinary volume was also reduced during the defunctioned period.

Pironi has also reported reduced calcium excretion during the defunctioned period. In this group, there were no abnormalities in serum levels of parathyroid hormone, calcitonin or vitamin D. The reduced urinary calcium was taken to be indicative of a combination of malabsorption of calcium, increased intestinal losses, and a degree of renal tubular reabsorption (Pironi *et al.*, 1989a).

Whilst no formal small intestinal resection is performed during the course of pouch–anal anastomosis, the defunctioning ileostomy excludes the pouch itself and a variable length of its afferent limb from the faecal stream. Exclusion of 60 cm of ileum during J-pouch–anal anastomosis is associated with a significant increase in faecal bile acids, particularly secondary and free bile acids. The degree of such increased losses was found to be proportional to the length of ileum excluded, and was associated with increased faecal bacterial counts, especially anaerobic organism counts (Natori *et al.*, 1989).

Using a standard 100 g of fat per day test diet, faecal fat excretion was elevated during the period of defunctioning. This was positively correlated with increased daily faecal weight (Guidetti *et al.*, 1989).

Consistently, we have demonstrated a fall in the immediate postoperative albumin level, from a mean preoperative value of 41.9 ± 5.5 g/l to 32.1 ± 7.4 g/l. After the period of defunctioning, no patient remained hypoalbuminaemic.

Protein-calorie status has been demonstrated to be low during the defunctioned state, in spite of an increased oral intake. These same workers found electrolyte depletion to be common. In particular, sodium and potassium were depleted during this period. Normal serum levels were maintained by reducing urinary excretion with secondary hyperaldosteronism (Miglioli, Pironi and Ruggeri, 1989).

Our serial assessments of trace minerals confirmed that the serum zinc, magnesium and copper remain normal during the defunctioned period. We have therefore concluded that the creation of an ileal reservoir is followed by few, if any, long-term metabolic sequelae. However, Max *et al.* felt that the most distal segment of ileum possible should be utilized for construction of the ileostomy, in order to allow for the maximum absorptive surface area to be utilized during this period of intense metabolic activity.

Radiological

Most groups performing the ileoanal pouch procedure utilize some form of radiological assessment of anastomosis integrity prior to closure of the temporary loop ileostomy. Usually these are static, lateral pelvic contrast studies. The radiological features of the ileal pelvic reservoir were discussed in the previous chapter.

The authors' studies have confirmed a role for the dynamic assessment of reservoir function during the period of defunctioning. Prior to closure of the ileostomy, we have performed defaecation pouchograms, which are recorded on videotape. A pad is placed over the ileostomy to act as a seal. Barium is placed endoanally within the pouch, allowing for assessment of the anastomosis and pouch integrity. Subsequently, recordings are taken during the act of defaecation. After prior instruction, patients can usually successfully evacuate their pouches at this initial attempt. Should difficulty be encountered, we have found this technique of fluoroscopic screening to be useful in aiding patient tuition. In addition, if late complications ensue, the ability to compare efficiency of emptying with earlier studies has similarly proved to be of value.

Manometric

In a study from the Mayo clinic, anal manometry was performed using a rigid, polyglass probe in 104 patients after ileal pouch–anal anastomosis prior to ileostomy closure, and again at 1 year post closure (Scott *et al.*, 1988a; Scott *et al*, 1989). Using the station pull-through technique, they found that a low resting pressure was associated with nocturnal incontinence and the need for antidiarrhoeal medication. In addition, a low pouch compliance prior to closure, correlated with a significantly increased nocturnal stool frequency at 1 year. Interestingly, neither anal canal length, maximal squeeze pressure nor reservoir capacity as assessed before ileostomy closure, appeared to affect ultimate functional outcome. They concluded that manometry in the defunctioned state was a good prognostic indicator of functional outcome at 1 year.

13

Metabolic sequelae of the ileoanal reservoir

The previous chapters of this book have documented that rectal replacement with a reservoir constructed from the terminal ileum is usually associated with very acceptable functional results. That pathophysiological sequelae are witnessed after pouch construction has also been discussed. In terms of allowing for disease excision and providing for anorectal continence, the pelvic pouch procedure is patently an advance over previous techniques. However, what of any other effects of constructing a terminal ileal reservoir?

It is well recognized that the most proximal segment of the jejunum differs markedly from the most distal segment of the ileum. Anatomical variations include a greater diameter of the jejunum; its villi also being more prominent than those in the ileum. Mechanically, the small bowel is more active distally than proximally, and is known to be stimulated by various bacterial metabolites, including short chain volatile fatty acids (see Chapter 8). The latter may also be important in intestinal growth. Physiologically, the ileum possesses a chloride-bicarbonate exchange pump, allowing bicarbonate to accumulate in the ileal lumen. The jejunum, on the other hand, has a more permeable mucosa than that of the ileum. Small nutrient molecules, such as amino acids and glucose, are absorbed passively throughout the small intestine. In contrast, the terminal ileum is important in the active absorption of both bile acids and vitamin B12. Whilst the proximal and distal limits of the small intestine vary considerably in their morphometric and physiological characteristics, their intermediate features merge imperceptibly.

Of greater significance is the fact that there are normally relatively efficient mechanisms for preventing bacterial overgrowth of the small bowel. In that clinical sequelae of such overgrowth are usually obvious, it is plainly important that bacterial contamination of the small intestine is best avoided. The normal jejunum is a virtually sterile region, whereas the terminal ileum represents an area of intermediate bacterial count prior to entry into the densely populated colon. The ileocaecal valve is likely to be one of several mechanisms avoiding coloileal reflux, and preventing the manifestations of small bowel overgrowth.

This chapter will be concerned with the metabolic sequelae of pouch construction for the individual. Other potential sequelae, such as those on the pouch itself or on the more proximal intestine, are considered in earlier chapters.

Haematological

The ileal pouch, whether it be utilized as a continent ileostomy, or as a pelvic reservoir, is constructed from the terminal ileum. This is a region well known for its specialized absorptive function. In particular, vitamin B12 and bile acids are actively absorbed within this region. Certain diseases of, and bacterial overgrowth within, the terminal ileum may be associated with deficiencies of these compounds. Similarly, resection of the terminal ileum may result in deficiencies leading to well recognized clinical syndromes.

Briefly, vitamin B_{12} is a highly charged molecule, consisting of two major component parts: a porphyrin-like ring with a cobalt atom at its centre, with a nucleotide bound to it. Depending upon the different ligands attached to the cobalt atom, it exists in four recognized forms. Of these, deoxyadenosylcobalamin (or coenzyme B_{12}) is the main dietary form of the vitamin, being present in animal tissue and in bacteria. Humans are entirely dependent upon dietary vitamin B_{12}, which is synthesized by bacteria present in the intestine or in water. Indeed, vitamin B_{12} is one of the largest water-soluble molecules that can be absorbed intact through the normal intestinal mucosa. Approximately $2\,\mu g$ per day is required by normal adults, with an average diet containing up to $30\,\mu g$. The total body pool of vitamin B_{12} is some $4\,\mu g$, of which approximately 0.1% (i.e. $4\,ng$) is lost every day. This loss is not obligatory, and in conditions in which the body pool is compromised, such as after partial gastrectomy, the losses may be reduced. There is an enterohepatic circulation of vitamin B_{12}, with some $4\,\mu g$ excreted daily into the bile. In deficiency states the enteric absorption of vitamin B_{12} is increased. Hence, there may be no physiological consequences of a reduced total pool.

Vitamin B_{12} is absorbed by two independent processes. First, there is a quantitatively unimportant and inefficient passive absorption within the jejunum and ileum, which is not dependent upon gastric intrinsic factor. In part, this inefficiency is due to the size of the vitamin B_{12} molecule. Secondly, there is a highly efficient active absorption of vitamin B_{12} within the terminal ileum. This requires the formation of a vitamin B_{12}–gastric intrinsic factor complex prior to its absorption. This complex subsequently becomes attached to a receptor situated in the ileal mucosa; such binding occurs passively, but requires calcium and an optimum pH of 7.0. Entry of the complex into the enterocyte occurs where the vitamin B_{12}–intrinsic factor complex is split, releasing the vitamin. Vitamin B_{12} is then converted to the coenzyme form (see above) and stored in the mitochondria of the enterocytes. This free form of vitamin B_{12} is released

into the portal blood some 4 hours after its oral administration, reaching a peak level within 8 hours or so, and disappearing completely after 12 hours. In the blood, the vitamin is bound to two plasma globulins, termed transcobalamins. Peripheral uptake of vitamin B_{12} is extremely rapid, particularly by the liver. Therefore, plasma levels of vitamin B_{12} are normally very small (300 ng/l). In spite of the efficiency of this active absorption, the oral requirement of vitamin B_{12} in pernicious anaemia, where there is an absence of intrinsic factor, is some 1000 to 10 000 times that normally required. Only by such oral doses can sufficient absorption be assured. Consequently, parenteral vitamin B_{12} is usually to be preferred in such circumstances.

Until recently, most studies of the haematological sequelae of intestinal pouches had been focused upon the continent ileostomy. There is good evidence that Kock pouches utilized as continent ileostomies continue to actively absorb vitamin B_{12} (Gadacz, Kelly and Phillips, 1977). Both serum vitamin B_{12} levels and the results of Schilling tests remain normal even on prolonged follow-up of such continent stomas (Jagenburg *et al.*, 1971; Nilsson *et al.*, 1984). Whilst impaired vitamin B_{12} absorption has been described (Nilsson *et al.*, 1979), it is likely that an associated ileal resection may be the causal factor in many of these patients.

Ileal resection may predispose some patients to subsequent deficiencies, however, Kelly and colleagues described the improvement in the Schilling test result after treatment with metronidazole in a group of four patients with abnormal Schilling tests after continent ileostomy formation. Only one of these patients had had an ileal resection (Kelly *et al.*, 1983). This would suggest that in some patients bacterial overgrowth may contribute to the malabsorption of vitamin B_{12}. This is certainly possible, as host dietary vitamin B_{12} is well known to be utilized by some intestinal microbial species.

Initial experience with the ileoanal reservoir is in line with the above. Increasing numbers of studies have begun to assess such factors in the very long term, and tend to support that there are few noteworthy metabolic sequelae to this procedure. Assessing the early sequelae in 14 patients, workers from St Mark's measured numerous haematological parameters, and performed Schilling tests in 12 patients (Nicholls *et al.*, 1981). One patient had a microcytic anaemia, with a low serum iron and transferrin saturation. Similarly low serum iron levels were observed in four other patients, without evidence of anaemia. Most of these were premenopausal women. In all patients except one (a strict vegetarian), the serum vitamin B_{12} level was normal, whilst serum folate was reduced in two patients. Red cell folate levels were normal in all patients. Schilling tests were between 5% and 10% in four patients, being marginally low. None had values of less than 5%, suggesting that there was no significant vitamin B_{12} malabsorption.

Further evidence of minor haematological abnormalities was found in 20 patients at a mean of 2 years after pouch construction (O'Connell *et al.*, 1986). Six patients had a mild microcytic anaemia, however the mean haemoglobin for the whole group was within normal limits. Five patients developed a mild thrombocytosis of greater than $370 \times 10^9/l$. Two patients had serum vitamin B_{12} levels slightly below the normal range. In one of these patients the Schilling test was marginally abnormal. In all patients, the serum folate concentration was within the normal range. More recently, Fiorentini recorded that numerous haematinnics remained normal in eight patients after ileal pouch–anal anastomosis (Fiorentini *et al.*, 1987).

In an ongoing study of the metabolic sequelae of pouch–anal anastomosis in the authors' department, patients are assessed prior to pouch formation, at the end of the period of defunctioning, and subsequently up until the present (mean follow-up 34.25 ± 20.92 months, range 6–84 months). In our patients, the mean preoperative haemoglobin concentration was $12.6 \pm 1.65\,g/l$, and the operative transfusion requirement was 3.08 ± 1.1 units. Two patients remained anaemic in the defunctioned period, however a normal haemoglobin was recorded in both within the first year thereafter. The mean follow-up haemoglobin was normal throughout the group. Seven patients were thrombocythaemic preoperatively (the mean for these seven patients was $703 \pm 99.1 \times 10^9/l$), and two of these remained so to a lesser extent in the defunctioned period. No patient remained thrombocythaemic at subsequent follow-up. Otherwise, full blood counts (including MCV, MCH, MCHC, red cell count and white cell count) were normal throughout the study. A low serum iron was common peroperatively, but improved during the defunctioned period and on long-term follow-up ($20.8 \pm 7.6\,\mu mol/l$). Serum ferritin, vitamin B_{12}, folate and red cell folate were normal in all patients throughout the study (Thomas and Taylor, 1989b).

Body water, electrolytes and renal function

Clarke has previously asserted that even the presence of a conventional ileostomy may be associated with chronic depletion of both water and salt (Clarke, Chirnside and Hill, 1967). However, this has remained somewhat controversial (Cooper, Laughland and Gunning, 1986). The position with regard to the pelvic pouch procedure has recently received attention (Christie, Knight and Hill, 1990).

Comparing body fluid compartments in controls and in patients after either conventional ileostomy or J-pouch–anal anastomosis, these workers assessed several postoperative metabolic indices. Basic measurements of body weight and height were supplemented by other body composition assessments, including total body protein, total body water, extracellular water volume and fat-free mass. Total body water was calculated by tritium dilution after an intravenous injection of tritiated water. Total body protein was assessed from gamma *in vivo* neutron activation analysis. Addition of both these values, incorporating an estimate of total body minerals and glycogen, allowed for the calculation of the fat-free mass. The technique of bromide dilution was used to measure the volume of the extracellular water. Forty-eight-hour collections of both urine and ileal effluent also were collected. The volumes, and sodium and potassium levels within both of these products were measured. Fourteen patients with well-functioning ileostomies and 20 patients with duplicated ileal pelvic reservoirs were assessed. The temporary loop ileostomies covering the pelvic pouches had been closed for an average of 18 months (6–40 months), whilst the permanent ileostomies had been present for 14 years (1.5–30 years). There was no information regarding possible ileal resection in the permanent ileostomy group, however all of the patients studied had suffered with ulcerative colitis prior to colectomy.

Correlating total body water with fat-free mass, this group did not find any evidence suggestive of chronic dehydration in either group of patients compared with the controls. Similarly, correlations between extracellular water volume and fat-free mass failed to demonstrate any evidence of depletion in extracellular volume in either group. No difference was found between the groups in stool or urine volumes. Stool electrolyte concentrations were unchanged postoperatively. However, urinary electrolyte output was significantly lower in both of the patient groups, suggesting urinary retention of sodium after colectomy. Whilst this group found that faecal volumes were similar in both colectomy groups, the outputs were approximately double those measured in controls. As a consequence, the kidneys conserve water and sodium. This study stresses that, whilst body stores of water and salt remain normal after colectomy, such patients rely heavily upon renal conservation to compensate for faecal losses. Hence, a propensity for the development of renal calculi might be expected.

At the moment, there is little evidence that there are any derangements of serum electrolyte concentrations after restorative proctocolectomy (Thomas and Taylor, 1989a).

Protein and fat metabolism

To date, there is little evidence that either protein or fat metabolism are affected adversely by ileal reservoir formation (Pironi *et al.*, 1989b).

Biliary metabolism

Bile acids are secreted by the liver as primary, conjugated bile acids (cholic and chenodeoxycholic acids). These conjugated acids (and those remaining in the ionized form) are actively reabsorbed in the terminal ileum, constituting the enterohepatic circulation of these substances. Whilst passive diffusion of bile acids occurs throughout the whole length of the small intestine, including the terminal ileum, the aforementioned energy-dependent active absorptive process ensures that more than 95% of the bile acids are reabsorbed within the terminal ileum. Of the small amount of bile acid entering the large intestine, some is passively reabsorbed; the rest is deconjugated and dehydroxylated by anaerobic bacteria and excreted as secondary bile acids (deoxycholic and lithocholic acids). Deconjugated bile acids may become bound to either dietary fibre or to bacteria within the colon, resulting in their impaired absorption. Faecal excretion of bile acids is of the order of 500 mg per day.

Should malabsorption of bile acids occur, the cycle is broken. Clinical consequences may ensue, including cholesterol gall stones, steatorrhoea and diarrhoea. Moderate malabsorption can be surmounted by increased hepatic synthesis. Therefore, fat digestion is unaltered. However, excessive amounts of bile acids pass into the colon where they inhibit water and salt absorption, resulting in a diarrhoea which may be ameliorated by cholestyramine. Clearly, this mechanism is unlikely to be important in patients who have undergone a previous colectomy. Severe malabsorption ultimately results in depletion of the bile acid pool, and in fat malabsorption, resulting in steatorrhoea. The substitution of long-chain with medium-chain triglycerides may reduce this symptom.

Concerning bile acid metabolism after surgery for ulcerative colitis, clearly there may be potential effects subsequent to the colectomy itself. Several studies have documented the effects of panproctocolectomy with Brooke ileostomy formation (Miettinen and Peltokallio, 1971; Kay *et al.*, 1979). Unfortunately, in most such studies patients with both ulcerative colitis and Crohn's disease are collated. Hence details of concomitant ileal resection, and its effects, are often ambiguous. In spite of such difficulties, it is clear that colectomy with conventional ileostomy formation is associated with values for bile acid excretion which are within the normal ranges of those found in patients with intact colons. Similar studies performed on patients after continent ileostomy formation have revealed similar difficulties in interpretation, and yielded similar results (Gadacz, Kelly and Phillips, 1977; Kay *et al.*, 1979). Again, it would appear that, in the absence of an ileal resection, bile acid excretion is no greater in such patients than in controls.

Bile acid excretion is, of course, only one definable 'end-product' of bile acid metabolism. As such, it probably provides little direct evidence of all the intervening processes. What of the ability of conventional ileostomies, and ileal pouches, both abdominal and pelvic, to actively reabsorb bile acids? In spite of relatively normal bile acid excretion, such a question is of more than academic interest. One secondary bile acid, lithocholic acid, has been incriminated in the pathogenesis of chronic liver disease. It is well recognized that the bacterial flora of reservoirs constructed from the terminal ileum undergoes transformation to one which is more colonic in nature (see Chapter 8). This may therefore allow the ileal pouch to function as a mini-colon. Gadacz and colleagues have demonstrated that both conventional and continent ileostomies metabolize bile acids in a similar fashion.

Prior to a discussion of the findings with regard to the ileal pelvic pouch, it is worth first studying the methods of assessing bile acid metabolism. Basically, two forms of study have been used to quantify bile acid absorption and excretion after pouch–anal anastomosis. Radiolabelled primary bile acids, or analogues thereof, can be measured in the faecal effluent after intravenous injection. One such compound, $[^{14}C]$cholic acid, has been used in this clinical context (Andersson, Fasth and Philipsson, 1979). However, these bile acids are deconjugated within the colon into secondary bile acids, and so may have dubious significance in patients who have undergone colectomy. In addition, they may be absorbed passively within the small intestine by non-ionic diffusion.

The other major technique for quantifying bile acid metabolism uses the ring-labelled bile acid $[^{75}Se]$homotaurocholate (SeHCAT). This is a gamma-emitting isotope, the activity of which can be measured using a whole-body counter. After oral administration of SeHCAT, whole-body counts are taken after 2 hours and again after 1 week. This compound is not metabolized significantly by bacteria, and so is probably a more reliable assessment of the capacity of the terminal ileum to absorb bile acids in an active manner. However, in the normal situation, colonic clearance of SeHCAT is slow. Therefore, in individuals

with intact colons, the precise significance of the results obtained for the whole-body retention of SeHCAT is uncertain. Differences between such normal controls may either reflect differences between colonic handling of the isotope, differences in ileal absorption, or both. Consequently, when comparing patients after colectomy with normal controls, it must be appreciated that, in some respects, this is not a totally valid comparison. If a mechanism could be found for providing for a 'colonic correction factor', allowing for the retention of SeHCAT within the colon, then such comparisons would become more meaningful.

In a controlled study after pouch–anal anastomosis, normal patients were compared with patients after S-pouches with long efferent limbs were constructed. The control group was found to excrete predominantly secondary bile acids, whereas the ileal pouch group excreted mainly primary bile acids. Overall, bile acid excretion was significantly greater within the pouch group. Interestingly, and perhaps surprisingly, the degree to which the intestinal flora approached that of the colon did not correlate with bile acid excretion. Similarly, bile acid excretion did not correlate with faecal fat excretion; the latter being similar in both groups of patients. The conclusion from this study was that terminal ileal dysfunction does occur after pouch–anal anastomosis, which is particularly manifest as abnormalities in bile acid metabolism (Hojlund et al., 1985).

In the study from Italy alluded to above, eight patients were assessed, of whom seven were found to demonstrate bile acid malabsorption. Other assessments of terminal ileal function were quantified, however, using SeHCAT, this group similarly found that abnormal bile acid metabolism was the most significant terminal ileal dysfunction after pouch–anal anastomosis (Fiorentini et al., 1987).

Nasmyth and his colleagues from Leeds have studied bile acid absorption in 10 healthy controls, and compared them with 15 patients after colectomy with conventional ileostomy formation, and 13 patients after pouch–anal anastomosis (five S-, six J-, and two lateral pouches). Of the conventional ileostomy group, nine patients were known to have less than 10 cm of terminal ileum resected, whereas the other six patients had undergone resection of 20 cm or more of terminal ileum. In this series, pelvic pouches had been functioning for 14 months (1–40 months); the ileostomies had been in place for a statistically longer period of 72 months (3–192 months). Importantly, these workers assessed both ileal excretion and ileal absorption of bile acids (Nasmyth *et al.*, 1989b). Ileal absorption was quantified using the whole-body SeHCAT technique, whilst bile acid excretion was performed using gas–liquid chromatographic analysis of processed effluent. The normal controls retained significantly more SeHCAT (33%) than any of the patient groups (pouches 9%; ileostomy without resection 15%; ileostomy with ileal resection 0.5%). Further, the results in both the pouches and the non-resection ileostomates were statistically different from those in the resection group. Regarding ileal effluent bile acids, lithocholic acid was found in all the samples analysed. However, deoxycholic acid was found in only 18% of ileostomy effluent, but in 88% of pouch effluent. As a percentage of the whole bile acid excretion, both primary and secondary, secondary bile acids exceded primary acids in only 9% of the ileostomates, but did so in half of the pouch patients.

These studies therefore demonstrate that bile acid metabolism is not normal after restorative proctocolectomy. Indeed, many workers have shown that it is probably the most deranged terminal ileal function after this procedure (Villanova *et al.*, 1989). Bacterial degradation of primary bile acids is significantly greater after pouch construction than it is after conventional ileostomy. Consequently, there is a greater concentration of the potentially harmful lithocholic acid within the absoptive terminal ileum. Whether this ultimately may result in chronic liver disease in these patients is yet to be shown. Increased bile acid excretion will result in an increase in the synthesis of bile acids within the liver. This may result in a reduction in the serum cholesterol. However, most series, including our own, have recorded normal values for serum cholesterol even on prolonged follow-up (Thomas and Taylor, 1989a).

Bile acid absorption is significantly reduced after colectomy, but the presence of an ileal pelvic reservoir does not appear to make this any worse. However, Nasmyth and colleagues point out that, in both pouch and ileostomy groups, there are patients who demonstrate SeHCAT retentions which are not significantly better than those recorded in ileostomates who have undergone a concomitant terminal ileal resection. As the length of ileum resected in these patients is equivalent to that used for pouch construction, it is clear that the pouch ileum continues to function relatively 'normally'. That is, normal within the context of the new conditions in which it finds itself after colectomy. It is only in patients after ileal resection that bile acid deficiency, supersaturation of bile and consequent cholesterol gall stones should ensue. There appears to be little data, at present, to suggest that patients after restorative proctocolectomy are more susceptible to this complication.

Use of isolated jejunal segments for neorectal formation

As stated above, bile acid malabsorption has been shown consistently to be the most deranged function of the terminal ileum after ileal pouch–anal anastomosis. In order to spare the terminal ileum from such surgical manipulations, isolated segments of jejunum for neorectal formation have received attention. Stringel (1985) was the first to report the use of such a straight jejunal segment to facilitate straight intestinal pull-through. In this case, a young female with ulcerative colitis had undergone an emergency subtotal colectomy with Brooke ileostomy formation at the age of 7 years. Two years later it was decided to perform a mucosal proctectomy and straight ileoanal anastomosis. However, the patient was keen to keep her satisfactorily functioning ileostomy to cover the ileoanal anastomosis. Therefore a conventional anastomosis could not be performed. An isolated jejunal loop was created, and the distal end anastomosed to the anal canal. The proximal end was brought out as a mucous fistula. After 6 months the ileostomy was closed by ileojejunostomy. Functional results of what might be termed 'jejunoileoanoplasty' were excellent.

Itoh and colleagues have reported their experimental experience with an isolated jejunal loop interposed between the terminal ileum and the anal canal. In dogs, gall bladder bile was sampled for both bile acid composition and lithogenic index peri- and 24 weeks postoperatively (Itoh *et al.*, 1989). Total bile

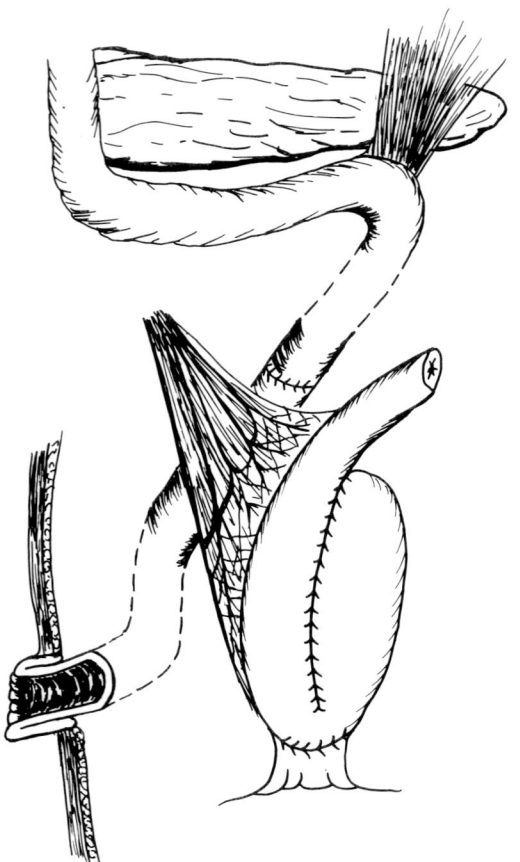

Figure 13.1 Isolated jejunal pouch

ileal function and with avoidance of bile acid malabsorption. The cholesterol saturation index was increased after this procedure. However, this appears to be a non-specific consequence of proctocolectomy, rather than of the form of intestinal restoration per se.

It has been suggested that jejunoanal anastomosis might be a viable alternative to conventional ileoanal anastomosis for several reasons. First, the jejunum has a better blood supply than the terminal ileum, and so ischaemia in the distal parts of the loop should be less of a problem. In addition, Stringel felt that as a result of the vascular arcade distribution, he had a better selection of bowel from which to select a loop. Thirdly, as the jejunum has a wider diameter when compared to the ileum, subsequent capacity should be greater and may reduce the necessity for a reservoir. He also postulated that as the bacterial count is less in the jejunum, subsequent overgrowth problems might be less. Finally, he proposed that should the pull-through not be successful, that the resection of the involved bowel would not result in loss of the terminal ileum. Obviously, there are potential disadvantages to jejunoanal anastomosis. Jejunal transit is quicker than that in the ileum, so that postoperative diarrhoea might be problematical. Secondly, operating time is likely to be longer due to the necessity for both jejunal isolation and subsequent intestinal reconstruction. The authors are presently assessing the possibilty of neorectal formation using doubly folded reservoirs using isolated jejunum, as depicted diagrammatically in Figure 13.1. In our studies performed in cadavers, such a 'jejunal-pouch-ileoanoplasty' appears to be technically quite feasible.

acid concentrations were unchanged after jejunoanal anastomosis, however the secondary bile acid concentration increased. Consequently, use of isolated jejunum as a neorectum is associated with preservation of terminal

14

Malignancy and the pelvic pouch procedure

The implications of colorectal malignancy for the pelvic pouch procedure

A few reports have reported the specific experience of patients with colorectal adeno-carcinoma undergoing the ileoanal reservoir procedure (Taylor *et al.*, 1988; Stelzner and Fonkalsrud, 1989). Ileal pouch construction has also been reported in an HIV-negative ulcerative colitic who had a Kaposi's sarcoma in the resected colon (Thompson *et al.*, 1989).

Taylor and colleagues described that in the 5 years to 1985, the Mayo clinic group had performed 518 ileal reservoir operations. Seventeen of these patients (3.3%) had a coexisting carcinoma. Of this subgroup of patients, 13 were previous colitics with an average length of history of 16 years, whilst four patients had polyposis coli (Taylor *et al.*, 1988). It is important to study this patient group carefully. Prior to pouch construction, four had undergone previous surgery. One patient had undergone a segmental colectomy for carcinoma of the splenic flexure, this patient also had a metachronous sigmoid carcinoma at the time of reservoir construction. Three patients had undergone a colectomy and ileorectal anastomosis. One of these had been performed 17 years previously for colitis, this patient subsequently developed a rectal tumour. The other two were performed for sigmoid and caecal neoplasms respectively; the latter patient having a metachronous rectal tumour at the time of restorative proctocolectomy. In the other 13 patients, colectomy and ileoanal reservoir formation were performed as the primary procedure. Therefore, in this group of 17 patients, a preoperative diagnosis of malignancy was reached in eight, three of whom had undergone a previous colectomy. In the other five patients, colonoscopic biopsies had provided evidence of cancer. The indications for surgery in the remaining nine patients were severe dysplasia (four), polyposis prophylaxis (three), intractable colitis (one), and a radiological stricture suggestive of malignancy in a colitic (one).

Twenty-two malignancies were present in this group of 17 patients, including the three which had previously been excised. One colitic patient had four synchronous neoplasms. In terms of histological grading, 36% were of grade I; 23% each were grade II or III; 18% were grade IV. Only one tumour was staged as being Duke's stage A; 32% were stage B_1; 18% were stage B_2 and 45% were staged as C (C_1 or C_2) tumours. One patient with a stage C_2 grade IV tumour at diagnosis died of metastatic disease 9 months postoperatively. The rest were well with no evidence of recurrent disease at a mean of 3 years post closure of ileostomy. Hospital stay was slightly prolonged compared with non-malignant cases, and postoperative morbidity, especially due to intestinal obstruction, was increased. Functional results were little different from the non-malignant group of patients operated on by the same group.

Fonkalsrud has reported that in the 177 patients on whom he has performed endorectal ileoanal anastomosis, approximately 7% had colorectal cancer at the time of the operation (Stelzner and Fonkalsrud, 1989). Of these 14 patients, 12 were colitics, whilst two had polyposis. Only one-third of these cancers were diagnosed postoperatively. In addition, some 40 patients had mucosal dysplasia, of which nine were severe, 18 moderate and 13 low grade. All the malignancies were adenocarcinomas, with two patients having multiple tumours. Nine of the colitis-associated cancers were advanced at the time of diagnosis, with regional metastatic lymphadenopathy in five patients. Contrary to such lesions in the general population, both rectal and colonic carcinomas were present with equal incidence. Importantly, the mean precolectomy duration of colitis in patients with cancer was 17 years compared to 8.5 years in those without cancer. Of the 14 malignancies, 10 patients are alive and well at a mean of some 2 years after colectomy.

These reports conclude that if the principles of radical surgery can be adhered to, then restorative proctocolectomy is not contraindicated should a carcinoma be found. Wiltz and colleagues have stated that in those patients known to have cancer at the time of colectomy, intraoperative staging may be difficult. Consequently, they advocate the use of initial resection, followed by pelvic pouch construction after an initial observation period (Wiltz *et al.*, 1990).

It is probably important that the mid or lower rectum is not severely involved in the malignant process. The prognosis is good and is related to the stage and grade of the tumour. The Mayo clinic group state that for more proximal colonic neoplasms it may well be better to perform a colectomy and ileorectal anastomosis, thus avoiding the necessity of a temporary ileostomy in patients whose life expectancy might not be prolonged. Fonkalsrud asserts that colitics should be referred at an earlier time for their surgery. Given the improved results for restorative proctocolectomy, such a policy should be more acceptable to both gastroenterologists and patients alike. He also states that as most cancers found in the retained rectum after ileorectal anastomosis are advanced (i.e. Dukes B or C), then such patients should be offered endorectal pull-through with complete excision of the rectal mucosa.

The implications of the pelvic pouch procedure for malignancy

Total extirpation of any colorectal mucosa with a potential for malignancy is achieved by complete mucosal proctectomy along any retained rectal cuff. However, as discussed in Chapter 7, the necessity for conventional mucosal proctectomy over the whole anal canal has now been questioned (Johnston *et al.*, 1987). There is evidence that the technique of stapled pouch–anal anastomosis, with retention of the whole of the anal canal mucosa intact, can result in improved continence. Although still contentious, this improvement may also be mirrored in better objective assessments of anal canal physiology (Williams *et al.*, 1989b). In spite of such studies, the role of the anal canal transition zone in discriminating between fluid and flatus (sampling) is not proven. Most reports documenting results of mucosal proctectomy to the dentate line have recorded very acceptable continence.

In a recent report, King and colleagues have described the histological features of the anal canal mucosa excised during mucosal proctectomy. In 16 consecutive ulcerative colitics undergoing pouch–anal anastomosis, a combined abdominal and endoanal mucosectomy was performed to the dentate line (King, Lubowski and Cook, 1989). Histological examination of these operative specimens revealed the mucosa to be totally columnar in nature down to the dentate line in three patients (20%). In the remaining 80% of patients, the proximal mucosa was columnar, becoming squamous in the transition zone. In almost 90% of specimens, chronic inflammatory changes consistent with ulcerative colitis were present. Four patients had evidence of moderate dysplasia, and one of these had poorly differentiated invasive adenocarcinoma extending down to the inferior limit of the specimen (i.e. to the dentate line). Subsequently, this patient underwent abdominoperineal excision of the ileal pouch and anal canal 2 weeks after pouch construction. Importantly, the excised rectum of this patient, whilst severely inflamed and showing mild dysplasia, was free from malignancy. It should be emphasized that this carcinoma was not suspected at the time of mucosectomy.

Nicholls' group from St Mark's Hospital have recently reported their results with the assessment of 132 mucosectomy specimens taken during restorative proctocolectomy (Tsunoda, Talbot and Nicholls, 1990). Only 2.5% of colitics had evidence of dysplasia within the mucosectomy specimens. Of those colitics who had carcinomas within their resected large bowels, 25% also had dysplasia in the excised anal mucosa. This compared with an incidence of only 0.9% in those colitics without cancer. In those patients in whom the duration of colitis was less than 10 years, dysplasia was not recorded in the mucosectomy specimen. The corresponding value in those with a history of longer than 10 years was 7.9%. Interestingly, in the polyposis group, dysplasia was significantly more common. Only 14% were free from dysplasia. Eighty-six per cent had some degree of dysplasia; 21% being severe, 65% being mild to moderate.

There is little doubt that the adoption of shorter rectal cuffs has resulted in fewer poor results following conventional hand-sewn anastomosis after complete rectal stripping. An important question which remains to be answered is whether there is a significant risk of islands of malignancy developing in the retained rectum. Cohen has seen one case of rectal cuff carcinoma (Cohen, 1989; Stern *et al.*, 1990). This patient had a pouch anastomosed through a 10–12-cm rectal cuff in 1984, after a 38-year history of colitis. Seven years previously, he had undergone subtotal colectomy and ileorectal anastomosis, when a carcinoma was found in the ascending colon. Three years after restorative proctocolectomy, he presented with diarrhoea, fatigue and weight loss. At laparotomy, a solid mass of tumour was invading the pouch, fixing it to the sacrum. The pouch was excised with end-ileostomy formation. Presumably, this neoplasm developed in residual rectal mucosa left after mucosal proctectomy. The presence of prolonged severe colitis prior to colectomy, implies a significant risk of developing cancer, and it is well recognized that adenomatous polyposis universally becomes malignant eventually. It is similarly recognized that mucosa can be retained after mucosectomy, but the significance of this has been questioned. It is

likely that such retention is more probable when long rectal cuffs are used.

It would therefore appear that there must be patients who have had rectal mucosa retained after their mucosectomy and pouch–anal anastomosis. It is perhaps surprising that more patients have not developed such malignancies. It would seem likely that risk is proportional to the amount of retained mucosa. Importantly, since the advent of restorative proctocolectomy, there has now been a lag period of 12 years or so. It is the experience with ulcerative colitis itself that such a lag period is recorded prior to the development of colorectal cancers. All patients with polyposis coli, and those colitics with either severe dysplasia in their mucosectomy specimen, a history of colitis of longer than 10 years, or a colorectal cancer at the time of colectomy are likely to be those most susceptible to the development of cuff carcinoma.

Concerning the ileal pouch itself, it has previously been stated that with time, the pouch mucosa tends to become more colonic in nature (see Chapter 8). It has also been noted that chronic inflammatory changes are extremely common within ileal pouches (Moskowitz, Shepherd and Nicholls, 1986).

Recurrent polyps occurring after colectomy are common in patients with adenomatous polyposis coli (see Chapter 3). Such polyposis patients have subsequently developed ileostomy cancers (Primrose, Quirke and Johnston, 1988). Similarly, colitics have undergone malignant degeneration within ileostomies (Suarez, Alexander-Williams and O'Connor, 1988; Coen, Lambert and Gray, 1988; Gadacz *et al.*, 1990). In the case reported by Coen, the aggressive nature of the tumour resulted in the ultimate demise of the patient. A mortality rate of some 25% would seem appropriate based upon the cases described to date. Approximately 20 such ileostomy cancers have been reported in the world literature. Whilst there is a wide range of durations between ileostomy formation and subsequent tumour development, the mean duration in 16 of these patients was 23.3 years (Gadacz *et al.*, 1990). The rarity of this complication has led Coen to suggest that ileostomy cancer is probably a primary tumour of the small intestine, rather than it arising in an area of colonic metaplasia. That these tumours are in fact of intestinal origin, and not a metastasis from an occult primary lesion, has been provided by the fact that most are carcinoembryonic antigen positive. It must be remembered, however, that the incidence of ileostomy carcinoma is increasing, perhaps because of the increasing number of patients who have had their stoma for more than a latent period of 20 years (Suarez, Alexander-Williams and O'Connor, 1988). However, might the mucosal changes seen in reservoirs have implications for the subsequent development of cancer within the terminal ileal reservoir; a region normally protected from malignant degeneration? If such chronic inflammatory changes were to prove to be significant, then a lag period would again be expected prior to the development of cancer. In ulcerative colitis, an exposure to this condition for 10–20 years is deemed important. It is now a little over a decade since the first pelvic pouch procedures were performed. To date, ileal pouch carcinoma has not been reported.

In an attempt to assess the potential for ileal reservoirs to develop malignancy, Heppell and his colleagues used a model incorporating a chemical carcinogen (Heppell *et al.*, 1990). In laboratory rats colectomy was followed by either straight ileorectal or ileal pouch–rectal anastomosis. In addition, a control group of sham-operated rats was included. A 3-month adaptation period was allowed. This ensured that faecal stasis and chronic mucosal changes had occurred. Thereafter, weekly doses of a carcinogen (1,2-dimethylhydrazine dihydrochloride) were administered over a 4-month period. One month after the last dose of carcinogen, the animals were sacrificed. In the controls, neither mucosal inflammation nor villous atrophy were seen in the ileal mucosa. Inflammatory changes were similarly absent in the ileum from the ileorectal anastomosis group. Villous atrophy was seen in one animal (5%). Within the reservoir group, the afferent limb was inflamed in 58%, and demonstrated villus atrophy in 21%. Comparable figures for the pouch were 76% and 67% respectively. In the efferent limb the values were 41% and 59% respectively. Fifty-eight per cent of the controls developed adenocarcinomas (only one tumour in the ileum), compared with 70% in the ileorectal anastomosis groups (none in the ileum). Twenty-five per cent of the pouch group developed cancers (two tumours occurred in the ileum). In the group, the rest of the

tumours occurred in the duodenum. Of the two reservoir cancers, one occurred in a moderately inflamed reservoir, the other in a pouch with mild villus atrophy. Comparing all the groups, tumour morphology (size, differentiation, invasion) was identical, as was the incidence of ileal tumours. This particular animal model therefore failed to demonstrate any predilection for the ileal reservoir to develop carcinoma, even if chronically inflamed.

Colonic pouch–anal anastomosis for rectal cancer

A few surgeons have applied sphincter-saving techniques after surgery for primary rectal malignancy. As with surgery for inflammatory bowel disease, that for malignant disease for the rectum has undergone a slower but equally significant series of changes. It is not so very long ago that anterior resection of the rectum was still regarded with suspicion by many. Convinced that local recurrence would prove all too common, they limited themselves to combined abdominoperineal excision of the rectum. Most would now regard anterior resection as one of the standard procedures to be employed in rectal cancer. Indeed, the lower limits of tumour clearance considered to be safe would now appear in principle to allow direct coloanal anastomosis.

Prior to his description of the ileal pelvic reservoir for colitis, the late Sir Alan Parks was the first to report the use of direct endoanal anastomosis of the colon to the anal sphincter apparatus (Figure 14.1) (Parks, 1972). The development of his techniques of mucosal stripping and pull-through sleeve anastomosis, along with his descriptions of new instruments for endoanal surgery, resulted in acceptable results and more widespread adoption of these methods. Subsequently, coloanal sleeve anastomosis has been utilized for many different rectal pathologies, both benign and malignant. In addition, coloanal anastomosis has been used in the management of rectovaginal fistula and radiation proctitis (Parks *et al.*, 1978; Gazet, 1985).

As with straight ileoanal anastomosis (see Chapter 2), the functional results can be extremely variable, and in some patients may be unacceptable. In particular, faecal urgency may be severe, and frequency excessive (Parks concluded that they did not feel that the addition of a J-pouch is justified at present. More prolonged follow-up is required before implications for local control of malignancy can be reported.

The use of a pelvic pouch constructed from colon has been reported in recent years (Figure 14.2) (Lazorthes *et al.*, 1986; Parc *et al.*, 1986; Drake *et al.*, 1987; Nicholls, Lubowski and Donaldson, 1988). Initial reports from France

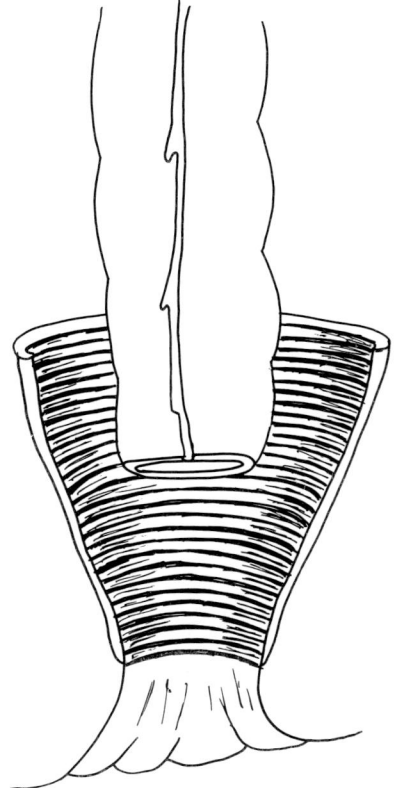

Figure 14.1 Straight coloanal anastomosis

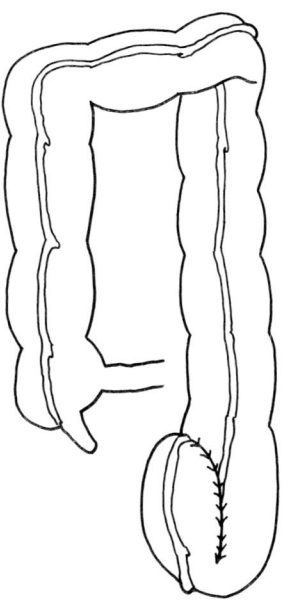

Figure 14.2 Colonic pouch construction

and Percy, 1982). It has been considered that the lack of any pelvic capacitance organ may be responsible for the poor results.

Recently preliminary experience with eight patients undergoing straight coloanal reconstruction after rectal excision for malignancy has been described (Cohen, Enker and Minsky, 1990). Invasive lesions, between 3 and 7 cm from the anal verge, were included. All patients underwent preoperative radiotherapy 4–6 weeks before laparotomy. After radical abdominal rectal resection, an endoanal mucosal proctectomy was performed to the dentate line. A hand-sewn coloanal anastomosis was then carried out which was protected for 2 months by a transverse colostomy. Primary healing occurred in all, and functional results at 1 year were excellent. Two patients suffered from infrequent soiling, and seven patients evacuated spontaneously between one and three times per day. One patient evacuated two to three times per week. This group

employed a posterior trans-sphincteric approach to facilitate direct anastomosis of a J-shaped colonic pouch to the anal sphincter. Of necessity, both sphincter division and subsequent reconstruction are required, adding to both operative time and potential morbidity (Lazorthes *et al.*, 1986). In addition, because a control group of straight coloanal anastomoses using this approach are not available, the precise benefits or otherwise of the interposed pouch are difficult to ascertain.

Consequently, and because of the now widespread use of endoanal techniques for ileal pouch–anal anastomosis, most workers utilize endoanal colonic pouch–anal anastomosis (Nicholls, Lubowski and Donaldson, 1988). This group compared straight coloanal versus colonic pouch–anal anastomosis in patients matched for age, sex, tumour level and proximal and distal resection margins. Pouches were constructed from two 10-cm lengths of colon using a two-layer continuous suture technique. An anterior defect was left 'wide enough to admit two fingers'; this was anastomosed to the anal canal endoanally. A proximal defunctioning stoma was used in all patients. The 13 patients who had undergone colonic J-pouch–anal anastomosis had a similar incidence of postoperative complications as in the 15 patients after a straight anastomosis. Continence performance was similar in both groups. Whilst resting anal pressure was similar in both groups, rectal sensitivity threshold volume was significantly greater in the pouch group. The pouch procedure should therefore be associated with somewhat greater threshold volumes, i.e. of the order of 75–100 ml, before the feeling of rectal distension commences. In addition, the mean maximal tolerable volume was significantly greater in the pouch group. This should be mirrored in the ability to defer defaecation for longer periods without urgency. Nicholls found that, even at a mean of only 7±4 months follow-up, stool frequency was less than two per 24 hours (mean 1.4) in all the pouch patients. This compared very favourably to the straight anastomosis group (more than two per 24 hours in 40% of patients at 47±23 months follow-up). Utilizing three different methods to assess 'neorectal' emptying, both groups performed similarly. However, on contrast proctography, three of the pouches failed to evacuate fully. Encouragingly, in only one of these patients was this apparent clinically, and in this individual suppositories were required to facilitate emptying. In 30% of the pouches assessed, the rectoanal inhibitory reflex remained intact postoperatively, this compared with a presence of 67% in the straight anastomosis group. This demonstrates, in accordance with the observations of Lane and Parks, that this reflex can persist after coloanal anastomosis (Lane and Parks, 1977).

Importantly, functional results after pouch–anal anastomosis have been found to be more predictable than after straight coloanal anastomosis. This has obvious implications for a procedure used for malignant disease, where further restorative surgery should be avoided if at all possible.

Continent caecostomy

In addition to his continent ileostomy, Kock has similarly described the use of a continent reservoir constructed from the caecum. This he performed in 30 patients requiring colonic excision for malignant disease. This group of patients would ordinarily have been given incontinent end-colostomies. Unfortunately, there was a high complication rate after this procedure, which even when successful proved to be functionally inadequate. The semisolid nature of the stool made emptying of the caecum somewhat difficult. Kock therefore concluded that, in those patients who could not tolerate an incontinent colostomy, that a continent ileostomy should be considered (Kock, Myrvold, Philipsson *et al* 1985).

15

Future trends in rectal replacement surgery

The preceding chapters have documented the developing role of the pelvic pouch procedure as an alternative to the formation of a permanent stoma. There can be little doubt that this operation represents a major advance in the management of certain diseases of the colon and rectum. However, the functional outcome after pouch–anal anastomosis continues to be variable and generally unpredictable. To some extent, it may be the pouch itself which increases the complexity of the procedure, and promotes the complications which may mar the success of the operation. Because of this, surgeons have continued to devise and develop new alternatives to permanent ileostomy. The primary aim of these is to obviate the need for such relatively complicated pouch constructions with long suture lines. As yet, some of the procedures described in Chapter 5 remain within the province of individual surgeons. Only time will tell whether they represent a serious challenge to the now readily accepted pelvic pouch procedure.

In spite of the advances in the avoidance of the permanent ileostomy discussed in Chapter 1, many patients have received, and continue to receive, permanent stomas. Whilst it is to the credit of the great majority that they accommodate readily to their new lifestyle, a small minority find a permanent stoma totally unacceptable. Rarely, such patients may demand that their stoma is reversed. Until recently, there was little to offer such patients. Williams has described a technique of creating not only an ileal pouch neorectum, but also a 'neo-anal sphincter' (Williams et al., 1989a). The neorectum employed was a conventional triplicated ileal pouch. A perineal track was created through the previously conjoined pelvic floor musculature and through the perianal skin. The efferent limb of the S-pouch was then anastomosed to the margins of the perineal cutaneous stoma. A temporary loop ileostomy was created. One month later, the left gracilis muscle was mobilized sparing the proximal neurovascular bundle, in a manner

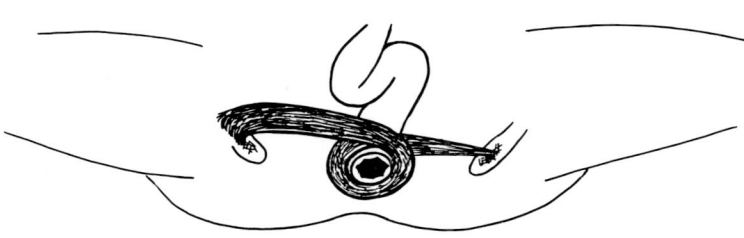

Figure 15.1 Neorectum and neosphincter (after Williams et al., 1989a)

analogous to that used in its mobilization as part of other gracilis transposition procedures used in faecal incontinence. An electrode plate was sewn over the main nerve supply to the muscle. A circumferential skin incision around the perineal ileostomy allowed the mobilized gracilis muscle to be wrapped around the efferent limb of the pouch (Figure 15.1). The receiver of an electronic nerve stimulator was placed in a supracostal subcutaneous compartment, and connected to the wires from the muscle electrode. Transcutaneous stimulation of the nerve stimulator allowed for the tetanic stimulation of the gracilis muscle. Per 'anum' insertion of a Silastic plug aided in the provision of continence. When this was satisfactory for synthetic stools, the ileostomy was closed. Even though only one patient was described after this formidable procedure, results were quite satisfactory. This procedure may then represent a potential course of action for ileostomates demanding closure of their stomas. However, it is unlikely that it will gain widespread popularity due to its present complexity.

Ryan and Fink have also described the construction of ileal pelvic reservoirs in two patients who had previously undergone procto-colectomy (Ryan and Fink, 1988). Whilst one patient had undergone a conservative procto-colectomy (see Chapter 1), and so retained the external sphincter, the other had undergone complete proctectomy 10 years prior to pouch construction. This patient therefore had neither intact external nor internal anal sphincter mechanisms. Electromyographic analysis demonstrated an intact pelvic floor mechanism. The plane between the levator ani and the vagina was mobilized, and a J-pouch brought down through this plane and through an incision made in the perineal skin, where it was sutured (Figure 15.2). A temporary loop ileostomy was fashioned. The functional outcome of this procedure, which is obviously less demanding than that described by Williams, was satisfactory. Perianal excoriation remained problematical, due in part to a degree of pouch mucosal prolapse. At 1 year post ileostomy closure bowel frequency was 12 per 24 hours, often with little or no nocturnal evacuation. In the absence of diarrhoea, continence was complete, and the patient returned to full-time employment. Whether this procedure will become popular amongst surgeons managing

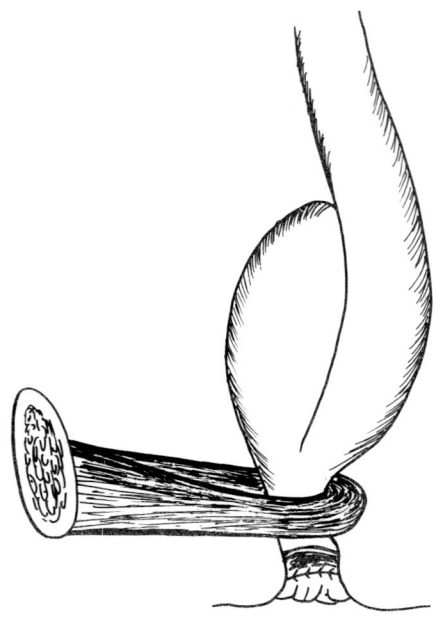

Figure 15.2 Pouch–'anal' anastomosis (after Ryan and Fink, 1988)

such patients remains to be answered.

Enthusiasm for the avoidance of the permanent stoma has even resulted in the development of a smooth muscle neosphincter, which is wrapped around a perineal colostomy after rectal excision for cancer (Fedorov, Odaryuk and Shelygin, 1989).

Accepting the above innovations and the continuing research into other neorectal constructions (see Chapter 2), the pelvic pouch procedure is likely to remain the procedure of choice when sphincter conservation is considered. Indeed, it may well become the new 'gold standard' against which all new procedures must be compared. However, what of the future of pouch–anal anastomosis? By definition, any such discussion is both somewhat personal and speculative. The on-going improvements in the design of stapling instruments, particularly the new Premium instrument and the Roticulator, are likely to encourage many more surgeons interested in colorectal disease to undertake pelvic pouch construction. In particular, many of the early teething problems have been ironed out, and the presently performed operation is very much less demanding than it was formally.

Many workers in this field feel that it is merely a matter of time before the first pouch carcinoma presents. Other pathophysiological consequences of reservoir construction are also likely to occupy much time and attention from workers. Pouchitis will be paramount in such studies. It may be that determined research into the aetiology of pouchitis may ultimately result in advances in our understanding of chronic ulcerative colitis itself.

Isolated jejunal segments may also attract attention for pelvic pouch construction. Should long-term terminal ileal insufficiency be demonstrable, particularly after pouch excision, such a trend might be encouraged (see Chapter 13).

In Chapter 8, the topic of the pacing of ileal pouches was briefly discussed. Manipulation of reservoirs, particularly those which fail to function adequately, may become more widespread. Such manipulations may not only be electronic, but may involve more widespread use of pharmacological agents, including intestinal prokinetic agents.

Of perhaps greatest interest is the opportunity which the ileal pouch provides for studying various aspects of intestinal physiology. Because it allows for easy access to a terminal ileal reservoir, it has become a powerful model. Such studies are presently in their infancy, but they will doubtless prove to be exceedingly fruitful.

References and Bibliography

Albert, V., Young, G.P., Morton, C.L. *et al.* (1990) Systemic factors are trophic in bypassed rat small intestine in the absence of luminal contents. *Gut,* **31**, 311–316.

Aly, A. and Fonkalsrud, E.W. (1988) Construction of ileal reservoir with longitudinal ileal myotomy. *Am. Surg.,* **54**, 475–478.

Aly, A., Hawkins, R.A., Snape, W.J. Jr and Fonkalsrud, E.W. (1987) Comparison of transit time in the J-shaped and the isoperistaltic lateral ileal reservoir – using an isotope technique in rabbits. *Arch. Surg.,* **122**, 1124–1127.

Ambrose, W.L., Bell, A.M., Pemberton, J.H. *et al.* (1989a) The effect of stool consistency on rectal and neorectal emptying. *Gastroenterology,* **96**, A11.

Ambrose, W.L., Dozois, R.R., Pemberton, J.H. and Kelly, K.A. (1990a) Familial adenomatous polyposis: comparison of results following ileal pouch–anal anastomosis and ileorectostomy. *Dis. Colon Rectum,* **33**, P5.

Ambrose, W.L., Pemberton, J.H., Bell, A.M. *et al.* (1989b) Fecal short chain fatty acids after ileal pouch–anal anastomosis. *Gastroenterology,* **96**, A11

Ambrose, W.L., Pemberton, J.H., Phillips, S.F. *et al.* (1990b) Fecal short chain fatty acid concentrations and effect on ileal-pouch function. *Gastroenterology,* **98**, A322

Andersson, H., Fasth, S. and Philipsson, S. (1979) Faecal excretion of intravenously injected ^{14}C-cholic acid in patients with conventional ileostomy and in patients with continent ileostomy reservoir. *Scand. J. Gastroenterol.,* **14**, 551–554.

Armstrong, D.M., Bilchik, A.J., Adrian, T.E. *et al.* (1989) PYY and Enteroglucagon levels are elevated after proctocolectomy and pelvic ileal–anal anastomosis. *Gastroenterology,* **96**, A15

Arn, E.R. (1931) Chronic ulcerative colitis: surgical treatment of refractory cases. *Ohio State Med. J.,* **27**, 121

Aylett, S.O. (1953) Conservative surgery in the treatment of ulcerative colitis. *Br. Med. J.,* **2**, 1348–1351.

Aylett, S.O. (1960) Diffuse chronic ulcerative colitis and its treatment by ileorectal anastomosis. *Ann. R. Coll. Surg. Engl.,* **27**, 260–284

Baba, S., Ekelund, G., Fischer, J. *et al.* (1990) Symposium: inflammatory bowel disease – spectrum. *Dis. Colon Rectum,* **33**, 232–240

Ballantyne, G.H., Graham, S.M., Hammers, L. and Modlin, I.M. (1987) Superior mesenteric artery syndrome following ileal J-pouch–anal anastomosis: an iatrogenic cause of early postoperative obstruction. *Dis. Colon Rectum,* **30**, 472–474

Ballantyne, G.H., Pemberton, J.H. and Beart, R.W. (1985) Ileal J-pouch–anal anastomosis: current technique. *Dis. Colon Rectum,* **28**, 197–202

Bank, E.R., White, S.J. and Coran, A.G. (1986) The radiographic appearance of the endorectal pull-through. *Pediatr. Radiol.,* **16**, 216–221

Bargen, J.A. (1928) Chronic ulcerative colitis associated with malignant disease. *Arch. Surg. Chicago,* **17**, 561.

Barkel, D.C., Pemberton, J.H., Pezim, M.E. *et al.* (1988) Scintigraphic assessment of the anorectal angle in health and after ileal pouch–anal anastomosis. *Ann. Surg.,* **208**, 42–49

Barnett, W.O. (1989) Current experience with the continent intestinal reservoir. *Surg. Gynecol. Obstet.,* **168**, 1–5

Barraza, R.P. (1988) A new device to facilitate intestinal pull-through procedures. *Surg. Gynecol. Obstet.,* **167**, 158–159

Barteau, J.A., Becker, J.M., Dunnegan, D.L. *et al.* (1990) Ileal pouch dysfunction following colectomy with ileal pouch–anal anastomosis. *Gastroenterology*, **98**, A158

Bartolo, D.C.C., Jarratt, J.A. and Read, N.W. (1983) The use of conventional electromyography to assess external sphincter neuropathy in man. *J. Neurol. Neurosurg. Psychiatr.*, **46**. 1115–1118

Bazzocchi, G., Di Falco, A. and Lanfranchi, G.A. (1990) Anorectal motility in patients with ulcerative colitis after colectomy and rectal pouch excision. *Gastroenterology*, **98**, A326

Beart, R.W. (1985) Familial polyposis. *Br. J. Surg.*, **72**, S31–32

Beart, R.W. (1986) Proctocolectomy and ileoanal anastomosis with a J-pouch. *Aust. N.Z. J. Surg.*, **56**, 467–469

Beart, R.W., Dozois R.R. and Kelly, K.A. (1982) Ileoanal anastomosis in the adult. *Surg. Gynecol. Obstet.*, **154**, 826–828

Becker, J.M. (1984) Anal sphincter function after colectomy, mucosal proctectomy and endorectal ileoanal pull-through. *Arch. Surg.*, **119**, 526–531

Becker, J.M., Dunnegan, D.L., Meinenger, T.A. and Soper, N.J. (1989) Loperamide improves functional results following ileal pouch–anal anastomosis. *Gastroenterology*, **96**, A36

Becker, J.M. and Raymond, J.L. (1986) Ileal pouch–anal anastomosis: a single surgeon experience with 100 consecutive cases. *Ann. Surg.*, **204**, 375–383

Bennett, R.C. and Duthie, H.B. (1964) The functional importance of the internal anal sphincter. *Br. J. Surg.*, **51**, 355–357

Berglund. B. and Kock, N.G. (1987) Volume, capacity and pressure characteristics of various types of intestinal reservoirs. *World J. Surg.*, **11**, 798–803

Bess, M.A., Adson, M.A. and Elveback, L.R. (1980) Rectal cancer following colectomy for polyposis. *Arch. Surg.*, **115**, 460–467

Best, R.R. (1952) Evaluation of ileoproctostomy to avoid ileostomy in various colonic lesions. *JAMA*, **150**, 637–642

Besterman, H.S., Mallinson, C.N. and Modigliani, R. (1983) Gut hormones in inflammatory bowel disease. *Scand. J. Gastroenterol.*, **18**, 845–852

Bodzin, J.H., Kestenberg, W., Kaufmann, R. and Dean, K. (1987) Mucosal proctectomy and ileoanal pull-through technique and functional results in 23 consecutive patients. *Am. Surg.*, **53**, 363–367

Bokey, E.L. (1984) Continent ileostomy without a reservoir. In *Alternatives to Conventional Ileostomy* (ed. R.R Dozois), Year Book Medical, Chicago, pp.199–207

Bokey, E.L., Chapuis, P.H., Dunn, D.W. *et al.* (1985) Continence following ileoanal anastomosis with an antiperistaltic terminal ileal segment. *Aust. N. Z. J. Surg.*, **55**, 507–511

Bokey, E.L., Hayward, P.J. and Johnson, S.E.

(1981) Experiments in the development of a continent ileostomy: a simplified technique without a reservoir in dogs. *Surgery*, **90**, 459–463

Bokey, E.L., Johnson, S.E., Chapuis, P.H. and Pheils, M.T. (1983) A 2-limb side-to-side reservoir for the continent ileostomy: an experimental study in dogs. *Aust. N.Z. J. Surg.*, **53**, 273–275

Brandberg, A., Kock, N.G. and Philipson, B. (1972) Bacterial flora in the intra-abdominal ileostomy reservoir. *Gastroenterology*, **63**, 413–416

Brooke, B.N. (1952) The management of an ileostomy including its complications. *Lancet*, **ii**, 102–104

Brough, W.A. and Schofield, P.F. (1989) An improved technique of J-pouch construction and ileoanal anastomosis. *Br. J. Surg.*, **76**, 350–351

Brown, J.J., Balfe, D.M., Heiken, J.P. *et al.* (1990) Ileal J-pouch: radiologic evaluation in patients with and without postoperative infectious complications. *Radiology*, **174**, 115–120

Brown, J.Y. (1913) The value of complete physiological rest of the large bowel in the treatment of certain ulcerative and obstructive lesions of this organ. *Surg. Gynecol. Obstet.*, **16**, 610–613

Bruun, E. and Hansen, L.K. (1990) Optimising the ileal S-reservoir. *Gastroenterology*, **98**, A161

Bubrick, M.P., Jacobs, D.M. and Levy, M. (1985) Experience with the endorectal pull-through and S-pouch for ulcerative colitis and familial polyposis in adults. *Surgery*, **98**, 689–696

Bulow, S. and Kirkegaard, P. (1987) Ileal pouch–anal anastomosis after failure of a straight ileoanal anastomosis. *Acta Chir. Scand.*, **153**, 463–464

Burns, T.W., Mathias, J.R., Carlson, G. *et al.* (1978) Effect of toxigenic *Escherichia coli* on myoelectrical activity of the small intestine. *Am. J. Physiol.*, **235**, 311–325

Burnstein, M.J., Schoetz, D.J., Coller, J.A. and Veidenheimer, M.C. (1987) Technique for mesenteric lengthening in ileal reservoir–anal anastomosis. *Dis. Colon Rectum*, **30**, 863–866

Bussey, H.R.J. (1975) *Familial Polyposis Coli*, John Hopkins University Press, Baltimore

Bussey, H.R.J., Eyers, A.A., Ritchie, J.M. and Thomson, J.P.S. (1985) The rectum in adenomatous polyposis: the St Mark's policy. *Br. J. Surg.*, **72**, Suppl., S29–31

Camilleri, M. (1989) Jejunal manometry in distal subacute mechanical obstruction: significance of prolonged simultaneous contractions. *Gut*, **30**, 468–475

Canty, T.G., Self T. and Bonaldi, L. (1983) The lateral reservoir technique of ileal endorectal pull-through for ulcerative colitis and familial polyposis in children. *J. Pediatr. Surg.*, **18**, 862–871

Caruso, C. and Buchthal, F. (1965) Refractory

period of muscle and E.M.G. findings in relatives of patients with muscular dystrophy. *Brain*, **88**, 29–50

Casanova-Diaz, A.S. (1954) Diffuse familial polyposis. *Bol. Asoc. Med. PR* **46**, 307–315

Cattell, R.B. (1948) The surgical treatment of ulcerative colitis. *Gastroenterology*, **10**, 63–66

Caudarella, R., Malavolta, N., Rizzoli, E. *et al.* (1989) Metabolic abnormalities promoting renal stones formation in patients undergoing ileal pouch–anal anastomosis. In *Symposium: New Trends in Pelvic Pouch Procedures, Bologna*, A9

Cerulli, M.A., Nikoomanesh, P. and Schuster, M.M. (1979) Progress in biofeedback conditioning for faecal incontinence. *Gastroenterology*, **76**, 742–746

Chaimoff, C., Kyzer, S., Karib, N. *et al.* (1989) New approach to surgical treatment of ulcerative colitis and polyposis coli without pelvic pouch: experimental study in dogs. *Dis. Colon Rectum*, **32**, 572–579

Charney, A.N. and Dansky, H.M. (1990) Additive effects of ileal secretagogues in the rat. *Gastroenterology*, **98**, 881–887

Chaussade, S., Denizot, Y., Nicoll, J. *et al.* (1990) Stool P.A.F.-Aceter (P.A.F.) is increased in patients with pouch ileo-anal anastomosis and pouchitis. *Gastroenterology*, **98**, A164

Chaussade, S., Merite, F., Hautefeuille, M. *et al.* (1989a) Motility of the jejunum after proctocolectomy and ileal pouch anastomosis. *Gut*, **30**, 371–375

Chaussade, S., Michopoulos, S., Hautefeuille, M. *et al.* (1989b) Ileoanal anastomosis with ileal pouch: evolution of the functional parameters before six months and twelve months after closure of the loop ileostomy. *Gastroenterology*, **96**, A84

Chaussade, S., Verduron, A., Hautefeuille, M. *et al.* (1989c) Proctocolectomy and ileoanal pouch anastomosis without conservation of a rectal muscular cuff. *Br. J. Surg.*, **76**, 273–275

Cherqui, D., Valleur, P., Perniceni, T. and Hautefeuille, P. (1987) Inferior reach of ileal reservoir in ileoanal anastomosis: experimental anatomic and angiographic study. *Dis. Colon Rectum*, **30**, 365–371

Chick, L.R., Brown, R.E. and Walton, R.L. (1988) Microvascular reconstruction of a devascularised ileal segment during ileoanal anastomosis. *J. Reconstr. Microsurg.*, **4**, 359–361

Christie, P.M. and Hill, G.L. (1990) Return to normal body composition after ileoanal J-pouch anastomosis for ulcerative colitis. *Dis. Colon Rectum*, **33**, 584–586

Christie, P.M., Knight, G.S. and Hill, G.L. (1990) Metabolism of body water and electrolytes after surgery for ulcerative colitis: conventional ileostomy versus J-pouch. *Br. J. Surg.*, **77**, 149–151

Christie, P.M., Schroeder, D. and Hill, G.L. (1988)

Persisting superior mesenteric artery syndrome following ileoanal J-pouch construction. *Br. J. Surg.*, **75**, 1036

Clarke, A.M., Chirnside, A. and Hill, G.L. (1967) Chronic dehydration and sodium depletion in patients with established ileostomies. *Lancet*, **ii**, 740–743

Coen, L.D., Lambert, W.G. and Gray, P.B. (1988) Adenocarcinoma at the ileocutaneous junction following subtotal colectomy for ulcerative colitis. *Acta Chir. Scand.*, **154**, 685–686

Cohen, A.M., Enker, W.E. and Minsky, B.D. (1990) Proctectomy and coloanal reconstruction for rectal cancer. *Dis. Colon Rectum*, **33**, 40–43

Cohen, A.M. and Minsky, B.D. (1990) A phase I trial of preoperative radiation, proctectomy, and endoanal reconstruction. *Arch. Surg.*, **125**, 247–251

Cohen, Z. (1989) Surgery in inflammatory bowel disease. *Curr. Opin. Gastroenterol.*, **5**, 514–519

Cohen, Z. and McLeod, R.S. (1988) Proctocolectomy and ileoanal anastomosis with J-shaped or S-shaped ileal pouch. *World J. Surg.*, **12**, 164–168

Cohen, Z., McLeod, R.S., Stern, H. *et al.* (1985) The pelvic pouch and ileoanal anastomosis procedure. *Am. J. Surg.*, **150**, 601–607

Cohen, Z., McLeod, R.S. and Lock, A.M. (1989) Quality of life of patients with ulcerative colitis preoperatively and postoperatively. *Symposium: New Trends in Pelvic Pouch Procedures*. Bologna A4

Cooper, J.C., Laughland, A. and Gunning, E.J. (1986) Body composition in ileostomy patients with and without ileal resection. *Gut*, **27**, 680–685

Coran, A.G. (1985) Straight endorectal pull-through of the ileum for the management of benign disease of the colon and rectum in children and adults. In: *Alternatives to Conventional Ileostomy* (ed. R.R. Dozois), Year Book Medical, Chicago, pp. 335–344

Coran, A.G., Sarahan, T.M. and Dent, T.L. (1983) The endorectal pull-through for the management of ulcerative colitis in children and adults. *Ann. Surg.*, **197**, 99–105

Corazza, G.R., Menozzi, M.G., Strocchi, A. *et al.* (1990) The diagnosis of small bowel bacterial overgrowth. *Gastroenterology*, **98**, 302–309

Corbett, R.S. (1945) A review of the surgical treatment of chronic ulcerative colitis. *Proc. R. Soc. Med.*, **38**, 277–290

Corbett, R.S. (1952) Recent advances in the surgical treatment of chronic ulcerative colitis. *Ann. R. Coll. Surg. Engl.*, **10**, 21–32

Coremans, G., Janssens, J., Vantrappen, G. *et al.* (1987) Migrating action potential complexes in a patient with secretory diarrhoea. *Dig. Dis. Sci.*, **32**, 1201–1206

Corfield, A.P., Warren, B.F. and Bartolo, D.C.C. (1990) Mucin metabolic labelling: with [^{35}S] sulphate and [³H] glucosamine to p monitor colonic metaplasia in the ileum following restorative proctocolectomy. *Br. J. Surg.*, **77**, A699

Corman, M.L., Veidenheimer, M.C. and Coller, J.A. (1978) Impotence after proctectomy for inflammatory disease of the bowel. *Dis. Colon Rectum*, **21**, 418–419

Counsell, P.B. and Dukes, C.E. (1952) The association of chronic ulcerative colitis and carcinoma of the rectum and colon. *Br. J. Surg.*, **39**, 485

Cranley, B. and McKelvey, S.T.D. (1982) The pelvic ileal reservoir: an experimental assessment of its function compared with that of normal rectum. *Br. J. Surg.*, **69**, 465–469

Cranley, B. and McKelvey, S.T.D. (1983) Ileal reservoir. *J. Surg. Res.*, **34**, 279–285

Crile, G. and Turnbull, R.B. (1954) Mechanism and prevention of ileostomy dysfunction. *Ann. Surg.*, **140**, 459–466

Crohn, B.B. and Rosenberg, H. (1925). The sigmoidoscopic appearance of chronic ulcerative colitis. *Am. J. Med. Sci.*, **170**, 220–225

Daly, D.E. and Brooke, B.N. (1967) Ileostomy and excision of the large intestine for ulcerative colitis. *Lancet*, **ii**, 62–64

Damgaard, B. and Kirkegaard, P. (1990) Creating a pelvic reservoir in the surgical treatment of ulcerative colitis and familial polyposis of the colon. *Ugeskr. Laeger*, **152**, 103–105

Davidson, B.R. and Thornton-Holmes, J. (1990) Restorative proctocolectomy: a procedure for the district general hospital? *Int. J. Color. Dis.*, **5**, 41–43

de Dombal, F.T. and Prantera, C. (1989) Sampling gastroenterologists' opinions at two world congresses and at ROMA 88. *Gastroenterol. Int.*, **2**, 62–66

Deitch, E.A., Bridges, W.M., Ma, J.W. *et al.* (1990) Obstructed intestine as a reservoir for systemic infection. *Am. J. Surg.*, **159**, 394–398

Delin, K., Fasth, S., Andersson, H. *et al.* (1984) Factors regulating sodium balance in proctocolectomized patients with various ileal resections. *Scand. J. Gastroenterol.*, **19**, 145–149

Denny-Brown, D. and Robertson, E.G. (1935) An investigation of the nervous control of defaecation. *Brain*, **58**, 256–310

de Silva, H.J., Ireland, A., Kettlewell, M. *et al.* (1989) Short-chain fatty acid irrigation in severe pouchitis (letter). *N. Engl. J. Med.*, **321**, 1416–1417

de Silva, H.J., Jones, M., Kettlewell. M. *et al.* (1990) Subsets of T-lymphocytes and macrophages in the mucosa of ileoanal pouches. *Gastroenterology*, **98**, A445

Deutsch, A.A., Gregoire, R., Cullen, J. *et al.* (1990) Results of the pelvic pouch procedure in patients with Crohn's disease. *Dis. Colon Rectum*, **33**, P4

Devine, H. (1943) Method of colectomy for desperate cases of ulcerative colitis. *Surg. Gynecol. Obstet.*, **76**, 136–138

Devine, J. and Webb, R. (1951) Resection of the rectal mucosa, colectomy and anal ileostomy with normal continence. *Surg. Gynecol. Obstet.*, **92**, 437–442

Di Febo, G., Miglioli, M., Lauri, A. *et al.* (1990) Endoscopic assessment of acute inflammation of the ileal reservoir after restorative ileoanal anastomosis. *Gastrointest. Endosc.*, **36**, 6–9

Diamant, N.E. and Harris, L.D. (1969) Comparison of objective measurement of anal sphincter strength with anal sphincter pressures and levator ani function. *Gastroenterology*, **56**, 110–116

Dimitriu, V. (1928) Crearea rectului din ansa subtire. *Spitalul*, **48**, 97–99

Dozois, R.R. (1985) Ileal J-pouch–anal anastomosis. *Br. J. Surg.*, **72**, S80–82

Dozois, R.R., Cohen, Z., Goldberg, S.M. *et al.* (1986) Symposium: restorative proctocolectomy with ileal reservoir. *Int. J. Color. Dis.*, **1**, 2–19

Dozois, R.R., Kelly, K.A. and Beart, R.W. (1980) Improved results with continent ileostomy. *Ann. Surg.*, **192**, 319–324

Dozois, R.R., Kelly, K.A., Welling, D.R. *et al.* (1989) Ileal pouch–anal anastomosis: comparison of results in familial adenomatous polyposis and chronic ulcerative colitis. *Ann. Surg.*, **210**, 268–273

Dragstedt, L.R., Dack, G.M. and Kirsner, J.B. (1941) Chronic ulcerative colitis. *Ann. Surg.*, **114**, 653–661

Drake, D.B., Pemberton, J.H., Beart, R.W. *et al.* (1987) Colo-anal anastomosis in the management of benign and malignant rectal disease. *Ann. Surg.*, **206**, 600–605

Drobni, S. (1967) One-stage proctocolectomy and anal ileostomy: report of 35 cases. *Dis. Colon Rectum*, **10**, 443–448

Dube, S. and Heyen, F.(1989) Pouchitis vs hypochlorhydria: cause or effect? In *Symposium: New Trends in Pelvic Pouch Procedures, Bologna.*, A55

Dunlop, M.G., Wyllie, A.H. and Steel, C.M. (1990) Presymptomatic diagnosis of familial adenomatous polyposis by DNA probe analysis. *Br. J. Surg.*, **77**, A698

Duthie, G.S. and Bartolo, D.C.C. (1990) Nocturnal leakage is related to high pressure pouch waves following restorative proctocolectomy. *Br. J. Surg.*, **77**, A699

Duthie, H.L. and Bennett, R.C. (1964) Anal sphincter pressure in fissure-in-ano. *Surg. Gynecol. Obstet.*, **119**, 19–21

Duthie, H.L. and Gairns, F.W. (1960) Sensory nerve endings and sensation in the anal region of man. *Br. J. Surg.*, **47**, 585–595

Duthie, H.L. and Watts, J.M. (1965) Contribution

of the external anal sphincter to the pressure zone in the anal canal. *Gut*, **6**, 64–68

Eckmann, H., Jacobsson, B., Kock, N.G. *et al.* (1964) The functional behaviour of different types of intestinal urinary bladder substitutes. *Congr. Soc. Int. Urol.*, **11**, 213–217

Edling, N.P.G. and Eklof, O. (1961) Radiological findings and prognosis in ulcerative colitis. *Acta. Chir. Scand.*, **121**, 299–308

Edwards, F.C. and Truelove, S.C. (1963) The course and prognosis of ulcerative colitis. Part III. Complications. Part IV. Carcinoma of the colon. *Gut*, **5**, 1–22

Emblem, R., Erichsen, A.A., Morkrid, L. *et al.* (1989) Failed ileoanal anastomosis: correlations between clinical function and anal canal neurophysiologic and histologic examinations. *Scand. J. Gastroenterol.*, **24**, 623–631

Emblem, R., Stien, R. and Morkrid, L. (1989a) Anal sphincter function after colectomy, mucosal proctectomy, and ileoanal anastomosis. *Scand. J. Gastroenterol.*, **24**, 171–178

Emblem, R., Stien, R. and Morkrid, L. (1989b) The effect of loperamide on bowel habits and anal sphincter function in patients with ileoanal anastomosis. *Scand. J. Gastroenterol.*, **24**, 1019–1024

Engel, B.T., Nikoomanesh, P. and Schuster, M.M. (1974) Operant conditioning of rectosphincteric responses in the treatment of faecal incontinence. *N. Engl. J. Med.*, **290**, 646–649

Everett, W.G. (1989) Experience of restorative proctocolectomy with ileal reservoir. *Br. J. Surg.*, **76**, 77–81

Everett, W.G. and Forty, J. (1989) The functional results of pelvic ileal reservoir in 10 patients with familial adenomatous polyposis. *Ann. R. Coll. Surg. Engl.*, **71**, 28–30

Everett, W.G. and Pollard, S.G. (1990) Restorative proctocolectomy without temporary ileostomy. *Br. J. Surg.*, **77**, 621–622

Failes, D.G. (1983) Proctocolectomy without ileostomy: ileoanal anastomosis with an ileal reservoir. *Aust. N.Z. J. Surg.*, **53**, 551–556

Faller, M.C., Welling, R.E. and Lambert, C.E. (1986) Nutritional implications and dietary management postproctocolectomy and ileal reservoir construction. *J. Am. Diet. Assoc.*, **86**, 1235–1236

Farnell, M.B., van Heerden, J.A. and Beart, R.W. (1980) Rectal preservation in non-specific inflammatory disease of the colon. *Ann. Surg.*, **192**, 249–253

Farrands, P.A., Shepherd, N.A. and Nicholls, R.J. (1988) Ileal reservoir inflammation (pouchitis) after restorative proctocolectomy. *Gut*, **29**, A1486

Fasth, S., Oresland, T., Ahren, C. and Hulten, L. (1985) Mucosal proctectomy and ileostomy as an alternative to conventional proctectomy. *Dis. Colon Rectum*, **28**, 31–34

Fasth, S., Scaglia, M., Nordgren, S. *et al.* (1986) Restoration of intestinal continuity (pelvic pouch) after previous proctocolectomy with distal mucosal proctectomy. *Int. J. Color. Dis.*, **1**, 256–258

Faxen, A., Kock, N.G. and Sundin, T. (1973) The long-term functional results after ileocystoplasty. *Scand. J. Urol. Nephrol.*, **7**, 127–130

Fazio, V.W. (1980). Toxic megacolon in ulcerative colitis and Crohn's colitis. *Clin. Gastroenterol.*, **9**, 389–407

Fedorak, R.N., Empey, L.R., MacArthur, C. and Jewell, L.D. (1990) Misoprostol provides a colonic mucosal protective effect during acetic acid-induced colitis in rats. *Gastroenterology*, **98**, 615–625

Fedorov, V.D., Odaryuk, T.S. and Shelygin, Y.A. (1989) Method of creation of a smooth-muscle cuff at the site of the perineal colostomy after extirpation of the rectum. *Dis. Colon Rectum*, **32**, 562–566

Feinberg, S.M., McLeod, R.S. and Cohen, Z. (1987) Complications of loop ileostomy. *Am. J. Surg.*, **153**, 102–107

Ferguson, G.H., Redford, J., Barrett, J.A. and Kiff, E.S. (1989) The appreciation of rectal distension in fecal incontinence. *Dis. Colon Rectum*, **32**, 964–967

Ferrari, B.T. and Fonkalsrud, E.W. (1978) Endorectal ileal pull-through operation with ileal reservoir after total colectomy. *Am. J. Surg.*, **136**, 113–120

Fiorentini, M.T., Locatelli, L., Ceccopieri, B. *et al.* (1987) Physiology of ileoanal anastomosis with ileal reservoir for ulcerative colitis and adenomatosis coli. *Dis. Colon Rectum*, **30**, 267–272

Fleshman, J.W., Cohen, Z., McLeod, R.S. *et al.* (1988a) The ileal reservoir and ileoanal anastomosis procedure: factors affecting technical and functional outcome. *Dis. Colon Rectum*, **31**, 10–16

Fleshman, J.W., McLeod, R.S., Cohen, Z. and Stern, H. (1988b) Improved results following the use of an advancement technique in the treatment of ileoanal anastomotic complications. *Int. J. Color. Dis.*, **3**, 161–165

Flotte, C.T., O'Dell, F.D. and Coller, F.A. (1956) Polyposis of the colon. *Ann. Surg.*, **144**, 165–169

Floyd, W.F. and Walls, E.W. (1953) Electromyography of the sphincter ani externus in man. *J. Physiol. (Lond.)*, **122**, 500–609

Fone, D.R., Horowitz, M., Read, N.W. *et al.* (1990) The effect of terminal ileal triglyceride infusion on gastroduodenal motility and the intragastric distribution of a solid meal. *Gastroenterology*, **98**, 568–575

Fonkalsrud, E.W. (1980) Total colectomy and endorectal ileal pull-through with internal ileal reservoir for ulcerative colitis. *Surg. Gynecol. Obstet.*, **150**, 1–8

Fonkalsrud, E.W. (1981) Endorectal ileal pull-through with lateral ileal reservoir for benign colorectal disease. *Ann. Surg.*, **194**, 761–766

Fonkalsrud, E.W. (1982) Endorectal ileal pull-through with ileal reservoir for ulcerative colitis and polyposis. *Am. J. Surg.*, **144**, 81–87

Fonkalsrud, E.W. (1984a) Endorectal ileoanal anastomosis with isoperistaltic ileal reservoir after colectomy and mucosal proctectomy. *Ann. Surg.*, **199**, 151–157

Fonkalsrud, E.W. (1984b) Colectomy and endorectal ileal pull-through with lateral ileal reservoir for ulcerative colitis and polyposis in children. *J. Pediatr. Surg.*, **19**, 541–546

Fonkalsrud, E.W. (1985) Endorectal ileal pull-through with isoperistaltic reservoir for colitis and polyposis. *Ann. Surg.*, **202**, 145–152

Fonkalsrud, E.W. (1987) Update on clinical experience with different surgical techniques of the endorectal pull-through operation for colitis and polyposis. *Surg. Gynecol. Obstet.*, **165**, 309–316

Fonkalsrud, E.W., Stelzner, M. and McDonald, N. (1988a) Construction of an ileal reservoir in patients with a previous straight endorectal ileal pull-through. *Ann. Surg.*, **208**, 50–55

Fonkalsrud, E.W., Stelzner, M. and McDonald, N. (1988b) Experience with the endorectal ileal pull-through with lateral reservoir for ulcerative colitis and polyposis. *Arch. Surg.*, **123**, 1053–1058

Fox, J.E., Daniel, E.E., Jury, J. and Robotham, H. (1984) The mechanism of motilin excitation of the canine small intestine. *Life Sci.*, **34**, 1001–1006

Fozard, J.B., Lowndes, R.H. and Young, H.L. (1990) Tissue oxygen measurement in ileal pouch construction. *Dis. Colon Rectum*, **33**, P32

Franceschi, D., Chen, P.F. and Yuh Jen-Nan (1986) Solitary J-pouch ulcer causing pouchitis-like syndrome. *Dis. Colon Rectum*, **29**, 515–517

Francois, Y., Dozois, R.R., Kelly, K.A. *et al.* (1989) Small intestinal obstruction complicating ileal pouch–anal anastomosis. *Ann. Surg.*, **209**, 46–50

Fujiwara, T., Kawarasaki, H. and Fonkalsrud, E.W. (1984) Endorectal ileal pull-through after chemical debridement of the rectal mucosa. *Surg. Gynecol. Obstet.*, **158**, 437–442

Gabriel, W.B. (1952) The surgical treatment of chronic ulcerative colitis. *Br. Med. J..*, **1**, 881–885

Gadasz, T.R., Kelly, K.A. and Phillips, S.F. (1977) The continent ileal pouch: absorptive and motor features. *Gastroenterology*, **72**, 1287–1291

Gadasz, T.R., McFadden, D.W., Gabrielson, E.W. *et al.* (1990) Adenocarcinoma of the ileostomy: the latent risk of cancer after colectomy for ulcerative colitis and familial polyposis. *Surgery*, **107**, 698–703

Galandiuk, S., Tsao, J., Ilstrup, D.M. *et al.* (1990a) Delayed ileo-pouch–anal anastomosis: complications and functional results. *Dis. Colon Rectum*, **33**, P6

Galandiuk, S., Wolff, B.G., Dozois, R.R. *et al.* (1990b) Ileo-pouch–anal anastomosis without ileostomy. *Dis. Colon Rectum*, **33**, P19

Gaston, E.A. (1948) The physiology of fecal continence. *Surg. Gynecol. Obstet.*, **87**, 280–290

Gazet, J-C. (1985) Parks' coloanal pull-through anastomosis for severe complicated radiation proctitis. *Dis. Colon Rectum*, **28**, 110–114

Ger, R., Ravo, B., Harris, M. *et al.* (1986) Mucosal destruction and regeneration of the colon by local hyperthermia: an experimental preliminary study. *Dis. Colon Rectum*, **29**, 177–181

Gerber, A., Apt, M.K. and Craig, P.H. (1983) The Kock continent ileostomy. *Surg. Gynecol. Obstet.*, **156**, 345–350

Gillespie, J.S. (1962) The electrical and mechanical responses of intestinal smooth muscle cells to stimulation of their extrinsic parasympathetic nerves. *J. Physiol. (Lond.)*, **162**, 76–92

Gilmore, I.T. (1990) Orocaecal transit time in health and disease. *Gut*, **31**, 250–251

Gingold, B.S., Jagelman, D.G. and Turnbull, R.B. (1979) Surgical management of familial polyposis and Gardner's syndrome. *Am. J. Surg.*, **137**, 54–56

Gionchetti, P., Paganelli, G.M., Tamagnini, N. *et al.* (1989) Macrophage sub-populations in normal pouch and pouchitis. In *Symposium: New Trends in Pelvic Pouch Procedures*, Bologna, A58.

Glass, R.E. and Mann, C.V. (1988) Anal anastomosis using the 'fish-hook' needle. *Surg. Gynecol. Obstet.*, **166**, 73

Glotzer, D.J. and Pihl, B.G. (1969) Preservation of continence after mucosal graft in the rectum and its feasibility in man. *Am. J. Surg.*, **117**, 403–409

Go, P.M.N.Y.H., Vaessen, N.H.J.J., van Durin, C.J. and Lens, J. (1986) A plastic rod to facilitate longitudinal incision of the bowel: an inexpensive and practical device. *Dis. Colon Rectum*, **29**, 674

Goligher, J.C. (1951) The functional results after sphincter-saving resections of the rectum. *Ann. R. Coll. Surg. Engl.*, **8**, 421–439

Goligher, J.C. (1961) Surgical treatment of ulcerative colitis. *Br. Med. J.*, **1**, 151–154

Goligher, J.C. (1971) Surgical treatment of ulcerative colitis: colectomy and ileorectal anastomosis. *Proc. R. Soc. Med.*, **64**, 973–977

Gorbach, S.L., Nakas, L. and Weinstein, L. (1976) Studies of intestinal microflora IV. The microflora of ileostomy effluent: a unique microbial ecology. *Gastroenterology*, **53**, 874–877

Gorenstein, L., Boyd, J.B. and Ross, T.M. (1988) Gracilis muscle repair of rectovaginal fistula after restorative proctocolectomy. Report of two cases. *Dis. Colon Rectum*, **31**, 730–734

Grant, D., Cohen, Z., McHugh, S. *et al.* (1986) Restorative proctocolectomy. Clinical results and manometric findings with long and short rectal cuffs. *Dis. Colon Rectum*, **29**, 27–32

Greenberg, G.R., Buchan, A.M.J., McLeod, R.S. *et al.* (1989) Gut hormone responses after reconstructive surgery for ulcerative colitis. *Gut*, **30**, 1721–1730

Griffen, W.O., Lillehei, R.C. and Wangensteen, O.H. (1963) Ileoproctostomy in ulcerative colitis: long-term follow-up extending to 20 years. *Surgery*, **53**, 705–710

Grundfest-Broniatowski, S., Moritz, A., Ilyes, L. *et al.* (1988) Voluntary control of an ileal pouch by coordinated electric stimulation: a pilot study in the dog. *Dis. Colon Rectum*, **31**, 261–267

Guidetti, C., Graziano, L., Poggioli, G. *et al.* (1989) Faecal fat excretion in patients with proctocolectomy and ileal pouch. In *Symposium: New Trends in Pelvic Pouch Procedures*, Bologna, A15.

Gustavsson, S., Weiland, L.H. and Kelly, K.A. (1987) Relationship of backwash ileitis to ileal pouchitis after ileal pouch–anal anastomosis. *Dis. Colon Rectum*, **30**, 25–28

Hallgren, T., Fasth, S., Nordgren, S. *et al.* (1989) Manovolumetric characteristics and functional results in three different pelvic pouch designs. *Int. J. Color. Dis.*, **4**, 156–160

Hancock, B.D. (1976) Measurement of anal pressure and motility. *Gut*, **17**, 645–651

Hancock, B.D. (1977) The internal sphincter and anal fissure. *Br. J. Surg.*, **64**, 92–95

Hancock, B.D. and Smith, K. (1975) The internal sphincter and Lord's procedure for haemorrhoids. *Br. J. Surg.*, **62**, 833–836

Handford, H. (1890) Disseminated polypi of the large intestine becoming malignant. *Trans. Pathol. Soc. Lond.*, **41**, 133–137

Hansen, L.K., Rosenkilde, O.P., Hebjorn, M. *et al.* (1982) The continent reservoir anal ileostomy with mucosal proctectomy. *Scand. J. Gastroenterol. Suppl.*, **78**, 1667

Hansen, L.K., Rosenkilde, O.P. and Simonsen, L. (1985) Total colectomy, mucosal proctectomy and endorectal ileal reservoir to an anal anastomosis. A comparison of short and long efferent legs. *Scand. J. Gastroenterol.*, **20**, 1091–1096

Hanson, P.A. (1990) Perianal skin care for persons with an ileoanal reservoir. *Ostomy Wound Management*, **27**, 16–20

Harig, J.M., Soergel, K.H., Komorowski, R.A. and Wood, C.M. (1989) Treatment of diversion colitis with short chain fatty acid irrigation. *N. Engl. J. Med.*, **320**, 23–28

Harms, B.A., Hamilton, J.W. and Starling, J.R. (1987) Management of chronic ulcerative colitis and rectovaginal fistula by simultaneous ileal pouch construction and fistula closure: report of a case. *Dis. Colon Rectum*, **30**, 611–614

Harms, B.A., Hamilton, J.W., Yamamoto, D.T. and Starling, J.R. (1987) Quadruple loop (W) ileal pouch reconstruction following proctocolectomy: analysis and functional results. *Surgery*, **102**, 561–567

Harms, B.A., Pahl, A.C. and Starling, J.R. (1990) Comparison of clinical and compliance characteristics between S and W ileal reservoirs. *Am. J. Surg.*, **159**, 34–40

Harms, B.A., Pellett, J.R. and Starling, J.R. (1987) Modified quadruple loop (W) ileal reservoir for restorative proctocolectomy. *Surgery* **101**, 234–237

Harms, B.A., Radosevich, D.G., Hamilton, J.W. and Starling, J.R. (1988) A new technique and catheter design for assessing capacity and compliance characteristics of ileal reservoirs. *Surg. Gynecol. Obstet.*, **166**, 468–470

Harris, L.D. and Pope, C.E. (1964) Squeeze vs resistance: an evaluation of the mechanism of sphincter competence. *J. Clin. Invest.*, **43**, 2272–2278

Harrison, R.C., Oka, H. and Owen, D.A. (1984) Experimental evaluation of the resistance of the skin grafted rectum to ileal contents. *Am. J. Surg.*, **147**, 624–628

Hatakeyama, K., Yamai, K. and Muto, T. (1989) Evaluation of ileal W-pouch–anal anastomosis for restorative proctocolectomy. *Int. J. Color. Dis.*, **4**, 150–155

Hautefeuille, P., Valleur, P. and Perniceni, T. (1988) Function and oncological results after coloanal anastomosis for low rectal cancer. *Ann. Surg.*, **207**, 61–64

Hawley, P.R. (1985) Ileorectal anastomosis. In *Frontiers in Colorectal Disease* (eds. R.C.G. Russell and J.P.S. Thomson), Butterworths, London, p.S75.

Haynes, W.G. and Read, N.W. (1982) Anorectal activity in man during rectal infusion of saline; a dynamic assessment of the anal continence mechanism. *J. Physiol.*, **330**, 45–56

Heald, R.J. and Allen, D.R. (1986) Stapled ileoanal anastomosis: a technique to avoid mucosal proctectomy in the ileal pouch operation. *Br. J. Surg.*, **73**, 571–572

Heimann, T.M., Bolnick, K. and Aufses, A.H. (1986) Results of surgical treatment for familial polyposis coli. *Am. J. Surg.*, **152**, 276–278

Heimann, T.M., Gelernt, I., Bauer, J. *et al.* (1983) Mucosal proctectomy without reservoir. *Am. J. Surg.*, **145**, 674–677

Heimann, T.M., Gelernt, I., Salky, B. *et al.* (1987) Familial polyposis coli: results of mucosal proctectomy with ileoanal anastomosis. *Dis. Colon Rectum*, **30**, 424–427

Heimann, T.M., Kurtz, R.J. and Aufses, A.H. (1985) Ultrasonic fragmentation. A new technique for mucosal proctectomy. *Arch. Surg.*, **120**, 1200–1203

Heimann, T.M., Kurtz, R.J., Shen-Schwarz, S. and Aufses, A.H. (1983) Mucosal proctectomy and endorectal pull-through using ultrasonic tissue fragmentation. *Surg. Forum*, **XXXIV**, 202–203

Heimann, T.M., Kurtz, R.J., Shen-Schwarz, S. and Aufses, A.H. (1984) Mucosal proctectomy using an ultrasonic scalpel. *Am. J. Surg.*, **147**, 803–806

Heimann, T.M., Kurtz, R.J., Shen-Schwarz, S. and Aufses, A.H. (1985) Ultrasonic mucosal proctectomy without endorectal pull-through. *Dis. Colon Rectum*, **28**, 336–340

Hennild, V., Kjaergard, H. and Hansen, L.K. (1986) Radiologic evaluation of the continent (S-pouch) ileal reservoir with anal anastomosis. *Acta Radiol. Diagn.*, **27**, 301–304

Henriksen, F.W. and Anthonisen, B. (1972) Measurement of the anal sphincter strength by a simple method suitable for routine use. *Scand. J. Gastroenterol.*, **7**, 555–558

Henry, M.M., Parkes, A.G. and Swash, M. (1982). The pelvic floor musculature in the descending perineum syndrome. *Br. J. Surg.*, **69**, 470–472

Heppell, J., Belliveau, P., Taillefer, R. *et al.* (1987) Quantitative assessment of pelvic ileal reservoir emptying with a semi- solid radionuclide enema: a correlation with clinical outcome. *Dis. Colon Rectum*, **30**, 81–85

Heppell, J., De Zubiria, M., Brais, M-F. *et al.* (1990) An assessment of the risk of neoplasia in long-term ileal reservoirs using the D.M.H. rodent model. *Dis. Colon Rectum*, **33**, 26–31

Heppell, J., Kelly, K.A., Phillips, S.F. *et al.* (1982) Physiologic aspects of continence after colectomy, mucosal proctectomy and endorectal ileoanal anastomosis. *Ann. Surg.*, **195**, 435–443

Heppell, J., Weiland, L.H., Perrault, J. *et al.* (1983) Fate of the rectal mucosa after rectal mucosectomy and ileoanal anastomosis. *Dis. Colon Rectum*, **26**, 768–771

Higham, S.E. and Read, N.W. (1990) Effect of ingestion of fat on ileostomy effluent. *Gut*, **31**, 435–438

Hill, G.L. (1987) Ileoanal anastomosis with J-pouch: an alternative to permanent ileostomy in ulcerative colitis and familial polyposis. *N.Z. Med. J.*, **100**, 659–661

Hill, J.R., Kelley, M.L., Schlegel, J.F. and Code, C.F. (1960) Pressure profile of rectum and anus of healthy persons. *Dis. Colon Rectum*, **3**, 203–209

Hillard, A.E., Mann, F.A., Becker, J.M. and Nelson, J.A. (1985) The ileoanal J-pouch: radiographic evaluation. *Radiology*, **155**, 591–594

Hines, J.R., Gore, R.M. and Ballantyne, G.H. (1984) Superior mesenteric artery syndrome. Diagnostic criteria and therapeutic approaches. *Am. J. Surg.*, **148**, 630–632

Hochenegg, J. (1900) Meine operationserfolge bei Rectumcarcinom. *Wien. Klin. Wochenschr.*, **13**, 399–404

Hojlund, P.B., Simonsen, L., Hansen, L.K. *et al.* (1985) Bile acid malabsorption in patients with an ileal reservoir with a long efferent leg to an anal anastomosis. *Scand. J. Gastroenterol.*, **20**, 995–1000

Holdsworth, P.J. and Johnston, D. (1988a) Anal sensation after restorative proctocolectomy for ulcerative colitis. *Br. J. Surg.*, **75**, 993–996

Holdsworth, P.J. and Johnston, D. (1988b) Use of the end-to-end anastomosis without mucosal stripping diminishes morbity and time in hospital after restorative proctocolectomy. *Br. J. Surg.*, **75**, 1232

Holgate, A.M. and Read, N.W. (1985) Effect of ileal infusion of Intralipid on gastrointestinal transit, ileal flow rate, and carbohydrate absorption in humans after ingestion of a liquid meal. *Gastroenterology*, **88**, 1005–1011

Hosie, K.B., Kmiot, W.A. and Keighley, M.R.B. (1990) Constipation: another indication for restorative proctocolectomy. *Br. J. Surg.*, **77**, 801–802

Hrabovsky, E.E., Watne, A.L. and Carrier, J.M. (1984) Changing management in familial polyposis. Role of ileoanal endorectal pull-through. *Am. J. Surg.*, **147**, 130–133

Hughes, E.S.R. (1965) The treatment of ulcerative colitis. *Ann. R. Coll. Surg. Engl.*, **37**, 191–206

Hughes, J.P., Bauer, A.R. and Bauer, C.M. (1988) Stapling techniques for easy construction of an ileal J-pouch. *Am. J. Surg.*, **155**, 783–785

Hulten, L. (1985) The continent ileostomy (Kock's pouch) versus the restorative proctocolectomy (pelvic pouch). *World J. Surg.*, **9**, 952–959

Hulten, L., Fasth, S., Nordgren, S. and Oresland, T. (1988) Kock's pouch converted to a pelvic pouch: report of a case. *Dis. Colon Rectum*, **31**, 467–469

Hurst, A.F. (1935) Ulcerative colitis. *Guys Hosp. Rep.*, **15**, 317–355

Hyman, N.H., Tuckson, W.B., Fazio, V.W. and Lavery, I.C. (1990) Consequences of ileal pouch–anal anastomosis for Crohn's disease. *Dis. Colon Rectum*, **33**, P4

Iida, M., Itoh, H., Matsui, T. *et al.* (1989) Ileal adenomas in postcolectomy patients with familial adenomatosis coli/Gardner's syndrome. *Dis. Colon Rectum*, **32**, 1034–1038

Ito, Y., Yokoyama, J., Namba, S. *et al.* (1981) Reappraisal of endorectal pull-through procedure. *J. Pediatr. Surg.*, **16**, 655–659

Itoh, H., Shosaku, N., Nakamura, K. *et al.* (1989) Bile composition after total proctocolectomy with interposed jejunal segment as neorectum. *Dis. Colon Rectum*, **32**, 711–715

Jagenburg, R., Dotevall, G., Kewenter, J. *et al.* (1971) Absorption studies in patients with 'intra-abdominal ileostomy reservoirs' and in patients with conventional ileostomies. *Gut*, **12**, 437

Jenkins, D., Goodall, A. and Scott, B.B. (1990) Ulcerative colitis: one disease or two? (Quantitative histological differences between distal and extensive disease.) *Gut*, **31**, 426–430

Johnson, G.P., Pemberton, J.H. and Kelly, K.A.

(1990) Parameters of anal–pouch function after W and J ileal pouch–anal anastomosis. *Dis. Colon Rectum*, **33**, P33

Johnson, G.P. and Wolff, B.G. (1990) Complications and functional outcome in patients with ileal pouch–anal anastomosis and Crohn's disease. *Dis. Colon Rectum*, **33**, P4

Johnston, D., Holdsworth, P.J., Nasmyth, D.G. *et al.* (1987) Preservation of the entire anal canal in conservative proctocolectomy for ulcerative colitis: a pilot study comparing end-to-end ileoanal without mucosal resection with mucosal proctectomy and endo-anal anastomosis. *Br. J. Surg.*, **74**, 940–944

Johnston, D., Holdsworth, P.J. and Smith, A.H. (1989) Preservation of ileocaecal junction and entire anal canal in surgery for ulcerative colitis – a 'two-sphincter' operation. *Dis. Colon Rectum*, **32**, 555–561

Johnston, D., Nasmyth, D.G., Williams, N.S. and Smith, A. (1985) The results of duplicated and triplicated reservoirs after mucosal proctectomy. *Br. J. Surg.*, **72**, S129

Johnston, D., Williams, N.S., Neal, D.E. and Axon, A.T.R. (1981) The value of preserving the anal sphincter in operations for ulcerative colitis and polyposis: a review of 22 mucosal proctectomies. *Br. J. Surg.*, **68**, 874–878

Karlan, M., McPherson, R.C. and Watman, R.N. (1959) An experimental evaluation of faecal continence – sphincter and reservoir – in the dog. *Surg. Gynecol. Obstet.*, **108**, 469–475

Kawakami, M. (1954) Electromyographic investigation of the human external sphincter muscle of the anus. *Jpn. J. Physiol.*, **4**, 196

Kawarasaki, H., Fujiwara, T. and Fonkalsrud, E.W. (1982) Endorectal ileal pull-through following chemical debridement of rectal mucosa. *Surg. Forum*, **XXXIII**, 196–198

Kawarasaki, H., Fujiwara, T. and Fonkalsrud, E.W. (1983) Electric activity and motility in the isoperistaltic side-to-side ileal reservoir. *Surg. Forum*, **XXXIV**, 199–202

Kawarasaki, H., Fujiwara, T. and Fonkalsrud, E.W. (1985) Electric activity and motility in the side-to-side isoperistaltic ileal reservoir. *Arch. Surg.*, **120**, 1045–1047

Kay, R.M., Cohen, Z., Siu, K.P. *et al.* (1979) Ileal excretion and bacterial modification of bile acids and cholesterol in patients with continent ileostomy. *Gut*, **21**, 128–132

Keighley, M.R.B. (1987) Abdominal mucosectomy reduces the incidence of soiling and sphincter damage after restorative proctocolectomy and J-pouch. *Dis. Colon Rectum*, **30**, 386–390

Keighley, M.R.B. (1989) Is permanent ileostomy an outmoded operation for colitis and polyposis coli? *Hosp. Update*, **15**, 717–719

Keighley, M.R.B., Hosie, K., Sakaguchi, M. *et al.*

(1990a) Mucosal blood flow following restorative proctocolectomy: pouchitis is associated with mucosal ischaemia. *Dis. Colon Rectum*, **33**, P5

Keighley, M.R.B. and Kmiot, W.A. (1988) A randomised comparison between the J or W-pouches for restorative proctocolectomy. *Gut*, **29**, A705

Keighley, M.R.B., Kmiot, W.A., Harding, L.K. *et al.* (1990b) Pouchitis following restorative proctocolectomy: an evaluation of [111]Indium labelled granulocytes for diagnosis. *Dis. Colon Rectum*, **33**, P33

Keighley, M.R.B., Kmiot, W.A. and Youngs, D.J. (1990) Recovery from pouchitis: the mechanism of adaptive ileal villous regrowth. *Dis. Colon Rectum*, **33**, P33

Keighley, M.R.B., Winslet, M.C., Flinn, R. and Kmiot, W. (1989) Multivariate analysis of factors influencing the results of restorative proctocolectomy. *Br. J. Surg.*, **76**, 740–743

Keighley, M.R.B., Winslet, M.C., Pringle, W. and Allan, R.N. (1987a) The pouch as an alternative to permanent ileostomy. *Br. J. Hosp. Med.*, **4**, 286–294

Keighley, M.R.B., Winslet, M.C., Yoshioka, K. and Lightwood, R. (1987b) Discrimination is not impaired by excision of the anal transition zone after restorative proctocolectomy. *Br. J. Surg.*, **74**, 1118–1121

Keighley, M.R.B., Yoshioka, K. and Kmiot, W. (1988) Prospective randomised trial to compare the stapled double lumen pouch and the sutured quadruple pouch for restorative proctocolectomy. *Br. J. Surg.*, **75**, 1008–1011

Keighley, M.R.B., Yoshioka, K., Kmiot, W. and Heyen, F. (1988) Physiological parameters influencing function in restorative proctocolectomy and ileo-pouch–anal anastomosis. *Br. J. Surg.*, **75**, 997–1002

Keller, R.J., Salky, B.A. and Gelernt, I.M. (1989) Mucosal proctectomy and ileoanal anastomosis. *Mt. Sinai J. Med.*, **56**, 36–40

Kelly, D.G., Phillips, S.F., Kelly, K.A. *et al.* (1983) Dysfunction of the continent ileostomy: clinical features and bacteriology. *Gut*, **24**, 193–201

Kerlin, P. and Phillips, S.F. (1982) Variability of motility of the ileum and jejunum in healthy humans. *Gastroenterology*, **82**, 694–700

Kerreman, R. (1968) Electrical activity and motility of the internal anal sphincter. *Acta Gastroenterol. Belg*, **31**, 465–482

Kestenberg, A. and Becker, J.M. (1985) A new technique of loop ileostomy closure after endorectal ileoanal anastomosis. *Surgery*, **98**, 109–111

Kestenberg, A., Becker, J.M. and Sharp, S.W. (1985) Electromechanical relationship of the internal anal sphincter of the cat. *Gastroenterology*, **88**, 1444

Kiff, E.S. (1983) The clinical use of anorectal

physiology studies. *Ann. R. Coll. Surg. Engl. (Sir Alan Parks Symposium)*, 27–29

Kiff, E.S. and Swash, M. (1984) Slowed conduction in the pudendal nerves in idiopathic (neurogenic) faecal incontinence. *Br. J. Surg.*, **71**, 614–616

King, D.W., Lubowski, D.Z. and Cook, T.A. (1989) Anal canal mucosa in restorative proctocolectomy for ulcerative colitis. *Br. J. Surg.*, **76**, 970–972

King, S.A. (1975) Quality of life: the continent ileostomy. *Ann. Surg.*, **182**, 29–32

Klein, K., Stenzel, P. and Katon, R.M. (1983) Pouch ileitis: report of a case with severe systemic manifestations. *J. Clin. Gastroenterol.*, **5**, 149–153

Kmiot, W.A., Harding, L.K., Hesselwood, S.R. *et al.* (1989a) Pouchitis following restorative proctocolectomy: an evaluation of ^{111}indium-labelled granulocytes for diagnosis. *Br. J. Surg.*, **76**, 1338

Kmiot, W.A. and Keighley, M.R.B. (1989a) Intussusception presenting as ileal reservoir ischaemia following restorative proctocolectomy. *Br. J. Surg.*, **76**, 148

Kmiot, W.A. and Keighley, M.R.B. (1989b) Totally stapled abdominal restorative proctocolectomy. *Br. J. Surg.*, **76**, 961–964

Kmiot, W.A., O'Brien, J.D. and Keighley, M.R.B. (1988) Breath hydrogen testing: an indicator of small bowel overgrowth following ileoanal pouch formation. *Gut*, **29**, A1467

Kmiot, W.A., O'Brien, J.D. and Keighley, M.R.B. (1989) Breath-hydrogen testing: an indicator of small bowel overgrowth following pouch formation. *Br. J. Surg.*, **76**, A644

Kmiot, W.A., Pinho, M., Yoshioka, K. and Keighley, M.R.B (1989b) Does anal sphincter function improve following restorative proctocolectomy? *Br. J. Surg.*, **76**, A636

Kmiot, W.A., Yoshioka, K., Pinho, M. and Keighley, M.R.B. (1990) Videoproctographic assessment after restorative proctocolectomy. *Dis. Colon Rectum*, **33**, 566–572

Kmiot, W.A., Youngs, D.J. and Keighley, M.R.B. (1989) Recovery from pouchitis: the mechanism of adaptive ileal villus regrowth. *Br. J. Surg.*, **76**, 1338

Kmiot, W.A., Youngs, D.J., Winslet, M.C. *et al.* (1989c) Ileal adaptation following restorative proctocolectomy. *Br. J. Surg.*, **76**, A625

Knill-Jones, R.P., Morson, B.C. and Williams, R. (1970) Prestomal ileitis: clinical and pathological findings in 5 cases. *Q. J. Med.*, **39**, 287–297

Kock, N.G. (1969) Intra-abdominal 'reservoir' in patients with permanent ileostomy. Preliminary observations on a procedure resulting in fecal 'continence' in five ileostomy patients. *Arch. Surg.*, **99**, 223–231

Kock, N.G. (1987) The use of surgically created reservoirs. *World J. Surg.*, **11**, 687–688

Kock, N.G., Darle, N. and Kewenter, J. (1974) The quality of life after proctocolectomy and ileostomy: a study of patients with conventional ileostomies converted to continent ileostomies. *Dis. Colon Rectum*, **17**, 287–292

Kock, N.G., Darle, N. and Hulton, L. (1977) Ileostomy. *Curr. Probl. Surg.*, **14**,(8), 1

Kock, N.G., Hulton, L. and Myrvold, H.E. (1989) Ileoanal anastomosis with interposition of the ileal 'Kock pouch'. *Dis. Colon Rectum*, **32**, 1050–1054

Kock, N.G., Myrvold, N.E. and Nilsson, L.O. (1980) Construction of a stable nipple valve for the continent ileostomy. *Ann. Chir. Gynaecol.*, **69**, 132–143

Kojima, Y., Sanada, Y. and Fonkalsrud, E.W. (1981) Comparison of endorectal ileal pull-through after colectomy with and without ileal reservoir. *Surg. Forum*, **XXXII**, 170–171

Kojima, Y., Sanada, Y. and Fonkalsrud, E.W. (1982a) Evaluation of techniques for chemical debridement of colonic mucosa. *Surg. Gynecol. Obstet.*, **155**, 849–854

Kojima, Y., Sanada, Y. and Fonkalsrud, E.W. (1982b) Comparison of endorectal ileal pull-through following colectomy with and without ileal reservoir. *J. Pediatr. Surg.*, **17**, 653–659

Koltun, W., Schoetz, D.J., Roberts, P.L. *et al.* (1990) Indeterminate colitis predisposes to perineal complications after ileal pouch–anal anastomosis. *Dis. Colon Rectum*, **33**, P4

Krausz, M.M. (1988) Loop ileostomy for complete fecal diversion following colectomy and ileoanal anastomosis. *Dis. Colon Rectum*, **31**, 819–820

Kremers, P.W., Scholz, F.J. and Schoetz D.J. Jr (1985) Radiology of the ileoanal reservoir. *AJR*, **145**, 559–567

Kumar, D., Waldron, D., Nicholls, R.J. and Williams, N.S. (1989) Motor function of the ileal reservoir following restorative proctocolectomy. *Gastroenterology*, **96**, A276

Kumar, D. and Williams, N.S. (1990) Surgical management of ulcerative colitis. *Hosp. Update*, **16**, 113–120

Kusunoki, M., Sakanoue, Y., Shoji, Y. *et al.* (1990a) Conversion of malfunctioning J-pouch to Kock's pouch. *Acta Chir. Scand.*, **156**, 179–181

Kusunoki, M., Shoji, Y., Ikeuchi, H. *et al.* (1990b) Usefulness of valproate sodium for treatment of incontinence after ileoanal anastomosis. *Surgery*, **107**, 311–315

Lane, R.H.S. and Parks, A.G. (1977) Function of the anal sphincters following colo-anal anastomosis. *Br. J. Surg.*, **64**, 596–599

Launer, D.P. and Sackier, J.M. (1990) One-stage proctocolectomy and J-pouch anal anastomosis without diverting ileostomy. *Dis. Colon Rectum*, **33**, P32

Lavery, I.C., Tuckson, W.B. and Easley, K.A.

(1989) Internal anal sphincter function after total abdominal colectomy and stapled ileal pouch–anal anastomosis without mucosal proctectomy. *Dis. Colon Rectum*, **32**, 950–953

Lawson, J.O.N. (1974a) Pelvic anatomy. I Pelvic floor muscles. *Ann. R. Coll. Surg. Engl.*, **54**, 244–252

Lawson, J.O.N. (1974b) Pelvic anatomy. II Anal canal and associated sphincters. *Ann. R. Coll. Surg. Engl.*, **54**, 288–300

Lawson, J.O.N. and Nixon, H.H. (1967) Anal canal pressures in the diagnosis of Hirschsprung's disease. *J. Pediatr. Surg.*, **2**, 544–552

Lazorthes, F., Fages, P., Chiotasso, P. *et al.* (1986) Resection of the rectum with construction of a colonic reservoir and colo-anal anastomosis for carcinoma of the rectum. *Br. J. Surg.*, **73**, 136–138

Lehur, P.A. and Leborgne, J. (1990) Totally stapled abdominal restorative proctocolectomy (letter). *Br. J. Surg.*, **77**, 594

Leijonmarck, C-E., Lofberg, R., Ost, A. and Hellers, G. (1990) Long-term results of ileorectal anastomosis in ulcerative colitis in Stockholm County. *Dis. Colon Rectum*, **33**, 195–200

Leijonmarck, C-E., Persson, P.G. and Hellers, G. (1990) Factors affecting colectomy rate in ulcerative colitis: an epidemiologic study. *Gut*, **31**, 329–333

Leite, J.F.M.S., Fausto-Pontes and Martins, M.I. (1990) Different ileoanal pouch designs with and without ileal valve in dogs. *Dis. Colon Rectum*, **33**, P32

Lennard-Jones, J.E., Melville, D.M., Morson, B.C. *et al.* (1990) Precancer and cancer in extensive ulcerative colitis: findings among 401 patients over 22 years. *Gut*, **31**, 800–806

Lennard-Jones, J.E., Morson, B.C., Ritchie, J.K. *et al.* (1977) Cancer in colitis: assessment of the individual risks by clinical and histological criteria. *Gastroenterology*, **73**, 1280–1289

Lerch, M.M., Braun, J., Harder, M. *et al.* (1989) Postoperative adaptation of the small intestine after total colectomy and J-pouch–anal anastomosis. *Dis. Colon Rectum*, **32**, 600–608

Lewis, P. and Bartolo, D.C.C. (1990) Closure of loop ileostomy after restorative proctocolectomy. *Ann. Royal Coll. Surg. Engl.*, **72**, 263–265

Lilienthal, H. (1903) Extirpation of the entire colon, the upper portion of the sigmoid flexure and four inches of the ileum for hyperplastic colitis. *Ann. Surg.*, **37**, 616

Liljeqvist, L. and Lindquist, K. (1985) A reconstructive operation on malfunctioning S shaped pelvic reservoirs. *Dis. Colon Rectum*, **28**, 506–511

Liljeqvist, L., Lindquist, K. and Ljungdahl, I. (1988) Alterations in ileoanal pouch technique, 1980 to 1987. Complications and functional outcome. *Dis. Colon Rectum*, **31**, 929–938

Lindquist, K. (1990) Anal manometry with microtransducer technique before and after restorative proctocolectomy. Sphincter function and clinical correlations. *Dis. Colon Rectum*, **33**, 91–98

Lindquist, K., Liljequist, L. and Sellburg, B. (1984) The topography of ileoanal reservoirs in relation to evacuation patterns and clinical functions. *Acta Chir. Scand.*, **150**, 573–579

Lindquist, K., Nilsell, K. and Liljequist, L. (1987) Cuff abscesses and ileoanal anastomotic separations in pelvic pouch surgery: an analysis of possible aetiological factors. *Dis. Colon Rectum*, **30**, 355–359

Lohmuller, J.L., Pemberton, J.H., Dozois, R.R. *et al.* (1990) Pouchitis and extraintestinal manifestations of inflammatory bowel disease after ileal pouch–anal anastomosis. *Ann. Surg.*, **211**, 622–627

Lontoft, E. (1986) *Salmonella typhimurium* infection after colectomy with mucosal proctectomy, a pouch and ileoanal anastomosis. *Dis. Colon Rectum*, **29**, 671–672

Lopez, R., Kemalyan, N., Mosely, S. *et al.* (1990) Problems in diagnosis and management of desmoid tumours. *Am. J. Surg.*, **159**, 450–453

Luukkonen, P. (1988) Manometric follow-up of anal sphincter function after an ileoanal pouch procedure. *Int. J. Color. Dis.*, **3**, 43–46

Luukkonen, P. and Jarvinen, H. (1987) Pelvic ileal reservoirs: experimental assessment of reservoir capacity in three reservoir designs. *Ann. Chir. Gynecol.*, **76**, 294–297

Luukonen, P., Jarvinen, H., Lehtola, A. and Sipponen, P. (1988a) Mucosal alterations in pelvic ileal reservoirs. A histological and ultrastructural evaluation in an experimental model. *Ann. Chir. Gynecol.*, **77**, 91–96

Luukkonen, P., Valtonen, V., Sivoren, A. *et al.* (1988b) Fecal bacteriology and reservoir ileitis in patients operated on for ulcerative colitis. *Dis. Colon Rectum*, **31**, 864–867

MacDougall, I.P.M. (1964) The cancer risk in ulcerative colitis. *Lancet*, **ii**, 655–658

McGowan, P.F., Postier, R.G. and Williams, G.P. (1987) Restorative proctocolectomy with the 'J' ileal reservoir in the management of ulcerative colitis and polyposis coli. *J.R. Coll. Surg. Edinb.*, **32**, 272–275

McHugh, S.M., Diamant, N.E., McLeod, R. and Cohen, Z. (1987) S-pouches versus J-pouches. A comparison of functional outcomes. *Dis. Colon Rectum*, **30**, 671–677

Madden, M.V., Farthing, M.J.G. and Nicholls, R.J. (1990) Inflammation in ileal reservoirs: 'pouchitis'. *Gut*, **31**, 247–249

Madigan, M.R. (1976) The continent ileostomy and the isolated ileal bladder. *Ann. R. Coll. Surg. Engl.*, **58**, 62–69

Mahida, Y.R., Gionchetti, P., Vaux, D. *et al.*

(1986) Macrophage subpopulations in inflammatory bowel disease. *Gut*, **27**, A1245

Mariani, P., Slors, F.J.M., Pietroletti, R. *et al.* (1989) Enteroglucagon and Peptide Tyrosin-Tyrosin plasma levels after total proctocolectomy and pouch construction in dog. *Gastroenterology*, **96**, A320

Marks, G., Mohiuddin, M., Basile, M. and Eitan, A. (1990) Experience with a new method of radical proctosigmoidectomy and coloanal anastomosis initiated by transanal dissection for rectal cancer post high-dose irradiation. *Dis. Colon Rectum*, **33**, P19

Martin, L.W. and Fischer, J.E. (1982) Preservation of anorectal continence following total colectomy. *Ann. Surg.*, **196**, 700–704

Martin, L.W., Le Coultre, C. and Schubert, W.K. (1977) Total colectomy and mucosal proctectomy with preservation of continence in ulcerative colitis. *Ann. Surg.*, **186**, 477–479

Martin, L.W. and Oldham, K.T. (1983) Staging of the endorectal pull-through operation for ulcerative colitis. *J. Pediatr. Surg.*, **18**, 453–456

Martin, L.W., Torres, A.M., Fischer, J.E. and Alexander, F. (1985) The critical level for preservation of continence in the ileoanal anastomosis. *J. Pediatr. Surg.*, **20**, 664–667

Marzouk, D., Williams, N.S. and Hallan, R.I. (1989) Function after stapled ileal pouch–anal anastomosis for ulcerative colitis. *Br. J. Surg.*, **76**, A627

Matikainen, M., Santavirta, J. and Hiltunen, K.M. (1990) Ileoanal anastomosis without covering ileostomy. *Dis. Colon Rectum*, **33**, 384–388

Max, E., Trabanino, G., Reznick, R.K. *et al.* (1987) Metabolic changes during the defunctionalized stage after ileal pouch–anal anastomosis. *Dis. Colon Rectum*, **30**, 508–512

Mayo, C.W. and Broders, C.W. (1957) The results of subtotal colectomy and ileoproctostomy in the treatment of chronic ulcerative colitis. *Surg. Gynecol. Obstet.*, **104**, 180–182

Mayo Robson, A.R. (1893) Case of colitis with ulceration treated by inguinal colostomy. *Trans. Clin. Soc. Lond.*, **26**, 213–215

Merton, P.A. and Morton, H.B. (1980) Stimulation of the cerebral cortex in the intact human subject. *Nature*, **285**, 227

Metcalf, A.M., Dozois, R.R., Beart, R.W. *et al.* (1986a) Temporary ileostomy for ileal pouch–anal anastomosis: function and complications. *Dis. Colon Rectum*, **29**, 300–303

Metcalf, A.M., Dozois, R.R., Beart, R.W. and Wolff, B.G. (1985) Pregnancy following ileal pouch–anal anastomosis. *Dis. Colon Rectum*, **28**, 859–861

Metcalf, A.M., Dozois, R.R. and Kelly, K.A.(1985) Ileal J-pouch–anal anastomosis: clinical outcome. *Ann. Surg.*, **202**, 735–739

Metcalf, A.M., Dozois, R.R., Kelly, K.A. and Wolff, B.G. (1986b) Ileal pouch–anal anastomosis without temporary, diverting ileostomy. *Dis. Colon Rectum*, **29**, 33–35

Meunier, P. and Mollard, P. (1977) Control of the internal anal sphincter. *Pflugers Archiv.*, **370**, 233–239

Mibu, R., Itoh, H. and Nakayama, F. (1987) Effect of total colectomy and mucosal proctectomy on intestinal absorptive capacity in dogs. *Dis. Colon Rectum*, **30**, 47–51

Miettinen, T.A. and Peltokallio, P. (1971) Bile salt, fat, water and vitamin B_{12} excretion after ileostomy. *Scand. J. Gastroenterol.*, **6**, 543–552

Miglioli, M., Barbara, L. and Di Febo, G. (1989) Topical administration of 5-aminosalicylic acid: a therapeutic proposal for the treatment of pouchitis (Letter). *N. Engl. J. Med.*, **320**, 257

Miglioli, M., Pironi, L., Ruggeri, E. *et al.* (1989) Digestive and systemic effects of ileal reservoir: nutritional consequences. In: *Symposium: New Trends in Pelvic Pouch Procedures, Bologna* A18

Miglioli, M., Stanghellini, V., Pironi, L. *et al.* (1989) The defunctionalized stage as a model for ileal-brake studies. In *Symposium. New Trends in Pelvic Pouch Procedures, Bologna*, A24

Mignon, M. and Bonfils, S. (1985) Altered physiology in ulcerative colitis patients with ileorectal anastomosis. In *Alternatives to Conventional Ileostomy* (ed. R.R. Dozois), Year Book Medical, Chicago, pp.61–80

Mignon, M., Bonnefond, A. and Vilotte, J. (1974) Les indications de la conservation du rectum dans les colectomies pour rectocolite hemorragique. *Arch. Fr. Mal. App. Dig.*, **63**, 541–553

Miller, R., Bartolo, D.C.C., Orrom, W.J. *et al.* (1990a) Improvement of anal sensation with preservation of the anal transition zone after ileoanal anastomosis for ulcerative colitis. *Dis. Colon Rectum*, **33**, 414–418

Miller, R., Orrom, W.J., Duthie, G. *et al.* (1990b) Ambulatory anorectal physiology in patients following restorative proctocolectomy for ulcerative colitis: comparison with normal controls. *Br. J. Surg.*, **77**, 895–897

Milligan, E.T.C. and Morgan, C.N. (1934) Surgical anatomy of the anal canal with special reference to anorectal fistulas. *Lancet*, **ii**, 1150–1156

Moertel, C.G., Hill, J.R. and Adson, M.A. (1970) Surgical management of multiple polyposis. *Arch. Surg.*, **100**, 521–526

Molnar, D., Taitz, L.S., Unwin, O.M. and Wales, J.K.H. (1983) Anorectal manometry results in defaecation disorders. *Arch. Dis. Child.*, **58**, 257–261

Moritz, A., Grundfest-Broniatowski, S., Ilyes, L. *et al.* (1989) Electrostimulation of ileum and jejunum reservoirs in an acute and chronic experiment. *Langenbecks Arch. Chir.*, **374**, 267–271

Morson, B. (1980) Use of dysplasia as an indicator of risk for malignancy in patients with ulcerative colitis. In *Colorectal Cancer: Prevention, Epidemiology and Screening* (eds S. Winawer *et al.*), Raven, New York

Morson, B. and Pang, L. (1967) Rectal biopsy as an aid to cancer control in ulcerative colitis. *Gut*, **8**, 423–434

Mortensen, N. (1988) Progress with the pouch – restorative proctocolectomy for ulcerative colitis. *Gut*, **29**, 561–565

Moskowitz, R.L., Shepherd, N.A. and Nicholls, R.J (1986) An assessment of inflammation in the reservoir after restorative proctocolectomy with ileoanal ileal reservoir. *Int. J. Color. Dis.*, **1**, 167–174

Myrhoj, T., Bulow, S. and Mogensen, A.M. (1989) Multiple adenomas in terminal ileum 25 years after restorative proctocolectomy for familial adenomatous polyposis: report of a case. *Dis. Colon Rectum*, **32**, 618–620

Myrvold, H.E. and Thoresen, J.E. (1989) The Kock pouch for ileoanal anastomosis. In *Symposium: New Trends in Pelvic Pouch Procedures, Bologna*, A68.

Naik, S.R., Pipalia, D.H., Plumber, S.T. *et al.* (1990) Adaptive changes in the terminal ileum after total colectomy, mucosal proctectomy and straight ileoanal anastomosis in chronic ulcerative colitis. *Ind. J. Gastroenterol.*, **9**, 69–72

Nakahara, S., Itoh, H., Iida. M. *et al.* (1985) Ileal adenomas in familial polyposis coli: differences before and after colectomy. *Dis. Colon Rectum*, **28**, 875–877

Nasmyth, D.G., Godwin, P.G.R., Dixon, M.F. *et al.* (1985) The relationship between mucosal structure and intestinal flora in ileal reservoirs. *Br. J. Surg.*, **72**, S129

Nasmyth, D.G., Godwin, P.G.R., Dixon, M.F. *et al.* (1989a) Ileal ecology after pouch–anal anastomosis or ileostomy. A study of mucosal morphology, fecal bacteriology, fecal volatile fatty acids and their interrelationship. *Gastroenterology*, **96**, 817–824

Nasmyth, D.G., Johnston, D., Godwin, P.G.R. *et al.* (1986) Factors influencing bowel function after ileal pouch–anal anastomosis. *Br. J. Surg.*, **73**, 469–473

Nasmyth, D.G., Johnston, D., Williams, N.S. *et al.* (1989b) Changes in the absorption of bile acids after total colectomy in patients with an ileostomy or pouch–anal anastomosis. *Dis. Colon Rectum*, **32**, 230–234

Nasmyth, D.G., Williams, N.S. and Johnston, D. (1986) Comparison of the function of triplicated and duplicated pelvic ileal reservoirs after mucosal proctectomy and ileoanal anastomosis for ulcerative colitis and adenomatous polyposis. *Br. J. Surg.*, **73**, 361–366

Nasmyth, D.G., Williams, N.S. and King, R.F.G.J. (1984) An investigation into the use of proximal transposition of the ileocaecal junction as an adjunct to total colectomy. *Eur. Surg. Res.*, **16**, 17–18

Natori, H., Kusunoki, M., Sakanoue, Y. *et al.* (1989) Changes of faecal bile acids and faecal bacterial flora after J shaped ileal pouch–anal anastomosis. In *Symposium: New Trends in Pelvic Pouch Procedures, Bologna*, A14.

Naylor, E.W., Gardner, E.J. and Richards, R.C. (1979) Desmoid tumours and mesenteric fibromatosis in Gardner's syndrome. *Arch. Surg.*, **114**, 1181–1185

Neal, D.E., Parker, A.J. and Williams, N.S. (1982) The long term effects of proctectomy on bladder function in patients with inflammatory bowel disease. *Br. J. Surg.*, **69**, 349–352

Neal, D.E., Williams, N.S. and Johnston, D. (1982) Rectal, bladder and sexual function after mucosal proctectomy with and without a pelvic reservoir for colitis and polyposis. *Br. J. Surg.*, **69**, 599–604

Nefzger, M.D. and Acheson, E.D. (1963) Ulcerative colitis in U.S. Army in 1944. Follow-up with particular reference to deaths in cases and controls. *Gut*, **4**, 183–192

Neill, M.E., Parks, A.G. and Swash, M. (1981) Physiological studies of the anal sphincter musculature in faecal incontinence and rectal prolapse. *Br. J. Surg.*, **68**, 531–536

Nelson, H., Dozois, R.R., Kelly. K.A. *et al.* (1989) The effect of pregnancy and delivery on the ileal pouch–anal anastomosis functions. *Dis. Colon Rectum*, **32**, 384–388

Nemer, F.D. and Rolstad, B.S. (1985) The role of the ileoanal reservoir in patients with ulcerative colitis and familial polyposis. *J. Enterostomal Ther.*, **12**, 74–83

Newton, C.R. and Baker, W.N.H. (1975) Comparison of bowel function after ileorectal anastomosis for ulcerative colitis and colonic polyposis. *Gut*, **16**, 785–791

Nicholls, R.J. (1983) Restorative proctocolectomy with ileal reservoir. *Ann. R. Coll. Surg. Engl.*, **66**, 42–45

Nicholls, R.J.(1987) Restorative proctocolectomy with various types of reservoir. *World J. Surg.*, **11**, 751–762

Nicholls, R.J. (1990) Restorative proctocolectomy with ileal reservoir: indications and results. *Schweiz. Med. Wochenschr.*, **120**, 485–488

Nicholls, R.J., Belliveau, P., Neill, M. *et al.* (1981) Restorative proctocolectomy with ileal reservoir: a pathophysiological assessment. *Gut*, **22**, 462–468

Nicholls, R.J. and Gilbert, J.M. (1990) Correction of the efferent ileal limb for disordered defaecation following restorative proctocolectomy with the S ileal reservoir. *Br. J. Surg.*, **77**, 152–154

Nicholls, R.J., Holt, S.D.H. and Lubowski, D.Z.,

(1989) Restorative proctocolectomy with ileal reservoir: comparison of two-stage vs. three-stage procedures and analysis of factors that might affect outcome. *Dis. Colon Rectum*, **32**, 323–326

Nicholls, R.J. and Kamm, M.A. (1988) Proctocolectomy with restorative ileoanal reservoir for severe idiopathic constipation. Report of two cases. *Dis. Colon Rectum*, **31**, 968–969

Nicholls, R.J. and Lubowski, D.Z. (1987) Restorative proctocolectomy: the four loop (W) reservoir. *Br. J. Surg.*, **74**, 564–566

Nicholls, R.J., Lubowski, D.Z. and Donaldson, D.R. (1988) Comparison of colonic reservoir and straight colo-anal reconstruction after rectal excision. *Br. J. Surg.*, **75**, 318–320

Nicholls, R.J., Moskowitz, R.L. and Shepherd, N.A. (1985a) Restorative proctocolectomy with ileal reservoir. *Br. J. Surg.*, **72**, 580–582

Nicholls, R.J., Pescatori, M., Motson, R.W. and Pezim, M.E. (1984) Restorative proctocolectomy with a three-loop reservoir for ulcerative colitis and familial polyposis. Clinical results in 66 patients followed for up to 6 years. *Ann. Surg.*, **199**, 383–389

Nicholls, R.J. and Pezim, M.E. (1985) Restorative proctocolectomy with ileal reservoir for ulcerative colitis and familial adenomatous polyposis: a comparison of three reservoir designs. *Br. J. Surg.*, **72**, 470–474

Nilsson, L.O., Andersson, H., Hulten, L. *et al.* (1979) Absorption studies in patients six to ten years after construction of ileostomy reservoirs. *Gut*, **20**, 499–503

Nilsson, L.O., Kock, N.G. and Kylberg, F. (1981) Sexual adjustment in ileostomy patients before and after conversion to continent ileostomy. *Dis. Colon Rectum*, **24**, 287–290

Nilsson, L.O., Myrvold, H.E., Swolin, B. and Ojerskog, B. (1984) Vitamin B$_{12}$ in plasma in patients with continent ileostomy and long observation time. *Scand. J. Gastroenterol.*, **19**, 369–374

Nissen, R. (1933) Demonstrationen aus der operativen Chirurgie zunachst einige Beobachtungen aus der plastischen Chirurgie. *Zentralbl. Chir.*, **60**, 888

Nivatvongs, S., Fang, D.T. and Kennedy, H.L. (1983) The shape of the buttocks. A useful guide for selection of anaesthesia and patient position in anorectal surgery. *Dis. Colon Rectum*, **26**, 85–86

Nivatvongs, S., Stern, H.S. and Fryd, D.S. (1981) The length of the anal canal. *Dis. Colon Rectum*, **24**, 600–601

Nugent, W. (1985) Surveillance of patients with ulcerative colitis: Lahey Clinic results. In *Alternatives to Conventional Ileostomy* (ed. R.R. Dozois), Year Book Medical, Chicago, p.275

O'Connell, P.R., Kelly, K.A. and Brown, M.L. (1986) Scintigraphic assessment of neorectal motor function. *J. Nucl. Med.*, **27**, 460–464

O'Connell, P.R., Pemberton, J.H., Brown, M.L. and Kelly, K.A. (1987a) Determinants of stool frequency after ileal pouch–anal anastomosis. *Am. J. Surg.*, **153**, 157–165

O'Connell, P.R., Pemberton, J.H. and Kelly, K.A. (1987) Motor function of the ileal J-pouch and its relation to clinical outcome after ileal pouch–anal anastomosis. *World J. Surg.*, **11**, 735–741

O'Connell, P.R., Pemberton, J.H., Weiland, L.H. *et al.* (1987b) Does rectal mucosa regenerate after ileoanal anastomosis? *Dis. Colon Rectum*, **30**, 1–5

O'Connell, P.R., Rankin, D.R., Weiland, L.H. and Kelly, K.A. (1986) Enteric bacteriology, absorption, morphology and emptying after ileal pouch–anal anastomosis. *Br. J. Surg.*, **73**, 909–914

O'Connell, P.R., Stryker, S.J., Metcalf, A.M. *et al.* (1988) Anal canal pressure and motility after ileoanal anastomosis. *Surg. Gynecol. Obstet.*, **166**, 47–54

Oh, C. and Kark, A.E. (1972) Anatomy of the external anal sphincter. *Br. J. Surg.*, **59**, 717–723

Ojerskog, B., Kock, N.G., Nilsson, L.O. *et al.* (1990) Long-term follow-up of patients with continent ileostomies. *Dis. Colon Rectum*, **33**, 184–189

O'Malley, V.P., Keyes, D.M., Cannon, J.P. and Postier, R.G. (1985) Longitudinal ileal myotomy: a new reservoir for use with ileoanal anastomosis. *Curr. Surg.*, **43**, 113–117

Oresland, T., Fasth, S., Akervall, S. *et al.* (1990a) Manovolumetric and sensory characteristics of the ileoanal J-pouch compared with healthy rectum. *Br. J. Surg.*, **77**, 803–806

Oresland, T., Fasth, S., Hulten, L. *et al.* (1988) Does balloon dilatation and anal sphincter training improve ileoanal–pouch function? *Int. J. Color. Dis.*, **3**, 153–157

Oresland, T., Fasth, S., Nordgren, S. *et al.* (1990b) Pouch size: the important functional determinant after restorative proctocolectomy. *Br. J. Surg.*, **77**, 265–269

Oresland, T., Fasth, S., Nordgren, S. and Hulten, L. (1989) The clinical and functional outcome after restorative proctocolectomy: a prospective study in 100 patients. *Int. J. Color. Dis.*, **4**, 50–56

Parc, R., Legrand, M., Frileux, P. *et al.* (1989) Comparative clinical results of ileal pouch–anal anastomosis and ileorectal anastomosis in ulcerative colitis. *Hepatogastroenterology*, **36**, 235–239

Parc, R., Tiret, E., Frileux, P. *et al.* (1986) Resection and colo-anal anastomosis with colonic reservoir for rectal carcinoma. *Br. J. Surg.*, **73**, 139–141

Parks, A.G. (1956) The surgical treatment of haemorrhoids. *Br. J. Surg.*, **43**, 337–351

Parks, A.G. (1972) Transanal technique in low rectal anastomosis. *Proc. R. Soc. Med.*, **65**, 975–976

Parks, A.G., Allen, C.L.O., Frank, J.D. and

McPartlin, J.F. (1978) A method of treating post-irradiation rectovaginal fistulas. *Br. J. Surg.*, **65**, 417–421

Parks, A.G. and Nicholls, R.J. (1978) Proctocolectomy without ileostomy for ulcerative colitis. *Br. Med. J.*, **2**, 85–88

Parks, A.G., Nicholls, R.J. and Belliveau, P. (1980) Proctocolectomy with ileal reservoir and anal anastomosis. *Br. J. Surg.*, **67**, 533–538

Parks, A.G. and Percy, J.P. (1982) Resection and sutured colo-anal anastomosis for rectal carcinoma. *Br. J. Surg.*, **69**, 301–304

Parks, A.G., Porter, N.H. and Melzack, J. (1962) Experimental study of the reflex mechanism controlling the muscles of the pelvic floor. *Dis. Colon Rectum*, **5**, 407–414

Parks, A.G., Swash, M. and Urich, H. (1977) Sphincter denervation in anorectal incontinence and rectal prolapse. *Gut*, **18**, 656–665

Passeri, D., Wright, H.K. and Kricker, M. (1979) Mechanism of increased ileal structure and function after colectomy. *Surg. Forum*, **XXX**, 373

Pearl, R.K., Nelson, R.L., Prasad, M.L. *et al.* (1985) Ileoanal anastomosis 24 years after total proctocolectomy for ulcerative colitis. *Dis. Colon Rectum*, **28**, 180–182

Peck, D.A. (1980) Rectal mucosal replacement. *Ann. Surg.*, **191**, 294–303

Peck, D.A. and Hallenback, G.A. (1964) Faecal continence in the dog after replacement of rectal mucosa with ileal mucosa. *Surg. Gynecol. Obstet.*, **119**, 1312–1320

Pemberton, J.H., Kelly, K.A., Beart, R.W. Jr *et al.* (1987) Ileal pouch–anal anastomosis for chronic ulcerative colitis: long term results. *Ann. Surg.*, **206**, 504–513

Pemberton, J.H., Phillips, S.F., Ready, R.R. *et al.* (1989) Quality of life after Brooke ileostomy and ileal pouch–anal anastomosis. Comparison of performance status. *Ann. Surg.*, **209**, 620–628

Perbeck, L., Lindquist, K. and Liljeqvist, L. (1985) The mucosal blood flow in pelvic pouches in man. A methodologic study of fluoroscein flowmetry. *Dis. Colon Rectum*, **28**, 931–936

Percy, J.P., Neill, M.E., Swash, M. and Parks, A.G. (1981) Electrophysiological study of motor nerve supply of pelvic floor. *Lancet*, **i**, 16–17

Perdue, M.H., Marshall, J. and Masson, S. (1990) Ion transport abnormalities in inflamed rat jejunum. *Gastroenterology*, **98**, 561–567

Pescatori, M. (1985) Myoelectric and motor activity of the terminal ileum after pelvic pouch for ulcerative colitis. *Dis. Colon Rectum*, **28**, 246–253,

Pescatori, M. (1988) A modified three-loop ileoanal reservoir. *Dis. Colon Rectum*, **31**, 823–824

Pescatori, M., Bartram, C., Manhire, A. and Ramcharan, J. (1984) Restorative proctocolectomy, radiology and physiology. *Ann. R. Coll. Surg. Engl.*, **66**, 45–47

Pescatori, M., Manhire, A. and Bartram, C.I. (1983) Evacuation pouchography in the evaluation of ileoanal reservoir function. *Dis. Colon Rectum*, **26**, 365–368

Pescatori, M., Mattana, C. and Castagneto, M. (1988) Clinical and functional results after restorative proctocolectomy. *Br. J. Surg.*, **75**, 321–324

Pescatori, M., Mattana, C., Maria, G. *et al.* (1989) A clinical and physiological comparison between standard and modified S-pouch for ulcerative colitis. In *Symposium: New Trends in Pelvic Pouch Procedures, Bologna*, A64

Pescatori, M. and Parks, A.G. (1984a) The sphincteric and sensory components of preserved continence after ileoanal reservoir. *Surg. Gynecol. Obstet.*, **158**, 517–521

Pescatori, M. and Parks, A.G. (1984b) Transmucosal myotomy of the small bowel after ileoanal anastomosis. *Dis. Colon Rectum*, **27**, 316–318

Pezim, M.E. (1984) Successful childbirth after restorative proctocolectomy with pelvic ileal reservoir. *Br. J. Surg.*, **71**, 292

Pezim, M.E. and Nicholls, R.J. (1985) Quality of life after restorative proctocolectomy. *Br. J. Surg.*, **72**, 31–33

Pezim, M.E., Pemberton, J.H., Beart, R.W. *et al.* (1989) Outcome of 'indeterminate' colitis following ileal pouch–anal anastomosis. *Dis. Colon Rectum*, **32**, 653–658

Pezim, M.E., Taylor, B.A., Davis, C.J. and Beart, R.W. Jr (1987) Perforation of the terminal ileal appendage of J pelvic ileal reservoir. *Dis. Colon Rectum*, **30**, 161–163

Philipson, B., Brandberg, A., Jagenburg, R. *et al.* (1975) Mucosal morphology, bacteriology and absorption in intra-abdominal ileostomy reservoir. *Scand. J. Gastroenterol.*, **10**, 1

Philipson, B.M., Kock, N.G., Jagerburg, R. *et al.* (1983) Functional and structural studies of ileal reservoirs used for continent urostomy and ileostomy. *Gut*, **24**, 392–396

Phillips, S.F. (1987) Biological effects of a reservoir at the end of the small bowel. *World J. Surg.*, **11**, 763–768

Pironi, L., Miglioli, M., Caudarella, R. *et al.* (1989a) Calcium-phosphorus balance in patients undergoing ileal pouch–anal anastomosis. In *Symposium: New Trends in Pelvic Pouch Procedures, Bologna*, A12

Pironi, L., Miglioli, M., Ruggeri, E. *et al.* (1989b) Protein-energy status in patients undergoing ileal pouch–anal anastomosis. In *Symposium: New Trends in Pelvic Pouch Procedures, Bologna*, A20

Porter, N.H. (1962) A physiological study of the pelvic floor in rectal prolapse. *Ann. R. Coll. Surg. Engl.*, **31**, 379–401

Prasad, M.L., Pearl, R.K., Orsay, C.P. and Abcarian, H. (1984) Rodless ileostomy: a modified loop ileostomy. *Dis. Colon Rectum*, **27**, 270–271

Primrose, J.N., Quirke, P. and Johnston, D. (1988) Carcinoma of the ileostomy in a patient with familial adenomatous polyps. *Br. J. Surg.*, **75**, 384

Quenu, J. (1933) L'ileo-coloplastie. *J. Chir.*, **42**, 15–48

Rabau, M.Y., Percy, J.P. and Parks, A.G. (1982) Ileal pelvic reservoir: a correlation between motor patterns and clinical behaviour. *Br. J. Surg.*, **69**, 391–395

Rabinovici, R. and Krausz, M.M. (1988) Use of a nylon sleeve for safe reservoir downpulling during ileoanal anastomosis. *Dis. Colon Rectum*, **31**, 821–822

Ramos, R. and Bode, W.E. (1988) A simple technique for construction of a J-pouch. *Dis. Colon Rectum*, **31**, 87–89

Ratelle, R., Kartheuser, A., Tiret, E. *et al.* (1990) Proctectomy and ileoanal anastomosis after ileorectal anastomosis for familial polyposis. *Gastroenterology*, **98**, A305

Ravitch, M.M. (1948) Anal ileostomy with sphincter preservation in patients requiring total colectomy for benign conditions. *Surgery*, **24**, 170–187

Ravitch, M.M. (1956) Total colectomy and abdomino-perineal resection (pan-colectomy) in one stage. *Ann. Surg.*, **144**, 758–764

Ravitch, M.M. and Sabiston, D.C. (1947) Anal ileostomy with preservation of the sphincter. *Surg. Gynecol. Obstet.*, **84**, 1095–1099

Raymond, J.L. and Becker, J.M. (1986) Ileoanal pull-through: a new surgical alternative to ileostomy and a new challenge to diet therapy. *J. Am. Diet. Assoc.*, **86**, 663–665

Read, N.W., Harford, W.V., Schmulen, A.C. *et al.* (1979) A clinical study of patients with faecal incontinence and diarrhoea. *Gastroenterology*, **76**, 747–756

Reinhoff, W.F. (1925) The surgical treatment of chronic ulcerative colitis by ileosigmoidostomy. *Ann. Clin. Med.*, **4**, 430–434

Ribet, M., Wurtz, A. and Paris, J.C. (1981) La conservation du rectum dans la rectocolite ulcero-hemorragique: etude a long term de 73 operes. *Gastroenterol. Clin. Biol.*, **5**, 1140–1145

Ribotta, G., Montesani, C., Pronio, A. and Catani, M. (1988) Restorative proctocolectomy with J reservoir in the treatment of ulcerative colitis. *Ital. J. Surg. Sci.*, **18**, 253–258

Riley, S.A., Mani, V., Goodman, M.J. and Lucas, S. (1990) Why do patients with ulcerative colitis relapse? *Gut*, **31**, 179–183

Ritchie, J.K. (1971) Ileostomy and excisional surgery for chronic inflammatory disease of the colon: a survey of one hospital region. *Gut*, **12**, 528–532

Ritchie, J.K., Powell-Tuck, J. and Lennard-Jones, J.E. (1978) Clinical outcome of the first ten years of ulcerative colitis and proctitis. *Lancet*, **ii**, 1140–1143

Roediger, W.E.W. (1988) Bacterial short-chain fatty acids and mucosal diseases of the colon. *Br. J. Surg.*, **75**, 346–348

Roediger, W.E.W. and Rae, D.A. (1982) Trophic effects of short chain fatty acids on mucosal handling of ions by the defunctioned colon. *Br. J. Surg.*, **69**, 23–25

Rogers, J., Laurberg, S., Misiewicz, J.J. and Henry, M.M. (1988) Validation of the motor and sensory tests of anorectal function: a repeatability study. *Gut*, **29**, A1456

Rosemurgy, A.S., Schraut, W.H. and Block, G.E. (1983) The physiological effects of ileal reservoirs and efferent conduits complementing ileoanal anastomosis: an experimental study in dogs. *Surgery*, **94**, 697–703

Rosenberg, A.J. and Vela, A.R. (1983) A new simplified technique for paediatric anorectal manometry. *Pediatrics.*, **71**, 240–245

Ross, J.E. and Mara, J.E. (1974) Small bowel polyps and carcinoma in multiple intestinal polyposis. *Arch. Surg.*, **108**, 736–738

Roth, J.A. and Logio, T. (1982) Carcinoma arising in an ileostomy stoma: an unusual complication of adenomatous polyposis coli. *Cancer*, **49**, 2180–2184

Rothenberger, D.A., Buls, J.G., Nivatvongs, S. and Goldberg, S.M. (1985) The Parks' S ileal pouch and anal anastomosis after colectomy and mucosal proctectomy. *Am. J. Surg.*, **149**, 390–394

Rothenberger, D.A., Vermeulen, F.D., Christenson, C.E. *et al.* (1983) Restorative proctocolectomy with ileal reservoir and ileoanal anastomosis. *Am. J. Surg.*, **145**, 82–88

Rothenberger, D.A., Wong, W.D., Buls, J.G. and Goldberg, S.M. (1985) The S ileal pouch–anal anastomosis. In *Alternatives to Conventional Ileostomy* (ed. R.R. Dozois), Year Book Medical, Chicago, pp.345–362

Ryan, P. and Fink, R. (1988) New rectum and new anal canal: two cases of ileal reservoir–cutaneous anastomosis. *Aust. N.Z. J. Surg.*, **58**, 161–165

Sackier, J.M. and Wood, C.B. (1988) Ulcerative colitis and polyposis coli. Surgical options. *Surg. Clin. North Am.*, **68**, 1319–1338

Saeger, H.D., Barth, H.O., Linder, M.M. and Trede, M. (1985) Experiences with ileoanal anastomosis and ileal pouch formation following colectomy and proctomucosectomy. *Langenbecks Arch. Chir.*, **366**, 477–480

Safaie-Shirazi, S. and Soper, R.T. (1973) Endorectal pull-through procedure in the surgical treatment of familial polyposis. *J. Pediatr. Surg.*, **8**, 711–715

Sagar, P.M., Holdsworth, P.J. and Johnston, D. (1989) Continuous pouch–anal manometry after restorative proctocolectomy. *Br. J. Surg.*, **76**, 1338

Sagar, P.M., Holdsworth, P.J. and Johnston, D.

(1990) Ileal pouch adaptation and anal canal recovery after restorative proctocolectomy. *Br. J. Surg.*, **77**, 700

Sagar, P.M., Salter, G., King, R.F.G.J. *et al.* (1990) Straight ileoanal anastomosis with myotomy: an alternative to restorative proctocolectomy. *Br. J. Surg.*, **77**, 698

Sakaguchi, M., Hosie, R., Tudor, R. *et al.* (1989) Mucosal blood flow following restorative procto-colectomy: pouchitis is associated with mucosal ischaemia. *Br J. Surg.*, **76**, 1331

Sawchuk, A., Nogami, W. and Goto, S. (1986) Reverse electrical pacing improves intestinal absorption and transit time. *Surgery*, **100**, 454–459

Scharli, A.F. and Keisewetter, W.B. (1970) Defaec-ation and continence: some new concepts. *Dis. Colon Rectum*, **13**, 81–107

Schjonsby, H., Halvorsen, J.F., Hofstad, T. and Hovdenak, N. (1977) Stagnant loop syndrome in patients with continent ileostomy (intra-abdominal ileal reservoir). *Gut*, **18**, 795

Schneider, S. (1955) Anal ileostomy: experiences with a new three-stage procedure. *Arch. Surg.*, **70**, 539–544

Schoetz, D.J., Coller, J.A. and Veidenheimer, M.C. (1984) Proctocolectomy with ileoanal reser-voir: an alternative to permanent ileostomy. *Postgrad. Med.*, **75**, 123–138

Schoetz, D.J., Coller, J.A. and Veidenheimer, M.C. (1986) Ileoanal reservoir for ulcerative colitis and familial polyposis. *Arch. Surg.*, **121**, 404–408

Schoetz, D.J., Coller, J.A. and Veidenheimer, M.C. (1988) Can the pouch be saved? *Dis. Colon Rectum*, **31**, 671–675

Schraut, W.H. and Block, G.E. (1980) Ileoanal anastomosis with ileal reservoir – experimental study in dogs. *Eur. Surg. Res.*, **12**, 37.

Schraut, W.H. and Block, G.E. (1982) Ileoanal anastomosis with proximal ileal reservoir: an experimental study. *Surgery*, **91**, 275–281

Schraut, W.H., Rosemurgy, A.S., Block, G.E. and Wang, C.H. (1981) Ileoanal anastomosis with ileal reservoir: function is determined by reservoir configuration. *Eur. Surg. Res.*, **13**, 43

Schraut, W.H., Rosemurgy, A.S. and Wang, C.H. (1983) Determinants of optimal results after ileoanal anastomosis: anal proximity and motility patterns of the ileal reservoir. *World J. Surg.*, **7**, 400–408

Scott, A.D. and Phillips, R.K.S. (1989) Ileitis and pouchitis after colectomy for ulcerative colitis. *Br. J. Surg.*, **76**, 668–669

Scott, N.A., Barkel, D.C., Wolff, B.G. (1988a) Anal manometry and pouch compliance measure-ments before ileostomy closure are related to functional outcome of the ileal pouch–anal anastomosis. *Br. J. Surg.*, **75**, 1270

Scott, N.A., Dozois, R.R., Beart, R.W. *et al.* (1988b) Postoperative intra-abdominal and pelvic sepsis complicating ileal pouch–anal anastomosis. *Int. J. Color. Dis.*, **3**, 149–152

Scott, N.A., Pemberton, J.H., Barkel, D.C. and Wolff, B.G. (1989) Anal and ileal pouch mano-metric measurements before ileostomy closure are related to functional outcome after ileal pouch–anal anastomosis. *Br. J. Surg.*, **76**, 613–616

Sene, A., Thomas, P.E., Gautam, V. *et al.* (1989) Juvenile polyp in an ileoanal J-pouch following restorative proctocolectomy for juvenile polyposis coli. *Br. J. Surg.*, **76**, 801–802

Sener, S.F., Miller, H.H. and De Cosse, J.J. (1984) The spectrum of polyposis. *Surg. Gynecol. Obstet.*, **159**, 525–532

Sharp, F.R., Bell, G.A., Seal, A.M. and Atkinson, K.G. (1987) Investigations of the anal sphincter before and after restorative proctocolectomy. *Am. J. Surg.*, **153**, 469–472

Shepard, J.A. (1971) Familial polyposis of the colon with special reference to regression of rectal polyposis after subtotal colectomy. *Br. J. Surg.*, **58**, 85–91

Shepherd, N.A., Hulten, L., Tytgat, G.N. *et al.* (1989) Pouchitis. *Int. J. Color. Dis.*, **4**, 205–229

Shepherd, N.A., Jass, J.R., Duval, I. *et al.* (1987) Restorative proctocolectomy with ileal reservoir: a pathological and histochemical study of mucosal biopsy specimens. *J. Clin. Pathol.*, **40**, 601–607

Simonsen, L., Hojlund, P.B., Hansen, L.K. *et al.* (1985) The defaecation pattern and diet in patients with an ileal reservoir and anal anastomo-sis with long efferent leg. *Scand. J. Gastroenter-ol.*, **20**, 1057–1061

Sjogren, R.W., Wardlow, M. and Charles, L.G. (1984) Stimulation of action potential complexes by fluid distension of rabbit small intestine – evidence that migrating action potential com-plexes are a non specific myoelectric response. In *Gastrointestinal Motility* (ed. C. Roman), MTP, Lancaster, pp.287–296

Skarsgard, E.D., Atkinson, K.G., Bell, G.A. *et al.* (1989) Function and quality of life results after ileal pouch surgery for chronic ulcerative colitis and familial polyposis. *Am. J. Surg.*, **157**, 467–471

Skinner, M.A., Tyler, D., Branum, G.D. *et al.* (1990) Subtotal colectomy for familial polyposis. *Arch. Surg.*, **125**, 621–624

Slaney, G. and Brooke, B.N. (1959) Cancer in ulcerative colitis. *Lancet*, **ii**, 694–698

Sloan, W.P., Bargen, J. and Gage, R. (1950) Life histories of patients with chronic ulcerative colitis: a review of 2000 cases. *Gastroenterology*, **16**, 25–38

Slors, J.F., Taat, C.W. and Brummelkamp, W.H. (1989) Ileal pouch–anal anastomosis without rectal muscular cuff. *Int. J. Color. Dis.*, **4**, 178–181

Slors, J.F., Taat, C.W. and Brummelkamp, W.H. (1990) Ileoanal anastomosis with ileum reservoir. *Ned. Tijdschr. Geneeskd.* **134**, 334–337

Smith, A.N. and Sircus, W. (1987) Ileal reservoir after colectomy and mucosal proctectomy for chronic ulcerative colitis and dysplasia. *J. R. Coll. Surg. Edinb.*, **32**, 276–280

Smith, L.E. (1985) Current status of sphincter saving operations for chronic ulcerative colitis. *South. Med J.*, **78**, 1304–1308

Smith, L., Friend, W.G. and Medwell, S.J. (1984) The superior mesenteric artery. The critical factor in the pouch pull-through procedure. *Dis. Colon Rectum*, **27**, 741–744

Snooks, S.J. and Swash, M. (1984) Perineal nerve and transcutaneous spinal stimulation: new methods for investigation of the urethral striated sphincter musculature. *Br. J. Urol.*, **56**, 406–409

Snooks, S.J., Swash, M., Setchell, M. and Henry, M.M. (1984) Injury to the innervation of pelvic floor sphincter musculature in childbirth. *Lancet*, **ii**, 546–550

Soave, F. (1964) Hirschprung's disease. A new surgical technique. *Arch. Dis. Child.*, **39**, 116–124

Soave, F. (1985) Endorectal ileal pull-through for ulcerative colitis and polyposis in children. *Dis. Colon Rectum*, **28**, 76–80

Soper, N.J., Chapman, N.J., Kelly, K.A. *et al.* (1990) The 'ileal brake' after ileal pouch–anal anastomosis. *Gastroenterology*, **98**, 111–116

Soper, N.J., Kestenberg, A. and Becker, J.M. (1988) Experimental ileal J-pouch construction: a comparison of three techniques. *Dis. Colon Rectum*, **31**, 186–189

Spigelman, A.D., Talbot, I.C. and Williams, C.B. (1989) Upper gastrointestinal cancer in patients with familial adenomatous polyposis. *Lancet*, **ii**, 783–785

Stahlgren, L.H. and Ferguson, L.K. (1959) Effects of abdominoperineal resection on sexual function in sixty patients with ulcerative colitis. *Arch. Surg.*, **78**, 604–610

Steichen, F.M. (1977) The creation of autologous substitute organs with stapling instruments. *Am. J. Surg.*, **134**, 659–673

Stelzner, M., Buddington, R.K., Fonkalsrud, E.W. and Diamond, J.M. (1989) Changes in mucosal nutrient transport as possible cause in ileal reservoir inflammation ('pouchitis'). In *Symposium: New Trends in Pelvic Pouch Procedures, Bologna*, A52

Stelzner, M. and Fonkalsrud, E.W. (1989) The endorectal ileal pull-through procedure in patients with ulcerative colitis and familial polyposis with carcinoma. *Surg. Gynecol. Obstet.*, **169**, 187–194

Stelzner, M. and Fonkalsrud, E.W. (1990) Assessment of anorectal function after mucosal proctectomy and endoanal ileal pull-through for ulcerative colitis. *Surgery*, **107**, 201–208

Stelzner, M., Fonkalsrud, E.W., Buddington, R.K. *et al.* (1990) Adaptive changes in ileal mucosa nutrient transport following colectomy and endorectal ileal pull-through with ileal reservoir. *Arch. Surg.*, **125**, 586–590

Stelzner, M., Fonkalsrud, E.W. and Lichtenstein, G. (1988) Significance of reservoir length in the endorectal ileal pull-through with ileal reservoir. *Arch. Surg.*, **123**, 1265–1268

Stelzner, M., Fonkalsrud, E.W. and Salehmoghaddam, S. (1989) Nephrolithiasis in patients with colitis undergoing colectomy and endorectal ileal pull-through. In *Symposium: New Trends in Pelvic Pouch Procedures, Bologna*, A10

Stern, H., Bernstein, M., Killam, S. *et al.* (1987) A stapled S-shaped ileoanal reservoir. *Dis. Colon Rectum*, **30**, 214–219

Stern, H., Walfisch, S., Mullen, B. *et al.* (1990) Cancer in an ileoanal reservoir: a new late complication? *Gut*, **31**, 473–475

Stoller, D.K., Coran, A.G., Drongowski, R.A. *et al.* (1987) Physiologic assessment of the four commonly performed endorectal pull-throughs. *Ann. Surg.*, **206**, 586–594

Stone, H.B. (1928) Interposition of a loop of ileum to repair defects in the colon. *Ann. Surg.*, **88**, 593–596

Stone, M.M., Lewin, K. and Fonkalsrud, E.W. (1986) Late obstruction of the lateral ileal reservoir after colectomy and endorectal ileal pull-through procedures. *Surg. Gynecol. Obstet.*, **162**, 411–417

Stone, M.M., Mulvihill, S.J., Snape, W.J. Jr and Fonkalsrud, E.W. (1986) Comparison of the myoelectric activity of the lateral and J shaped ileal reservoir. *J. Pediatr. Surg.*, **21**, 500–505

Strauss, A.A. and Strauss, S.F. (1944) Surgical treatment of ulcerative colitis. *Surg. Clin. North Am.*, **24**, 211–224

Stringel, G. (1985) Pull-through with isolated jejunal loop for ulcerative colitis. *J. Pediatr. Surg.*, **20**, 661–663

Stryker, S.J., Borody, T.J., Phillips, S.F. *et al.* (1985a) Motility of the small intestine after proctocolectomy and ileal pouch–anal anastomosis. *Ann. Surg.*, **201**, 351–356

Stryker, S.J., Carney, J.A. and Dozois, R.R. (1987) Multiple adenomatous polyps arising in a continent reservoir ileostomy. *Int. J. Colorect. Dis.*, **2**, 43–45

Stryker, S.J., Daube, J.R., Kelly, K.A. *et al.* (1985b) Anal sphincter electromyography after colectomy, mucosal rectectomy and ileoanal anastomosis. *Arch. Surg.*, **120**, 713–716

Stryker, S.J., Kelly, K.A., Phillips, S.F. *et al.* (1986) Anal and neorectal function after proctocolectomy and ileal pouch–anal anastomosis. *Ann. Surg.*, **203**, 55–61

Stryker, S.J., Telander, R.L. and Perrault, J. (1985)

Anoneorectal evaluation after colectomy and endorectal ileoanal anastomosis in children and young adults. *J. Pediatr. Surg.*, **20**, 656–660

Suarez, V., Alexander-Williams, J. and O'Connor, H.J. (1988) Carcinoma developing in ileostomies after 25 or more years. *Gastroenterology*, **95**, 205–208

Subramani, K., Sachar, D.B., Harpaz, N. *et al.* (1990) Resistant pouchitis: does it reflect underlying Crohn's disease? *Gastroenterology*, **98**, A205

Sullivan, E.S. and Garnjobst, W.M. (1982) Advantage of initial transanal mucosal stripping in ileoanal pullthrough procedures. *Dis. Colon Rectum,* **25**, 170–171

Summers, W., Anuras, S. and Green, J. (1983) Jejunal manometry patterns in health, partial obstruction, and pseudo-obstruction. *Gastroenterology*, **85**, 1290–1300

Taillefer, R., Heppell, J., Derbe-Ryan, V. *et al.* (1986) Radionuclide assessment of ileoanal anastomosis emptying: preliminary results. *J. Nucl. Med.*, **27**, 1010

Takamatsu, H., Albert, A., Mulvihill, S.J. *et al.* (1985) Electrical activity and motility in the isoperistaltic side-to-side ileal reservoir. *Surg. Gynecol. Obstet.*, **161**, 425–430

Talbot, R.W., Ritchie, J.K. and Northover, J.M.A. (1988) Conservative proctocolectomy – is it an option in ulcerative colitis. *Gut*, **29**, A1474–1475

Talbot, R.W., Ritchie, J.K. and Northover, J.M.A. (1989) Conservative proctocolectomy – a dubious option in ulcerative colitis. *Br. J. Surg.*, **76**, 738–739

Taverner, D. and Smiddy, F.G. (1959) An electromyographic study of the normal function of the external anal sphincter and pelvic diaphragm. *Dis. Colon Rectum*, **2**, 153–160

Taylor, B.A., Beart, R.W., Dozois, R.R. *et al.* (1983a) Straight ileoanal anastomosis versus ileal pouch–anal anastomosis after colectomy and mucosal proctectomy. *Arch. Surg.*, **118**, 696–701

Taylor, B.A., Beart, R.W., Dozois, R.R. *et al.* (1984) The endorectal ileal pouch–anal anastomosis. Current clinical results. *Dis. Colon Rectum*, **27**, 347–350

Taylor, B.A., Beart, R.W. and Phillips, S.F. (1984) Longitudinal and radial variations of pressure in the human anal sphincter. *Gastroenterology*, **86**, 693–697

Taylor, B.A., Cranley, B., Kelly, K.A. *et al.* (1983b) A clinico-physiological comparison of ileal pouch–anal and straight ileoanal anastomosis. *Ann. Surg.*, **198**, 462–468

Taylor, B.A. and Dozois, R.R. (1987) The J ileal pouch–anal anastomosis. *World J. Surg.*, **11**, 727–734

Taylor, B.A., Wolff, B.G., Dozois, R.R. *et al.* (1988) Ileal pouch–anal anastomosis for chronic

ulcerative colitis and familial polyposis coli complicated by adenocarcinoma. *Dis. Colon Rectum*, **31**, 358–362

Taylor, T.V. (1986) *A Colour Atlas of Mucosal Proctectomy and Ileal Reservoir Formation*, Wolfe Medical/Year Book Medical, Chicago

Taylor, T.V. (1987) Experience with mucosal proctectomy and a J shaped ileal reservoir in ulcerative colitis. *Ann. R. Coll. Surg. Engl.*, **68**, 12–15

Taylor, T.V. and Thomas, P.E. (1987) *Mucosal Proctectomy and Ileal Reservoir Formation in the Treatment of Ulcerative Colitis*, Beecham Medical Research

Telander, R.L. and Perrault, J. (1981) Colectomy with rectal mucosectomy and ileoanal anastomosis in young patients. *Arch. Surg.*, **116**, 623–629

Templeton, J.L. and McKelvey, S.T.D. (1985) The pelvic ileal reservoir: an experimental comparison of the three-loop and two-loop systems. *Dis. Colon Rectum*, **28**, 782–785

Thayer, M.L., Madoff, R.D., Jacobs, D.M. and Bubrick, M.P. (1990) Comparative intrinsic and extrinsic compliance characteristics of S, J, and W ileoanal pouches. *Dis. Colon Rectum*, **33**, P6

Thoeni, R.F., Fell, S.C., Engelstad, B. and Schrock, T.B. (1990) Ileoanal pouches: comparison of CT, scintigraphy, and contrast enemas for diagnosing postsurgical complications. *Am. J. Roentgenol.*, **154**, 73–78

Thomas, P.E., Hobbis, J.H. and Taylor, T.V. (1990) Closed loop obstruction in an ileal pelvic pouch. In preparation.

Thomas, P.E., Hosker, G. and Taylor, T.V. (1989a) There is evidence of abnormal neural innervation to the external anal sphincter after restorative proctocolectomy. In *Symposium: New Trends in Pelvic Pouch Procedures, Bologna*, A5

Thomas, P.E., Hosker, G. and Taylor, T.V. (1989b) Anomanometric studies and anal canal motility after restorative proctocolectomy. In *Symposium: New Trends in Pelvic Pouch Procedures, Bologna*, A37

Thomas, P.E., Seehra, H.K., Sene, A. and Taylor, T.V. (1990) Psoas-hitch 'pouchopexy' for a malfunctioning long J-pouch. In preparation.

Thomas, P.E. and Taylor, T.V. (1989a) Mineral status and serum biochemistry remain normal on long term follow-up after restorative proctocolectomy. In *Symposium: New Trends in Pelvic Pouch Procedures, Bologna*, A11

Thomas, P.E. and Taylor, T.V. (1989b) There are few long-term haematological sequelae of restorative proctocolectomy. In *Symposium: New Trends in Pelvic Pouch Procedures, Bologna*, A21

Thomas, P.E. and Taylor, T.V. (1990a) Clinical experience with J-pouch-anal anastomosis. Submitted.

Thomas, P.E. and Taylor, T.V. (1990b) Use of the

DePezzer catheter to facilitate endoanal pull-through during restorative proctocolectomy. Submitted.

Thompson, G.B., Pemberton, J.H., Morris, S. *et al.* (1989) Kaposi's sarcoma of the colon in a young HIV-negative man with chronic ulcerative colitis. *Dis. Colon Rectum*, **32**, 73–76

Thompson, J.S. (1989) Alopecia after ileal pouch–anal anastomosis. *Dis. Colon Rectum*, **32**, 457–459

Thomson, W.H.F. and O'Kelly, T.J. (1988) Ileal salvage from failed pouches. *Br. J. Surg.*, **75**, 1227

Thomson, W.H.F., Simpson, A.H.R.W. and Wheeler, J.L. (1987) Mathematical prediction of ileal pouch capacity. *Br. J. Surg.*, **74**, 567–568

Thow, C.B. (1985) Single stage colectomy and mucosal proctectomy with stapled antiperistaltic ileoanal reservoir. In *Alternatives to Conventional Ileostomy* (ed. R.R. Dozois), Year Book Medical, Chicago, pp.420–432

Tsunoda, A., Talbot, I.C. and Nicholls, R.J. (1990) Incidence of dysplasia in the anorectal mucosa in patients having restorative proctocolectomy. *Br. J. Surg.*, **77**, 506–508

Turnage, R.H., Coran, A.G. and Drongowski, R.A. (1990) The value of intestinal myotomy and myectomy in improving the reservoir capacity of the endorectal pull-through. *Ann. Surg.*, **211**, 463–469

Turnbull, R.B., Weakley, F.L., Hawk, W.A. and Schofield, P. (1970) Choice of operation for the toxic megacolon phase of non-specific ulcerative colitis. *Surg. Clin. N. Am.*, **50**, 1151

Tytgat, G.N.J. and van Deventer, S.J.H. (1988) Pouchitis. *Int. J. Color. Dis.*, **3**, 226–228

Tzu-Chi Hsu (1989) Traumatic perforation of ileal pouch: report of a case. *Dis. Colon Rectum*, **32**, 64–66

Ustach, T.J., Tobson, F. and Hambrecht, T. (1970) Electrophysiological aspects of human sphincter function. *J. Clin. Invest.*, **49**, 41–48

Utsunomiya, J. and Iwama, T. (1985) The J ileal pouch–anal anastomosis: the Japanese experience. In *Alternatives to Conventional Ileostomy* (ed. R.R. Dozois), Year Book Medical, Chicago, pp.371–383

Utsunomiya, J., Iwama, T., Imajo, M. *et al.* (1980) Total colectomy, mucosal proctectomy and ileoanal anastomosis. *Dis. Colon Rectum*, **23**, 459–466

Utsunomiya, J., Oota, M. and Iwama, T. (1986) Recent trends in ileoanal anastomosis. *Ann. Chir. Gynaecol.*, **75**, 56–62

Utsunomiya, J., Yamamura, T., Kusonoki, M. and Iwama, T. (1988) The current technique of ileoanal anastomosis. *Dig. Surg.*, **5**, 207–214

Valiente, M.A. and Bacon, H.E. (1955) Construction of a pouch using 'pantaloon' technique for pull-through of ileum following total colectomy: report of experimental work and results. *Am. J. Surg.*, **90**, 742–750

Van de Pavoordt, H.D., Fazio, V.W., Jagelmann, D.G. *et al.* (1987) The outcome of loop ileostomy closure in 293 cases. *Int. J. Color. Dis.*, **2**, 214–217

Varma, J.S., Browning, G.G.P., Smith, A.N. *et al.* (1987) Mucosal proctectomy and coloanal anastomosis for distal ulcerative proctocolitis. *Br. J. Surg.*, **74**, 381–383

Vasilevsky, C., Rothenberger, D.A. and Goldberg, S.M. (1987) The S ileal pouch–anal anastomosis. *World J. Surg.*, **11**, 742–750

Vignolo, Q. (1912) Nouveau procede operatoire pour retablir la continuite intestinale dans les resections recto-sigmoidiennes etendues. *Arch. Gen. Chir.*, **6**, 621–643

Villanova, N., Mazzella, G., Aldini, R. *et al.* (1989) Bile acid metabolism after ileo-anal pouch. *Gastroenterology*, **96**, A671

Wangensteen, O.H. (1943) Primary resection (closed anastomosis) of the colon and rectum. *Surgery*, **14**, 403–432

Wangensteen, O.H. and Toon, R.W. (1948) Primary resection of the colon and rectum with particular reference to cancer and ulcerative colitis. *Am. J. Surg.*, **75**, 384–404

Warren, N. and McKittrick, L.S. (1951) Ileostomy for ulcerative colitis. *Surg. Gynecol. Obstet.*, **93**, 555–567

Watne, A.L., Core, S.K. and Carrier, J.M. (1975) Gardner's syndrome. *Surg. Gynecol. Obstet.*, **141**, 53–56

Watts, J., de Dombal, F.T. and Goligher, J.C. (1966a) The early results of surgery for ulcerative colitis. *Br. J. Surg.*, **53**, 1005–1013

Watts, J., de Dombal, F.T. and Goligher, J.C. (1966b) Long-term complications and prognosis following major surgery for ulcerative colitis. *Br. J. Surg.*, **53**, 1014–1023

Waugh, J.M., Harp, R.A. and Spencer, R.J. (1964) The surgical management of multiple polyposis. *Ann. Surg.*, **159**, 149–154

Weakley, F.L. and Farmer, R.G. (1964) Ileitis after colectomy and ileostomy for nonspecific ulcerative colitis: report of 35 cases. *Dis. Colon Rectum*, **7**, 427–435

Weir, R.F. (1902) quoted by Corbett (1945)

Wexner, S.D., Jensen, L., Rothenberger, D.A. *et al.* (1989a) Long-term functional analysis of the ileoanal reservoir. *Dis. Colon Rectum*, **32**, 275–281

Wexner, S.D., Rothenberger, D.A., Jensen, L. *et al.* (1989b) Ileal pouch vaginal fistulas: incidence, etiology, and management. *Dis. Colon Rectum*, **32**, 460–465

Wexner, S.D., Wong, W.D., Rothenberger, D.A. and Goldberg, S.M. (1990) The ileoanal reservoir. *Am. J. Surg.*, **159**, 178–185

White, J.C., Verlot, M.G. and Ehrentheil, O. (1940) Neurogenic disturbances of the colon and their investigation by the colonmetrogram. *Ann. Surg.*, **112**, 1042–1057

Whitehead, W.E., Engel, B.T. and Schuster, M.M. (1980) Irritable bowel syndrome: physiological and psychological differences between diarrhoea predominant and constipation predominant patients. *Dig. Dis. Sci.*, **25**, 404–413

Williams, N.S. (1989a) Stapling technique for pouch–anal anastomosis without the need for purse-string sutures. *Br. J. Surg.*, **76**, 348–349

Williams, N.S. (1989b) Restorative proctocolectomy is the first choice elective surgical treatment for ulcerative colitis. *Br. J. Surg.*, **76**, 1109–1110

Williams, N.S., Hallan, R.I., Koeze, T.H. and Watkins, E.S. (1989a) Construction of a neorectum and neoanal sphincter following previous proctocolectomy. *Br. J. Surg.*, **76**, 1191–1194

Williams, N.S. and Johnston, D. (1985a) The current status of mucosal proctectomy and ileoanal anastomosis in the surgical treatment of ulcerative colitis and adenomatous polyposis. *Br. J. Surg.*, **72**, 159–168

Williams, N.S. and Johnston, D. (1985b) Mucosal proctectomy and ileoanal anastomosis. In *Progress in Surgery 1*, (ed. I. Taylor), Churchill Livingstone, Edinburgh, pp.95–113.

Williams, N.S. and King, R.F.G.J. (1985) The effect of a reversed ileal segment and artificial valves on intestinal transit and absorption following colectomy and low ileorectal anastomosis in the dog. *Br. J. Surg.*, **72**, 169–174

Williams, N.S., Marzouk, D.E.M.M., Hallan, R.I. and Waldron, D.J. (1989b) Function after ileal pouch and stapled pouch–anal anastomosis for ulcerative colitis. *Br. J. Surg.*, **76**, 1168–1171

Williams, N.S. and Nasmyth, D.G. (1988) Ileostomy or ileal pouch for the surgical treatment of ulcerative colitis? *Postgrad. Med. J.*, **64**, 596–602

Wiltz, O., Hashmi, H., Schoetz, D.J. *et al.* (1990) Cancer and the ileal pouch–anal anastomosis. *Dis. Colon Rectum*, **33**, P5

Winslet, M.C., Flinn, R. and Keighley, M.R.B. (1987) Factors influencing the outcome of restorative proctocolectomy. *Gut*, **28**, A1365–1366

Wolfstein, H., Bat, L. and Neumann, G. (1982) Regeneration of rectal mucosa and recurrent polyposis coli after total colectomy and ileoanal anastomosis. *Arch. Surg.*, **117**, 1241–1242

Wong, W.D., Rothenberger, D.A. and Goldberg, S.M. (1985) Ileoanal pouch procedure. *Curr. Probl. Surg.*, **22**, 9–78

Wood, B.A. (1985) Anatomy of the anal sphincters and pelvic floor. In *Coloproctology and the Pelvic Floor. Pathophysiology and Management* (eds. M.M. Henry and M. Swash), Butterworths, Guildford, pp.3–21

Wunderlich, M. and Swash, M. (1983) The overlapping innervation of the two sides of the external anal sphincter by the pudendal nerves. *J. Neurol. Sci.*, **59**, 97–109

Yoshioka, K., Kmiot, W.A. and Keighley, M.R.B. (1988) Factors influencing motor function after restorative proctocolectomy. *Gut*, **29**, A702–703

Index